Bloomsbury Healthcare Library
151 Gower St.
London WC1E 6BA

Tel: 0171 380 9097

£15.00

Behavioral Concepts and Nursing Intervention

D1390624

Br 5/95 Books are to be returned on or before the last date below

8/12/00

Contributors

Betty Blackwell, R.N., M.S.
Private practice, Sedona, Arizona
Dorothy W. Bloch, R.N., Ph.D.
Professor of Nursing, University of Colorado, Denver, Colorado
Carolyn E. Carlson, R.N., Ph.D.
Associate Professor of Nursing, University of Illinois, Chicago, Illinois
Evelyn Char, R.N., M.S.
Recently completed M.S. in Mental Health Nursing at University of Hawaii, Honolulu, Hawaii
Sister M. Martha Kiening, R.N., M.S.
Professor Emeritus, University of San Francisco, California
Silvia Prodan Lange, R.N., M.N.
Clinical Specialist, Department of Psychological and Social Medicine, Pacific Medical Center, San Francisco, California
Catherine M. Norris, R.N., Ed.D.
Clinician-Consultant, Tucson, Arizona
Vera M. Robinson, R.N., Ph.D.
Associate Professor, Nursing Program, California State University, Fullerton, California
Sandra S. Sweeney, R.N., M.A.
Assistant Professor, College of Nursing, University of Iowa, Iowa City, Iowa
Mary D. Thomas, R.N., M.S.N., Ph.D.
Recently received Ph.D. in Anthropology, University of Hawaii, Honolulu, Hawaii

Bloomsbury Healthcare Library
151 Gower St.
London WC1E 6BA

Tel: 0171 380 9097

Behavioral Concepts and Nursing Intervention

Second Edition

Edited by

CAROLYN E. CARLSON

and

BETTY BLACKWELL

ST. PETER'S HOSPITALS.
TEACHING DIVISION.
THE SHAFTESBURY HOSPITAL.
LONDON. W.C.2.

J. B. Lippincott Company

Philadelphia

WLM 120
~~S.1396~~
15156

Bloomsbury Healthcare Library
151 Gower St.
London WC1E 6BA

Tel: 0171 380 9097

Copyright © 1970, 1978 by J. B. Lippincott Company

This book is fully protected by copyright and, with the exception of brief excerpts for review, no part of it may be reproduced in any form by print, photoprint, microfilm, or by any other means without the written permission of the publishers.

ISBN 0-397-54217-8

Library of Congress Catalog Card Number 78-8761

Printed in the United States of America
4 6 8 9 7 5 3

Library of Congress Cataloging in Publication Data
Main entry under title:

Behavioral concepts and nursing intervention.

Bibliography: p.
1. Nursing—Psychological aspects. I. Carlson, Carolyn E. II. Blackwell, Betty.
[DNLM: 1. Nurse-patient relations. 2. Psychology—Nursing texts. WY87 B419]
RT86.B39 1978 610.73 78-8761
ISBN 0-397-54217-8

CONTENTS

Introduction vii

Section I: FUNDAMENTAL CONCEPTS IN ILLNESS AND DISABILITY

Introduction 1

1. **Body Image: Its Relevance to Professional Nursing** *Catherine M. Norris* 5
2. **Stigma** *Betty Blackwell* 37
3. **Shame** *Silvia Prodan Lange* 51
4. **Loss** *Carolyn E. Carlson* 72
5. **Grief** *Carolyn E. Carlson* 87

Section II: RESPONSES TO CHANGES IN HEALTH STATUS: CONCEPTS WITH NEGATIVE CONNOTATIONS

Introduction 113

6. **Alienation** *Dorothy W. Bloch* 116
7. **Hostility** *Sister M. Martha Kiening* 128
8. **Restlessness** *Catherine M. Norris* 141
9. **Boredom** *Evelyn Char* 154

Section III: RESPONSES TO CHANGES IN HEALTH STATUS: CONCEPTS WITH POSITIVE CONNOTATIONS

Introduction 161

10. **Trust** *Mary Durand Thomas* 164
11. **Hope** *Silvia Prodan Lange* 171
12. **Humor** *Vera M. Robinson* 191
13. **Denial of Illness** *Sister M. Martha Kiening* 211
14. **Privacy** *Dorothy W. Bloch* 226
15. **Relaxation** *Sandra S. Sweeney* 240

Section IV: EXAMPLE OF APPLYING CONCEPTS FROM A THEORY TO NURSING: TRANSACTIONAL ANALYSIS CONCEPTS

Introduction 253

16. **Transactional Analysis and Nursing** *Silvia Prodan Lange* . 255

Dedicated to Catherine M. Norris
for her:

Knowledge of the past;
Vision into the future;
Encouragement in the present.

C. C. and B.B.

INTRODUCTION

The second edition of this book, like the first,[1] includes concepts which the authors have developed independently, from their own frames of reference. This can be viewed as both a strength and a weakness. There may be advantages to developing concepts from a common perspective. Such an approach might facilitate making statements about the interrelationships of concepts, developing constructs and strengthening a particular nursing theory. A unified, systematic approach would probably lead more directly to questions which could be researched to test the theory. Presently, there are many conceptual frameworks underlying nursing curricula, practice and research. But despite these different frameworks, there are many common topics. For example, most programs will include content on body image, grief, privacy, relaxation, and hostility. Terminology may differ, but common areas of content are covered regardless of the conceptual framework. The concepts included in this edition are those likely to be included in various orientations to nursing. The generality of the concepts or their wide applicability might be viewed as strengths.

The second edition focuses primarily on substantive rather than process-oriented concepts. Attempts have been made both to update and strengthen concepts developed for the first edition and to present new concepts. Six new concepts are presented: loss, alienation, boredom, hope, restlessness and relaxation. Restlessness, based on an article originally published in *Nursing Outlook,* has been modified for the second edition.

Ten of the original set of concepts are included here: trust, shame, body image, stigma, grief, hostility, denial, transactional analysis, humor and privacy. The chapters on shame and trust are essentially the same in content as in the first edition, but many topics have been added to the chapter on body image, such as obesity, women's changing body image, the sexual revolution and body image and problems created by medical technology. The chapter on hostility has been revised to include discussion of more definitive differences among such phenomena as anger, hostility, aggression and violence. Denial has been revised to include alcoholism, studies on specific conditions in which denial is common and more emphasis on denial as it relates to death and dying. The chapter on humor has been updated and a new section on cultivating the use of humor added. The chapter on privacy has been expanded to include recent nursing literature and research on privacy, new clinical examples and discussion of legal and group efforts to protect people's privacy (that is, the Federal Privacy Act of 1974 and the American Hospital Association Patient's Bill of Rights). Grief has been completely redeveloped, using literature on numerous types of crises and placing greater emphasis on nursing process and nursing research. A guide for assessment of loss and grief is included. Revisions in the chapter on stigma include the introduction of labeling and deviance theory from a sociological framework. Public deviant identity as differentiated from private and consensual deviant identities is defined and applied to nursing situations. The role of essences as moral identifiers and modes of adaptation to deviance are noted and applied to nursing. Finally, the following changes have been made in the chapter on transactional analysis: definitions and descriptions of basic concepts are more precise; application of definitions and descriptions to nursing are clearer; sections on ego states, strokes, life positions, and scripts are expanded; such new material as a chart of ego state behaviors, egograms, the drama triangle, cultural scripting of women and men, and the script of nurse is included; and references are updated.

In the second edition the editors begin an attempt to show relationships between concepts. The material has been divided into four sections. Introductions show some of the relationships between these concepts.

CHANGES IN NURSING

In the years since the first publication of this book, there have been many dramatic changes in the practice of nursing and in nurses' relationships with each other, other professionals and organizations. Among those affecting the utilization and further development of behavioral concepts in the practice of nursing are (1) proliferation in types of specialization; (2) return to the apprenticeship system in certain agency orientations and specializations; (3) increased focus on power; (4) changes in organizational practice; and (5) intraprofessional struggles for legitimization of position, status, prestige and power. In the following paragraphs, each of these topics will be discussed in greater detail.

Questions about quality as well as quantity are raised when the proliferation in types of specialized nursing is at issue. Identification of nurses by formal education and licensure obtained, such as LPN (LVN), RN (technical or professional), does little to inform the employer about the tasks a particular nurse can perform, the information obtained by assessing patient behavior and her or his abilities to function in a bureaucratic institution or work successfully with patients and coworkers. Similar questions are raised for patients and other professionals with the use of profession-ascribed titles such as nurse clinician, clinical specialist, independent nurse practitioner, physician's assistant or associate, or primary care nurse.

Despite the confusion for consumers, coprofessionals and other professional coworkers over the proliferation of specializations and expansion of the nurse's role, some generalizations about nurse specializations may be made. It is generally accepted that nurses with these new titles will utilize instruments, skills, pathophysiological knowledge and problem-solving procedures traditionally viewed as within the physician's purview. In the narrower fields, such as the care of the physically, acutely ill patient, the nurse specialist is expected to have thorough knowledge of specific pathophysiological disorders, to exercise considerable judgment in treatment alterations and also to be comfortable with and efficient in the use of complex instruments and machinery. In the broader fields, such as family health, knowledge of pathophysiology is usually limited to statistically common malfunctions for age groups; patient teaching is seen as a basic treatment modality; and the instruments used are usually simple. For the practitioners in both narrow and broad fields, the institution of or alteration in pharmacological treatments and certain diagnostic procedures is bounded by physician or cooperatively derived protocols. In discussing the different types of nurse specialists, most authors emphasize the importance of psychosocial concepts in assessing patient problems and planning comprehensive nursing care.

One of the topics most persistently discussed in the letters-to-the-editor sections of professional journals and the research findings on recent nursing graduates is the lack of technical skills exhibited by the new nurse. Health care institutions have met this perceived lack by reintroducing apprentice or formal educational programs. For both health care and educational institutions, the intellectual, economic and ethical implications of this development have proved to be a dilemma. For the health care institutions, the old questions about the effectiveness of apprenticeships and cost to the patient of more formal educational programs are raised. For the educational institutions, educational balance, proper curriculum planning for future practice and recent reductions in college and university budgets are issues. Though individual authors differ on the solution for the problem, most suggest patience, pragmatic and formal testing, adherence to efforts for improved patient care and assurance of patient safety as measures that are necessary before dramatic changes can be made.

Identical questions are raised about the apprentice/formal education procedures used to prepare nurses to function as physicians' assistants or associates, family health practitioners, and so forth. As university nursing faculties have gained the skills and knowledge needed for teaching these new nurse practitioners, it has become possible to alleviate some of the problems of cost to the patient or the total population of patients.

Another persistent theme in nursing publications and practice is power. There are at least four recurring subthemes under this topic. These are (1) the women's liberation effort; (2) power relations between nurses, doctors and other agency administrators; (3) sporadic and limited, though significant, reports on increased militancy over economic issues and definitions of nursing function (patient care standards); and (4) the place of men in nursing.

The first of the themes mentioned above seems to be of major importance. Long before the formalization of a women's liberation effort, prominent nurses have been commenting on the subservience of nurses (female) to physicians (male). The rationale for this subservience most frequently mentioned by these nurses involves the military and religious origins of the nursing profession. More recent authors have seen the socialization process of men and women, based on male superiority, as a significant factor in the difficulties women face in any profession.

Although some authors have argued that nurses have always exercised some control over both their own actions and the health care of patients, they suggest that the strategies the nurse uses are evidences of further degradation for her as a female and a human being.

Other authors, analyzing power relationships between nurses, physicians and health care administrators, note the disparities in power allocation as a consequence of the nurse's status as an employee. Suggestions for new methods of supplying nursing personnel to health care agencies and the individual patient are frequently supplemented by noting the need for individual nurses to be more assertive in their function of patient advocate and their interactions with physicians and agency administrators.

The third theme of increased militancy in battles for better economic recompense and improved control over the practice of nursing is most frequently found in the newspapers and news columns of professional journals. The role of professional organizations in providing expert labor relations counsel and educative programs on employee-employer relationships continues to provoke considerable discussion over the appropriateness of a professional organization undertaking what many see as union functions. The American Nurses' Association's inability to recruit the majority of practicing nurses as active members continues to be a major obstacle to its effective use of power, not only in single institution negotiations, but also in providing nursing input into state and national health care planning.

Both female and male practitioners are ambivalent over the increased recruitment of men into nursing. Some male practitioners have found it necessary to demonstrate through research that men are as empathetic and nurturing as women. Some female practitioners have looked upon male nursing recruits as messiahs who will bring the whole profession increased prestige and economic rewards. What seems undeniable is the ability of male practitioners to achieve positions of prestige and economic reward in proportionately greater numbers than their female colleagues.

Throughout this discussion of power, the significance of past and present socialization processes that divide the sexes and allocate position and status may be noted. Catherine Norris comments on the consequences of the women's liberation efforts on the changes in female body image, and it may also be hypothesized that pervasive and long-lasting changes are occurring in female nurses' perceptions of their profession, their interactions with physicians and agency administrators and their commitment to improve both nursing and total health care.

The fourth type of change in nursing practice which affects the use and further development of behavioral concepts in nursing is in organizational practices. Specific topics to be discussed are (1) changes in job titles; (2) changes in methods of patient assignment; (3) changes in intraagency communications systems; and (4) the effects of recent interpretations of the Taft-Hartley Act vis-à-vis supervisors.

The proliferation of clinical appellations previously mentioned is matched by a proliferation of job titles within the health agencies. For example, the traditional titles of director, supervisor, head nurse and staff nurse have been supplanted in many places by titles such a president, vice-president, assistant clinical director, associate clinical director, clinical specialist, team leader and primary care nurse. These titles are frequently followed by appropriate designations or descriptions of positions, such as "of nursing service," "of nursing education," "of medical-surgical nursing" or "of pediatric nursing."

It should be noted that in many instances these title changes tend to reflect concomitant changes in organization, the most optimistic of these organizational changes being the attempts to shift from vertical (supervisory) to horizontal (collegial) relationships and communication systems among nurses and between nurses and other personnel. Changes in titles may be seen by the profession as reflecting the state of flux and climate for improvement in patient care. In many instances, however, they may only symbolize the mysteries of present health care practices for the recipient of nursing care.

Equally problematic for clients, and to some extent for nurses, are the modifications of nursing personnel assignment procedures for care of patients. Presently, at least three systems are in use: functional, team and primary nursing assignments. Pragmatic observations and philosophical preferences frequently conflict with economic considerations in selecting the system of care. Because of the cogency of the latter consideration and the continuing difficulty in distinguishing and explaining the differences in the skills and knowledge of different levels of nursing personnel, the argument for economic accountability is often the ascendant one.

In recent years, intraagency communication systems have become a focus of intra- and interprofessional discussion. The legal demands for formal and written systems of communication have frequently interfered with the ability of nurses to communicate effectively with each other or with other professionals. The development of interprofession care plans and progress notes has been one innovation directed to the correction of this problem. The dissemination of information about Problem Oriented Medical Records (POMRs) and the decision by many nurses across the country to develop a nomenclature of nursing diagnoses have been an integral part of this innovation.

The suggested improvements in written communications have been supplemented by the continuing efforts to make oral communications among nurses and between nurses and other professionals more effective. Recent authors, in discussing the use of interprofession conferences, have noted the reluctance of higher status professionals to accept the nurses' contributions as being noteworthy and the resultant games nurses play when they recognize their observations and suggestions are considered unworthy.

The fourth factor noted as significant to organizational practice is the effect of Taft-Hartley Act interpretations on supervisory nursing personnel. It can be speculated that some of the organizational and title changes mentioned above have the latent objective of circumventing some of the definitions within the Act or in recent interpretations of it. Most nursing writers familiar with the Act and its interpretations see the elimination of nursing supervisory personnel from participation in labor negotiations as severely weakening the power of these nurses to act as professionals as well as lessening the power of all nurses in individual institutions to exercise control over their personal and professional destinies.

The final discussion of this section approaches the proliferation in types of nurses from a different frame of reference, that of the profession's efforts to police itself, to make more clear to its clients the distinctions between different levels of nurse practitioners and to develop methods from within the profession to accord status and prestige to some of its practitioners. The present efforts to legalize the educational requirements for different levels of nurses and enforce continuing education as a part of licensure may be listed under the rubric of self-policing and clarifying of distinctions for clients. The intensity of the arguments for and against each of these endeavors indicates not only the debators' attachment to the status quo but also real ambivalence about the differences in quality of the separate types of formal nursing education. Equally at question are the effectiveness of formal education in contrast to informal on-the-job learning and the efficiency of any type of testing introduced to date in measuring individual accomplishments.

The recent move to create academies of nursing where the individual nurse may gain recognition for excellence in practice marks the profession's efforts to award prestige and status in a manner recognizable not only to one's colleagues, but also clients, health care agencies and other professionals. There is presently a general lack of understanding of the meaning of various types of recognition. The most significant aspect of this change in nursing is the acknowledgment of the need to recognize excellence in nursing.

NURSING THEORY AND RESEARCH

The abundance of recently published material on nursing theory and research was considered as justification for not discussing particular theories in detail in this book. In the bibliography following this introduction, the reader will find representative books and articles that treat these subjects in detail.

USE OF THIS BOOK

The second edition should be useful to the same people as the first. The concepts are relevant to students at any point in their education, including graduate school. They also apply to any area of nursing practice, and can therefore be used by any practicing nurse. Chapters may serve many purposes for the reader. The reader may be interested in learning the content, the process of concept development, or research ideas. The second edition should serve these specific interests better than the first since the concepts are more carefully defined, application is generally more precise and there is greater emphasis on research.

The chapters in this volume illustrate the applications of concepts from single or from several academic disciplines. For example, Betty Blackwell's chapter on stigma is based almost completely on a sociological frame of reference; Silvia Lange's on shame and Dorothy Bloch's on privacy combine sociological, psychological and psychiatric viewpoints; Norris's on body image adds to these three disciplines concepts from medicine and natural science.

Using these four typical articles to demonstrate one possible method of application of the content reveals the following features:

1. The concepts are universally applicable. They are not restricted by type or severity of illness or by specific social contexts.
2. Definitions of each concept involve discussion of what it is not. For instance, Lange must define guilt in order to clearly delineate the features of shame.
3. Individually, the concepts do not explain fully any everyday occurrence. Although individual concepts are universally applicable, each of the authors, in suggesting application to nursing practice, discusses the influence of other concepts in what occurs in actual situations.
4. Elaboration of the concept does not clarify the circumstances under which that particular concept would best explain the phenomena under observation or predict specific behavior resulting from its application.

A careful reading of these four articles will demonstrate these first two features. The interrelatedness of the selected concepts is demonstrated by the inability of any one of them to be fully persuasive without consideration of the other three. One cannot imagine any everyday situation in which shame is present without the concepts of stigma, privacy and body image being involved, although, as Lange points out, these three concepts are not all of the explanatory concepts presently available to the practitioner.

The fourth feature mentioned above perhaps best demonstrates the state of tested knowledge in both nursing and the behavioral sciences. Norris[2] has previously stressed that adequate conceptualization is one of the first steps in developing nursing knowledge. The authors of this volume have endeavored to achieve such adequate conceptualizations.

The reader is advised to view the content as explicated and the concepts as defined and applied as unfinished. More is unknown than is known. As Norris points out in her chapter on restlessness, difinitive descriptions of the phenomena we are trying to study and understand in nursing are needed. This is true of all of the concepts described in this volume. What are the relevant behaviors and how do they relate to the respective concepts? Each chapter includes attempts at definitive descriptions which may need further refinement. Hopefully, questions that are generated will lead to research, more questions and more answers. Teachers, practitioners, students and researchers are all faced with the problems of trying to work with the knowledge presently available while realizing its inadequacies. Clients need to be taught and cared for now. Students are in educational programs now. Education and practice go on despite gaps, uncertainties and controversies. As long as the researchers, teachers, students and practitioners continue to ask questions and keep track of the progress made by others in the profession, the knowledge base of nursing will grow. Satisfaction with current knowledge, on the other hand, can only lead to contentment with current practices, blindness to the efforts of some to improve nursing care and indifference to the development of nursing concepts and theory. Both knowledge and practice then would rapidly become obsolete.

ORGANIZATION OF THE SECOND EDITION

The sixteen concepts in the second edition are divided into four sections: Section I includes body image, loss, stigma, shame and grief. These might be viewed as higher order concepts or constructs that are relevant to almost any illness or disability. Body image is the aspect of self most commonly attacked, threatened or altered by illness and disability. Loss includes objective and subjective perceptions of changes occurring in one's life. Loss is perceived when changes cause disruption in the achievement of important goals. The chapter on stigma includes a discussion of social processes that compound losses resulting from behavior, appearance, abilities and the like not in keeping with social norms or expectations. The stigmatized individual is judged to have less social worth than expected. Chapters on shame and grief include descriptions of painful emotions that commonly accompany stigma and loss. Shame refers to negative emotions such as disgrace, humiliation and embarrassment. Grief refers to a complex set of emotions that commonly follows a major loss perceived by the individual. Guilt, hopelessness, fear and anxiety are but a few of these emotions. All of these concepts are considered relevant to patients and patient care wherever the patient may be.

The second section includes four concepts: boredom, hostility, restlessness and alienation. All of these seem to have a general negative connotation. Alienation has many dimensions, such as powerlessness, normlessness, social isolation, self-estrangement and meaninglessness. Alienation and other concepts in the section have many commonalities and are related to concepts included in the first section.

The third section includes six concepts that cover feelings, thoughts, processes and states commonly related to comfort or well-being. Trust and hope are positive attitudes. Humor and denial of illness tend to decrease discomfort or increase comfort. Privacy and relaxation involve the goal of comfort or relief of tension.

The fourth section consists of just one chapter, Transactional Analysis. This chapter is very different from the others. Lange shows how a theory can be taken from another discipline and applied to nursing.

Certainly there are many ways to organize and apply the contents of the second edition, and the reader is encouraged to do so. Such efforts are taxing but very stimulating.

REFERENCES

1. A four-year project supported in part by Grant Number 5T31MH-9509 from the National Institute of Mental Health, Public Health Service, U.S. Department of Health, Education and Welfare, awarded to the Department of Continuing Education in Medicine and Health Sciences, University of California, Los Angeles, led to the first edition.
2. Norris, C. M.: The professional nurse and body image. *In* Carlson, C. E. (coord.): Behavioral Concepts and Nursing Intervention. 1st ed. Philadelphia, Lippincott, 1970.

BIBLIOGRAPHY

Changes in Nurse Roles and Organizational Practice

Alford, D. M., and Jensen, J. M.: Primary health care—reflections on private practice. Am. J. Nurs. 76:1966-68, December 1976.

Anderson, E. M. et al.: Epigenesis of the nurse practitioner role. Am. J. Nurs. 74:1812-16, October 1974.

Anderson, M.: Primary nursing in day-by-day practice. Am. J. Nurs. 76:802-05, May 1976.

Ashley, J. A.: This I believe about power in nursing. Nurs. Outlook. 21:637-41, October 1973.

Bakke, K.: Primary nursing perceptions of a staff nurse. Am. J. Nurs. 74:1432-34, August 1974.

Bullough, B.: Influences on role expansion. Am. J. Nurs. 76:1476-81, September 1976.

Ciske, K. L.: Primary nursing evaluation. Am. J. Nurs. 74:1436-38, August 1974.

Clark, T. P.: Primary health care—counseling victims of rape. Am. J. Nurs. 76:1964-66, December 1976.

Crandall, S. G.: Primary health care—how an FNP won over the bureaucracy. Am. J. Nurs. 76:1963-64, December 1976.

Craven, R.: Primary health care—in a nursing home. Am. J. Nurs. 76-1958-60, December 1976.

D'Addio, D. L., et al.: The clinical coordinator, a multifaceted role. Nurs. Clin. North Am. 8:247-55, June 1973.

Davis, M. Z.: Rehabilitative care in the skilled nursing facility: the mismatch of organizational structure and patient needs. J. Nurs. Admin. 22-27, January 1977.

Fagin, C. M.: Nurses' rights. Am. J. Nurs. 75:82-85, January 1975.

Group, T. M., and Roberts, J. I.: Exorcising the ghosts of Crimea. Nurs. Outlook. 22:368-72, June 1974.

Hanson, E. T.: Nurse practitioner in ambulatory psychiatric care. Nurs. Clin. North Am. 8:313-23, June 1973.

Hartley, L. M.: Complemental nursing—nurse's viewpoint. Am. J. Nurs. 77:985-87, June 1977.

Heimann, C. G.: Four theories of leadership. J. Nurs. Admin. 18-24, June 1976.

Keller, N. S.: The nurse's role: is it expanding or shrinking? Nurs. Outlook. 21:236-40, April 1973.
Kelly, L. Y.: Institutional licensure. Nurs. Outlook. 21:566-72, September 1973.
Kramer, M., and Schmalenberg, C. E.: Conflict: the cutting edge of growth. J. Nurs. Admin. 19-25, October 1976.
———: The first job . . . a proving ground basis for empathy development. J. Nurs. Admin. 12-20, January 1977.
Lambertson, M. M.: Primary health care—adult nurse clinician on a psychiatric unit. Am. J. Nurs. 76:1961-63, December 1976.
Leininger, M. M., et al.: Primex—the professional nurse responsible, accountable, reaching out and taking an active, frontline position in primary health care. Am. J. Nurs. 72:1274-77, July 1972.
Lewis, M. A., and Lewis, C. E.: Protocols for the nurse practitioner: uses and problems. Am. J. Nurs. 76-1312-23, August 1976.
Logsdon, A.: Why primary nursing? Nurs. Clin. North Am. 8:283-91, June 1973.
Lynch, C. C.: Management of nursing care on a psychiatric unit—nursing care coordinator. Nurs. Clin. North Am. 8:293-303, June 1973.
Mauksch, I.: Pro—nursing is coming of age through the practitioner movement. Am. J. Nurs. 75:1835-43, October 1975.
O'Shaughnessy, C.: Diary of an angry nurse practitioner. Am. J. Nurs. 76:1165-68, July 1976.
Page, M.: Primary nursing—perceptions of a head nurse. Am. J. Nurs. 74:1435-36, August 1974.
Rogers, M. E.: Con—nursing is coming of age through the practitioner movement. Am. J. Nurs. 75:1834-43, October 1975.
Schmalenberg, C. E., and Kramer, M.: Dreams and reality: where do they meet? J. Nurs. Admin. 35-43, June 1976.
Schutt, B. G.: Spot check on primary care nursing. Am. J. Nurs. 72:1996-2003, November 1972.
Simms, L. L.: Administrative changes and implications for nursing practice in the hospital. Nurs. Clin. North Am. 8:227-34, June 1973.
Stitely, D. M.: The role of the division head in a decentralized nursing service system. Nurs. Clin. North Am. 8:247-55, June 1973.
Styles, M. M.: In the name of integration. Nurs. Outlook. 24:738-44, December 1976.
Whitson, B. J.: Complemental nursing—patient's viewpoint. Am. J. Nurs. 77:985-87, June 1977.
Wolford, H. G.: Complemental nursing—originator's viewpoint. Am. J. Nurs. 77:985-87, June 1977.

Power

Ashley, J. A.: This I believe about power in nursing. Nurs. Outlook. 21:637-41, October 1973.
Bowman, R. A., and Culpepper, R. C.: Power: RX for change. Am. J. Nurs. 74:1053-56, June 1974.
Bush, P. J.: The male nurse: a challenge to traditional role identities. Nurs. Forum. 15:390-405, 1976.
Group, T. M., and Roberts, J. I.: Exorcising the ghosts of the Crimea. Nurs. Outlook. 22:368-72, June 1974.
Haase, P. T.: Pathways to practice; parts I and II. Am. J. Nurs. 76:806-09 and 76:950-54, May and June 1976.
Hopping, B.: Professionalism and unionism: conflicting ideologies. Nurs. Forum. 15:372-83, 1976.
Hott, J.R.: The struggles inside nursing's body politic. Nurs. Forum. 15:324-39, 1976.
Kalisch, B. J.: Of half gods and mortals: Aesculapian authority. Nurs. Outlook. 23:22-28, January 1975.
———: An analysis of the sources of physician-nurse conflict. J. Nurs. Admin. 51-57, January 1977.
———, and Kalisch, P. A.: A discourse on the politics of nursing. J. Nurs. Admin. 29-34, March-April 1976.
Lawrence, J. C.: Confronting nurses' political apathy. Nurs. Forum. 15:363-71, 1976.
McBride, A. B.: A married feminist and her job. Am. J. Nurs. 76:754-57, May 1976.

Powell, D. J.: The struggles outside nursing's body politic. Nurs. Forum. 15:341-61, 1976.
Raheja, K.: Nursing in transition. Nurs. Forum. 15:413-18, 1976.
Ramphal, M.: Clinical and administrative judgment. Am. J. Nurs. 72:1606-11, September 1972.
_____: Peer review. Am. J. Nurs. 74:63-67, January 1974.
Shapiro, B.: The dead end of altruism: a note to a nurse. Nurs. Forum. 15:384-89.
Sills, G. M.: Nursing, medicine and hospital administration. Am. J. Nurs. 76:1432-34, September 1976.
Styles, M., and Gottdank, M.: Nursing's vulnerability. Am. J. Nurs. 76:1978-80, September 1976.
Zimmerman, A.: ANA: its record on social issues. Am. J. Nurs. 76:588-90, April 1976.

Taft-Hartley

Cleland, V.: Taft-Hartley amended: implications for nursing—the professional model. Am. J. Nurs. 75:288-92, February 1975.
Despres, L. M.: What the National Labor Relations Act really says. Am. J. Nurs. 76:790-94, May 1976.
Herzog, T. P.: The National Labor Relations Act and the ANA: a dilemma of professionalism. J. Nurs. Admin. 34-36, October 1976.
Leininger, M.: Taft-Hartley amended: implications for nursing—conflict and conflict resolution. Am. J. Nurs. 75:292-96, February 1975.
Zimmerman, A.: Taft-Hartley amended: implications for nursing—the industrial model. Am. J. Nurs. 75:284-88, February 1975.

Concepts

Aiken, L., and Aiken, J. L.: A systematic approach to the evaluation of interpersonal relationships. Am. J. Nurs. 73:863-67, May 1973.
Barnett, K.: A theoretical construct of the concepts of touch as they relate to nursing. Nurs. Res. 21:102-10, March-April 1972.
Bolin, R. H.: Sensory deprivation: an overview. Nurs. Forum. 13:240-51, 1974.
Clark, C. C.: Reframing. Am. J. Nurs. 77:840-41, May 1977.
Ebersole, P.: Reminiscing. Am. J. Nurs. 76:1304-05, August 1976.
Fagerhaugh, S. Y.: Pain expression and control on a burn care unit. Nurs. Outlook. 22:645-50, October 1974.
Gordon, M: Nursing diagnosis and the diagnostic process. Am. J. Nurs. 77:598-601, April 1977.
Gunderson, K. et al.: How to control professional frustration. Am. J. Nurs. 77:1180-83, July 1977.
Jones, S. L.: Orthopedic injuries: illness as deviance. Am. J. Nurs. 75:2030-33, November 1975.
Kalisch, B.: The stigma of obesity. Am. J. Nurs. 1124-27, June 1972.
_____: What is empathy? Am. J. Nurs. 73:1548-52, September 1973.
Kinlein, M. L.: Self care concept. Am. J. Nurs. 77:598-601, April 1977.
Macdonald, M. R.: How do men and women students rate in empathy? Am. J. Nurs. 77:998, June 1977.
Mansfield, E.: Empathy: concept and identified psychiatric behavior. Nurs. Res. 22:525-29, November-December 1973.
McCorkle, R.: Effects of touch on seriously ill patients. Nurs. Res. 23:125-32, March-April 1974.
Meleis, A. I.: Role insufficiency and role supplementation: a conceptual framework. Nurs. Res. 24:264-65, July-August 1975.
Rose, M. H.: Coping behavior of physically handicapped children. Nurs. Clin. North Am. 10:329-39, June 1975.
Schmidt, J.: Availability: a concept of nursing practices. Am. J. Nurs. 72:1087-89, June 1972.
Shusterman, L. R.: Death and dying: a critical review of the literature. Nurs. Outlook. 21:465-71, July 1973.
Strauss, A. et al.: Pain: an organizational-work-interactional perspective. Nurs. Outlook. 22:560-66, September 1974.
Vincent, P.: Some crucial terms in nursing—a second opinion. Nurs. Outlook. 23:46-48, January 1975.
Wiener, C. L.: Pain assessment on an orthopedic ward. Nurs. Outlook. 23:508-16, August 1975.
Wolff, I. S.: Acceptance. Am. J. Nurs. 72:1412-15, August 1972.

Books:

Byrne, M. L., and Thompson, L. F.: Key Concepts for the Study and Practice of Nursing. St. Louis, Mosby, 1972.

Roberts, S. L.: Behavioral Concepts and the Critically Ill Patient. Englewood Cliffs, N.J., Prentice-Hall, 1976.

Theory

Berthold, J. S.: Theoretical and empirical clarification of concepts. Nurs. Sci. 406-22, October 1964.

Duffey, M., and Muhlenkamp, A. F.: A framework for theory analysis. Nurs. Outlook. 22:570-74, September 1974.

Books:

Auger, J. R.: Behavioral Systems and Nursing. Englewood Cliffs, N.J., Prentice-Hall, 1976.

Hardy, M. E. (ed.): Theoretical Foundations for Nursing. New York, Mss Information, 1974.

King, I. M.: Toward a Theory for Nursing: General Concepts of Human Behavior. New York, John Wiley, 1971.

Norris, C. M. (ed.): Proceedings First Nursing Theory Conference. University of Kansas Medical Center, Department of Nursing Education, 1969.

Orem, D. E.: Nursing: Concepts of Practice, New York, McGraw-Hill, 1971.

Paterson, J. G., and Zderad, L. T.: Humanistic Nursing. New York, John Wiley, 1976.

Riehl, J. P., and Roy, Sister C.: Conceptual Models for Nursing Practice. New York, Appleton-Century-Crofts, 1974.

Walter, J. B. et al.: Dynamics of Problem-Oriented Approaches: Patient Care and Documentation. Philadelphia, Lippincott, 1976.

Research

Gortner, S. R., et al.: Contributions of nursing research to patient care. J. Nurs. Admin. 23-28, March-April 1976.

———, and Nahm, H.: An overview of nursing research in the United States. Nurs. Res. 26:10-33, January-February 1977.

Schlotfeldt, R. M.: Nursing research: reflection of values. Nurs. Res. 26:4-9, January-February 1977.

Smoyak, S. A.: Is practice responding to research? Am. J. Nurs. 76:1146-50, July 1976.

Additional Readings

Christman, L.: Editorial—Where are we going? J. Nurs. Admin. 15-16, February 1976.

Editors: Nurses and nursing's issues. Am. J. Nurs. 75:1848-59, October 1975.

Norris, C. M.: Delusions that trap nurses . . . Nurs. Outlook. 21:18-21, January 1973.

Welch, C. A.: Health care distribution and third-party payment for nurses' service. Am. J. Nurs. 75:1844-47, October 1975.

Section I Fundamental Concepts in Illness and Disability

INTRODUCTION

Each of the five chapters in this section emphasizes the interpersonal and social aspects of processes frequently encountered in nursing practice. The influence of age or developmental task accomplishment is delineated in chapters on body image, loss, grief and shame. In Stigma, the major focus is on society's contribution to feelings and behaviors associated with the health-illness continuum and to the treatment and prevention of illness.

Catherine Norris defines body image as the constantly changing total of conscious and unconscious information, feelings and perception about one's body and responses to sensations originating from inner regions of the body as one copes with a kaleidoscopic variety of living activities. The body image is basic to identity and has been referred to as the somatic ego. Norris operationally defines body image as a social creation, noting that definitions of normality, sanctions for deviations, and approval and acceptance for compliance with societal norms act as interfaces with the individual's bodily and personality development, behavior and experiences.

She further explicates and discusses in detail body image problems stemming from pathophysiological processes; medical and nursing activities; threats to the continuity and stability of body image arising from normal development; cultural differences; interruptions to patterns of adaptation; degree and rate of change. Some common adaptations to alterations in body image are anxiety, humor, testing, experimentation, grief, rage and denial.

In her discussion of nursing intervention, Norris suggests variables deemed significant in history-taking and assessment. Inferences from these variables about nursing care planning are deducible and are developed further in later chapters.

Betty Blackwell defines stigma as the condition in which expectations about a person's social identity are judged by cointeractants as less than what that person or someone of a similar social identity should be. Such devaluations lead to a decrease in the individual's feelings of self-worth as well as in the cointeractants' estimation of his or her social worth.

The author distinguishes between the consensual deviant identity (discredited), the private deviant identity (discreditable) and the public deviant identity. The development of a stigma mythology and the use of essences as moral identifiers are discussed.

Blackwell further develops Erving Goffman's categories of own, wise and normals into categories of own, professional and intimate wise, and nonafflicted audience. The nurse's role as one of the professional wise is discussed. Blackwell also comments on aspects of relationships with the own, intimate wise and nonafflicted audiences which are relevant to the stigmatized.

Possible responses to stigmatization are discussed in detail. Nine modes of adaptations are suggested: acquiescence, repudiation, flight, channeling, evasion, modification, reinterpretation, redefinition and alteration. Blackwell summarizes recent nursing literature's conclusions and recommendations about conditions ordinarily carrying some stigma.

Following Goffman's conclusions, Blackwell discusses tension management as the task of the discredited. She notes that the main task of the discreditable is information control. For those with a public deviant identity, she suggests, the main task may be information manipulation. Implications for nursing education and practice in each category are discussed.

Shame is the basic feeling arising from the individual's deviations from social or personal expectations. As noted in the discussion of the chapter on stigma, the stigmatized individual's recognition of being classified as inferior results in the experiencing of shame. Silvia Lange notes the effect of others on both the development and monitoring of discrepancies between the ego and ego-ideal.

Lange defines shame as a discrepancy between ego and ego-ideal. It may arise from within the self or be induced by others. It involves the uncovering of such features as weakness, failure, physical defect, passivity, misplaced confidence or lack of recognition. Shame is generated when a goal or ideal is not being reached; concerns the more basic, unalterable aspects of the self in comparison with the ideal; contains a threat of abandonment; may involve the feeling of having loved the wrong person or being inadequate for the person one loves; and refers mostly to visual exposure.

Distinctions are drawn between shame and guilt, and it is noted that pride may be seen as the feeling opposite to shame. Specific observable responses are listed. Lange further discusses the development of shame and comments on the role of parents in developing standards; the role of disgust in developing body image; and the role of sociocultural values in developing the ego-ideal. Specific age-related conditions relevant to the origination of shame experiences are noted.

Lange suggests that shame may alert the ego to some impulse, thought, fantasy or act that has failed or may fail to meet its standards. Such a warning, if heeded, permits the individual to escape the discomfort of extreme shame. Lange notes that even extreme feelings of shame may lead not only to fuller understanding of oneself, but also to a better understanding of human behavior in general. In sharing one's shame with another, a trusting relationship may develop and lead to further growth in self-confidence and confidence in others.

Shaming as a technique in child-rearing and other interpersonal contexts is discussed. Lange comments on the individual techniques of responding to shaming by others. She notes the practices commonly used to avoid shaming as well as those initiated by shaming of another. Specific application to nursing practice is made. Noted among the common nursing situations in which shame can be anticipated are (1) modesty situations; (2) regressive behavior under stress; (3) reactions of the patient and family to critical situations; (4) body changes; (5) failure to meet social values; or (6) another's behavior or condition.

Feelings of loss and grief frequently are consequences of alterations in body image and stigma. Carolyn Carlson defines loss as any change in the individual's situation that reduces the probability of achieving implicit or explicit goals. It is assumed that a person's goals, ends or hopes exist to satisfy his or her needs. Severity of loss is related to the salience of goals that have become less accessible and the extent of goal disruption, displacement or extinction.

Carlson suggests that there are individual variations in aspects of specific goals (clarity, concreteness, numbers of paths available), in the relationships between goals (hierarchical arrangement, centrality) and in the effects on goal achievement (facilitation, obstruction, independence). In addition, she states that there are major objective characteristics of situations that disrupt goal achievement. These are: visibility of a change; duration; abruptness; extent of change in physical structure or function; time required for treatment, relearning and reconstruction; and financial requirements.

Included in Carlson's discussion are person characteristic variables which influence responses to loss, such as clarity of goals, openness, coping mechanisms, flexibility, motivation, education, age, past experiences with loss, attitudes and internal-external control orientation.

After discussion of the differences between objective and subjective definitions of loss, Carlson elaborates on and illustrates the consequences of the loss of people, body parts or function, inanimate objects, and abstract notions such as loss of freedom, happiness, hope, dreams, certainty or predictability.

In discussing nursing intervention, suggestions are made about variables requiring investigation for thorough nursing assessment. Nursing care actions, discussed further in later chapters, can be deduced from the assessment.

In the final chapter, Carlson defines grief as a complex combination of numerous emotions at the time of loss. The complex emotions include anxiety, indifference, guilt, hope, hopelessness, helplessness, despair, ambivalence, anger and possibly many more. Grief begins with the awareness of loss.

Carlson describes the phases of grief as precrisis, impact and shock, realization or initial awareness, retreat, acknowledgment, acceptance and adaptation. Within the discussion of each phase, clinical examples and nursing interventions are suggested. In addition, pathological patterns of grief, their manifestations and current therapies are delineated.

Carlson notes that variables such as suddenness of, anticipation of, and preparation for loss and the relationship of the grieving person to the lost object influence the intensity and duration of the grief process. Other variables discussed include age, sex, beliefs and values, personality characteristics, prior experience, socioeconomic status, social networks and cultural variations.

As noted by both Norris and Carlson, individual responses to changes in body image, loss and grief are influenced by the response of intimate others and the expectations arising from social values held by all interactants. In the discussion of stigma, Blackwell suggests that an understanding of stigma emphasizes the importance of society's contribution to one's behavioral responses to an alterated health status.

In each of the chapters in this section, internal and external conditions which affect both the healthy and ill are discussed. Such discussions alert the nurse to observe for situations in which the occurrence of any of the concepts is probable and hence preventable; is in process and therefore open to mediation; or has occurred and therefore demands treatment. As noted previously, the focus of the chapters is primarily on history-taking and assessment in the nursing process, although planning and intervention are also discussed.

It is believed that each of the chapters provides background and bibliographical data which suggest critical and needed research topics. Some of the authors have made the research needs explicit. Others, in presenting deductive and theoretical information, implicitly suggest the necessity of field research on the concepts.

1 BODY IMAGE
Its Relevance to Professional Nursing

Catherine M. Norris

WHAT IS BODY IMAGE?

Body image is the ever-changing total of conscious and unconscious information, perceptions and feelings about one's body as different and apart from all others. It is a social creation, developed through reflected perceptions of the surface of one's body, investments one makes in parts or the whole of the body and responses to sensations originating at the inner regions of the body as the individual experiences a kaleidoscopic variety of activities. The body image is basic to identity and has been referred to as the somatic ego.

Body image evolves slowly through the process of growth and development. Once identity tasks are completed in adolescence, it becomes more rigid, but still incorporates the sum of significant experiences and changes over time at a slower rate. One of its functions is to provide a sense of personal existence in time and space. Its rigidity processes and defends against change, devaluation and attack. It acts as a standard or frame of reference which influences people's ability to perform and the ways in which they perceive themselves, measure their continuity through life, and identify their mastery of the world. Once established, body image defines and places demands and limitations on what a person is capable of in life. Interpersonally, it expresses an individual's personality in many ways and with vivid representation.

Ultimately, body image is an intrapersonal experience of our feelings and attitudes toward our bodies and the way we organize these experiences. Much of the auditing of subjective experiences that makes and modifies the body image is unconscious, and no one can describe his or her own total body image. Much can be learned about one's own body image and that of others by observing how people use their bodies and listening to what they say. It is not uncommon for a person to recognize body image expressions in others which have communication value. A character trait of "weakness" may be assigned to someone with a receding chin. If a man is prematurely bald, he may be labeled "virile." Someone with knock knees may not be taken seriously; or a person who is flat-footed may be considered "tactless" or even "not very bright." If one has a big nose, he or she may be labeled as a member of a "minority group." Certain kinds of posturing are called "effeminate" in men or "masculine" in women. Certain hairstyles make the person look like a "hippie."

OPERATIONAL DEFINITION

The following outline constitutes an attempt to develop an operational definition of "body image." It is an oversimplified definition of a very complex concept. This definition was created within the framework of the growth and development process. It is based on some of these ideas:

1. Body image is a social creation.
   a. Normality is judged by appearance, ways of gesturing or posturing, and other ways of using the body that are prescribed by society.
   b. Painful sanctions are imposed for deviations from normality, whether behavioral or structural.
   c. Approval and acceptance are given for normal appearance and proper behavior.
   d. Body image emerges from an almost infinite variety and number of approvals and sanctions and an individual's response to them. Experience is integrated into the personality in terms of the satisfaction or dissatisfaction that the individual has had with it.
   e. Body development continually enlarges the individual's world, mastery of it, interaction with it (including interpersonal interaction) and ability to respond to the wide variety of experience it offers.
   f. This integration, which is largely unconscious, is constantly evolving and can be identified in the person's values, attitudes and feelings about him or herself.
2. There is very close interdependence between body image and personality, ego, self-image and identity.
3. Body image is an important determinant of behavior.
4. The impact of any experience on the human being is determined by the interplay of its reality level or meanings, the level of conscious fantasy and feeling about it, and unconsciously motivated fantasies and feelings.

STEPS IN THE DEVELOPMENT OF BODY IMAGE

1. At birth there is no physical body image except at the feeling level—comfort, discomfort, hunger, rage, pain and so on.

2. Mother is perceived as external source of comfort and discomfort—experienced but not interpreted by infant. Polyphasic rhythm of body functioning in terms of time cycle is learned through mother's response to needs.

3. Self is explored, with an ever-increasing number of variables involved—sensory impressions, motility, kinesthetic and touch sensations, ego development and sociocultural stimuli; pleasure, pain, shame or doubt are experienced, with concomitant learning of body attitudes, values and boundaries.

4. Opportunities are provided for exploring and manipulating environment—bathing, eating, toys, tools, water play, snow play, jungle gym and rhythmic activities, with concomitant learning of attitudes and values of

power, pleasure, fear, doubt, helplessness and so on. Beginning of adaptation to diurnal sleep-rest pattern and other adult structured circadian rhythms.

5. One becomes aware of separateness of one's own body from mother and all others.

6. Opportunities arise for learning about various parts of body and their functions, to be discovered with joy and pride or to be hidden in shame.

7. Opportunities occur for learning mastery of the body—to do, to protect self, to protect others, with internalized feelings of pleasure, power, confidence which fosters self-esteem, or to learn feelings of helplessness, pain, inadequacy, doubt and guilt.

8. Opportunities for manipulating self and tools of environment are provided.

9. One learns to use and master environment—e.g., running, skipping, skating, swimming, with concomitant learning of pleasure, competence and worth, or feelings of inadequacy.

10. One learns to relate to others of the same sex, with concomitant feelings of pleasure, power, warmth and anticipation, or pain, doubt and fear.

11. Opportunities arise for learning to audit or listen to the body with the potential for developing internalized feelings of pleasure and power.

12. There is praise, blame, derogation or criticism in relation to body, body part, or usage of body or body part, with internalized pleasure or pain, doubt and guilt.

13. The body and its function are appraised comparatively and competitively at level of peer group, with concomitant learning of values and attitudes about the body as strong, competent and powerful, or weak and helpless.

14. One learns to relate to persons of the opposite sex, with concomitant learning of values, attitudes and use of the body.

15. One accepts one's body without undue preoccupation with its function, or the control of these functions, so that one is free for other living activities.

16. The residuum of unresolved experiences, misconceptions, distortions and fears in relation to body image that persists from childhood is recognized.

17. One learns to see the personality as a whole, with less emphasis on the physical self and greater emphasis on the inner or psychic self, in preparation for aging and developing mature acceptance of self and full human potential for living.

HOW DOES BODY IMAGE DEVELOP?

The psychoanalytic concept, typified by Freud, is the most complex of the theories formulated. In psychoanalytic theory, the body is essentially divided into three areas or zones. The tools and tasks of these three areas, developing in succession—oral, anal, genital—are the focus of this theory. The success of the individual in coping with the changing demands of each area as it comes into its period of dominance is considered necessary to the development of a mature body image. If the individual is not able to integrate the functioning of each of these body zones in its turn into the total body scheme, his or her body image will retain some immature aspects. These immature images will interfere with securing adult satisfactions, which interference may be evidenced by personality disturbance. For example, in the anal phase, in which mastery of body and environment is the task, children who do not learn who they are in relation to the world, how they can manipulate their environment, and how they can manage or control their bodies, may be left with an "all thumbs" body image or may rationalize that physical activity is for the common people and esthetic activities are reserved for the elite.

Using the developmental approach, we can state that the body image develops pre- and postnatally by means of successive sequential steps in differentiation. Its goals are manipulation, mastery and control of relationships with self, others and environment, within a time-space context or rhythm. It is dynamic—ever-changing, evolving, expanding or contracting, progressive or regressive, but goal-directed in terms of forming newer, more stable systems in the organism. As new neural functions develop, they are integrated into the total individual, building on top of and inhibiting earlier and more primitive nervous structures. However, under stress, older ways of interpreting and functioning in relation to the body image may be revived. The human body image develops through sensory messages from the inner surface of the body and from the outer surface in contact with the environment. These sensations, which are received as the organism audits, experiments with, and manipulates the body and the environment, are of several kinds. They may be tactile, thermal or painful. Sensations come from the muscles, organs and nerves of the body in response to inner functioning or contact of the body with the environment. These experiences of the body may be interpreted in terms of feelings, view of self, by comparing and contrasting with other persons and comparing and contrasting with group or cultural value systems. Experiences, the use to which the organism puts them, and their storage in the form of memory provide a sense of body unity. Thus, each individual has a three-dimensional perception of form and position which functions as the somatic ego. Like the psychic ego, the somatic ego is developed as the result of experience (considering that the id is inherited and the superego is culturally determined).

The infant receives many internal perceptions which can only be interpreted as satisfying or painful. Many of these messages originate in the mucosa of the mouth and the nervous structures of the body periphery. Severe maternal anxiety would be first experienced peripherally, but the full perception would be in the deep layers of the infant's body, with several organs potentially involved. The first component of body image to emerge, then, is the group of sensations felt in relation to the inner workings of the body and the way in which these workings communicate to the total organism. The second phase develops as the child explores the environment and works at mastering it. Impressions are made as to how one's body compares with others and whether one's body is attractive to others. With time, more stable impressions of sensation, mastery and normality are formed: the ego identity base being strong, there are more integrations with the psychic components of the ego, in which intellectual and emotional development are more in focus. The individual's intelligence, emotional health, social and interpersonal adequacy and general satisfactions in living will influence to a great extent awareness of his or her body and preoccupation with it. It is possible for many people to rather skillfully monitor or "listen" to their bodies without morbid preoccupation, while others are fully preoccupied with their bodies and get most of their satisfactions at this level. The healthy person is aware of how the body feels, how it works and the effect of the physical self on others. One teacher makes this point about a student:

> I have one very attractive little student. Others see her as little, but she has never in the world thought of herself as little. She is very short, but she is very capable and this does not seem to get in her way. Once there were two big patients slugging it out with each other and she rushed in and put her hands on each of their chests and said, "Now, stop it you guys!" And, fortunately, they stopped it. Several people talked to her about it; her interpretation was that she felt big enough to cope with it and she did.

THE DYNAMIC NATURE OF BODY IMAGE

In illness and health there is a wide variety of messages about the body being constantly fed into the system, either for interpretation-acceptance with integration into the self or for rejection and revision. The infant responds to inner and outer experience at the sensory level with screaming, raging or cooing. Success in achieving comfort and relief from pain and anxiety prepares his or her body for the task of mastering the environment. Children in the two-to-four-year group, struggling with this task, are still uncertain of bodily boundaries and experience extreme apprehension about having their nails and hair cut. They have difficulty seeing body productions, namely feces, as separate and, given the chance, tend to resist having them flushed away.

After a sudden growth spurt, adolescents, not knowing how to manage their changed bodies, are very preoccupied with the changes in terms of cultural and social norms and attractiveness and study their bodies, comparing various aspects of them with those of their peers.

An occasional maternity patient describes the experience of delivering a baby as having her insides torn out. We need to study this type of reaction and to determine its meaning for a newborn infant's acceptance and integration into the family, the relationships between husband and wife, and its influence on family planning.

Every nurse is familiar with the disturbances in the person's body image following loss of a major part. A classic example is the phantom leg of the amputee patient. Although we may not be able to explain it on either a physiological or a psychological basis, we recognize it as a common phenomenon following amputation. It is so real that patients often act as if they still have both their legs, and end up falling to the floor, and we realize that this phantom may persist for years. We are somewhat aware that loss of certain other body parts—hair, teeth, one eye or both, the nose or a breast—necessitates adjustment of the person's body image. But, we are often not sure of how patients perceive their body images as the result of the loss and what the relationship of this perception is to their emotional experience.

We are less familiar with other events in which the body image of patients is disturbed. Patients' responses to these disturbances are less subject to recognition and study because the cause-and-effect aspect of the other events is not always as obvious as in the case of the loss of a limb. An obvious loss is only one experience in which a person's concept of his or her body image is affected. There are, in addition, surgical procedures in which the relationship of body parts is disturbed, such as colostomy, ileostomy, ureteroenterostomy or gastrostomy. A person living with a colostomy can no longer ignore what may have been conceived as the dirty or unpleasant part of bodily existence, for it is right under his or her eyes and nose.

In other surgical procedures the loss of body parts, even if invisible to others, may necessitate a revision of the patient's body image. A woman often has a difficult time physically and emotionally after a hysterectomy. There is a wide variety of changes in perception of the body image which play a part in this emotional response. What does the loss of a lung, gallbladder, larynx or stomach do to the patient's own body image? It is a natural tendency among many nurses to assume that removal of the diseased organ is a complete solution to the patient's original problem.

The literature provides us with some evidence that repair procedures, such as are done in plastic surgery, may not produce the change in the body image that either the patient or surgeon assumed would occur. To what extent or how nurses could foster the hoped-for result is not known, and this possibility has been little explored. For example, a patient feels inferior because of an unusually large nose or ears that protrude to an abnormal extent and goes to a plastic surgeon who does a plastic repair. The patient cannot reconstruct his or her body image to take in the improvements, but feels the same—inferior to others—as before the surgery. How would the nurse go about studying this problem and identifying the steps in intervention? What are the risks in trying to help change a patient's concept of his or her body image?

We usually think of a surgical procedure when we think of the problem of integrating change in a body part into the total body scheme. Actually, equally dramatic physical changes occur in human pathophysiology. Can we, as nurses, study the various ways in which patients deal with changes in body size and proportion such as in the development of obesity, emaciation, acromegaly or gigantism? Other changes in the external surfaces of the body may be caused by the development of characteristics common to the opposite sex, as the development of mammary glands in men or hirsutism in women. People respond to color changes in the skin, such as in Addison's disease or chronic dermatitis. Skin texture also changes in such conditions as exfoliative and excoriative dermatitis, in thyroid conditions or in scar formation. In both atrophic and hypertrophic arthritis an almost infinite variety of changes, often grotesque, occur not only in the joints, but also in the muscles, which atrophy for lack of use. Body posture may be distorted, and the face may take on the appearance of chronic suffering. Crippling changes occur in multiple sclerosis and Parkinson's disease.

Another problem of body image with which we are confronted is failure of a body part to function. Loss of function is usually accompanied by atrophy if the failure lasts a long time or is permanent. The rising rate of automobile accidents, along with military casualties, has increased the number of paraplegic patients. Nurses usually know a great deal more about the "acting out" behavior of the paraplegic than they do about how the patient's change in body image is perceived and interpreted. With the increasing number of older people among the population, more patients are seen who have had cerebrovascular accidents with accompanying loss of function of one or more body parts.

Although heart attacks, asthmatic attacks and pneumonia do not leave a body part functionless, the symbolism of these diseases in terms of life and death may cause distorted notions of structure, function or significance. The organ may have a special image, even independent of the body, with special needs and a name of its own, such as "Burpy" or "Ticker."

Side effects of drug therapy such as moon face, hirsutism, striated skin, or changes in body contour can be very threatening to the body image.

Violence is an evolving social theme. Both patients and nurses have problems dealing with the purposeless attacks on the body image that rape, shooting and knifing represent. In psychiatric nursing, schizophrenic patients often have very poorly organized concepts of their bodies. If asked to draw a picture of themselves, they may draw parts of their bodies separate from their torsos or place parts of the body in incorrect relationship to each other. They may deny the existence of one or more body parts. We all know the patient who cannot eat because he or she "hasn't any stomach." We are familiar, too, with the patient who has anorexia nervosa, in which the maintenance of a particular kind of body image is a major component of the illness. In hypochondriasis, fantasies of somatic attack occur. In malingering there is conscious direction of concern to an organ or part through simulation of illness. Hysteria, a subconscious phenomenon, represents the dissociation of emotional content, displacement of the problems, isolation of a body target and projection of the problem onto the organ that symbolizes the problem.

The patient who has tuberculosis and is isolated in the hospital receives the communication that his or her body is unacceptable and undesirable. This communication is reinforced by the amount of time he or she is actually left alone. The patient's input system picks these up in addition to whatever is felt and perceived to be happening in the chest. A patient whose condition is unavoidably malodorous may have considerable difficulty integrating this body concept into a total sense of identity.

We have been relating body images to illness and pathology, but as we become sensitive listeners we also become aware of the interactive nature of body parts and feelings in all interpersonal experience. There are literally thousands of idioms describing feeling behavior that people use every day. Nurses can learn to identify, by the theme in patients' use of body idioms, organs that feel, are sensitive, or may be possible targets for the individual under extreme stress. Many of these terms draw dramatic word pictures, such as "chicken-hearted," "yellow bellies," "lost my head," "blood-curdling," "jump out of my skin," "get my teeth into," "broken-hearted" and so on. Others, although not as pungent, are still descriptive of a certain physical experience, such as "pain in the neck," "knees turned to water," "big mouth," "can't stomach any more," "have a belly full of," "knocked my eye out" or "put my finger on."

Intuitively, we are aware that body posture or functioning tells us a great deal concerning how we feel about ourselves, how we feel today, how we approach people, and how we function. However, there have not been a great many systematic studies documenting how behavior or feelings participate in shortening of muscles, depositing or invading of muscle tissue by fatty tissue, reducing function of the joints, or affecting coordination of the body in action.

BODY IMAGE DYNAMICS: ACCELERATION AND CHANGE

Dramatic social changes between 1960 and 1977 have had an impact on the body image of almost everyone in Western civilization, if not everyone in the world. These changes influence every aspect of culture and the lives of each of us. The years between 1965 and 1975 have been called the decade of the body.

The women's movement and the sexual revolution have had an impact on the body image and body integrity of almost every woman. Obesity has become our number-one health problem. When one in three Americans is overweight, it means that one-third of the population has adjustments to make in or problems with body image. Medical technology has reached the point where organ transplants between humans are commonplace and mechanical and animal transplants are anticipated for the future. Medical technology saves persons who previously would not have survived. For example, patients with 90 percent second- and third-degree burns can be saved even though they may look like monsters. Technology also keeps people alive when there is no hope for recovery. In response, the theme of the right to control one's body when it has become unserviceable or unbearable to contemplate has emerged. The aging population, 25,000,000 people over 65, has to cope with great changes in body image and integrate chronic diseases into an already deteriorating body image. The sexual revolution has not only been influential in people's body image but also in the removal of homosexuality from the disease nomenclature of the American Psychiatric Association and the acceptance of transexualism with its accompanying surgery as a reasonable option, forcing society to modify its ideas about the static nature of body image. Increasing use of drugs has increased body awareness and changed definitions of body boundaries for the millions of people who take or experiment with them. The use of trail bikes, Hondas, motor boats, dune buggies and snow mobiles, as well as automobiles, from childhood on has added the concept of speed to body image, and the space program promises increases in body speed. People incorporate their vehicles' speed into their body image. They say, "I go 60 miles an hour," "I almost got hit" or "I barely squeezed through." Immobilization may mean something very different for people who have adapted to the body speeding through space than for people of earlier times.

Touching with hands, lips and arms has increased as patting, kissing and embracing are used in both public and private situations. Touching is also more available to nurses as a means of actively reaching out to people to decrease isolation and loneliness.

Increased attention on violence has brought out the problems of child-battering, incest, rape and wife-beating. The effects of people's bodies being misused and violated is being studied within and without the health care system. Increasingly, victims are recognized by nurses or go to nurses for help.

Surgical technology that maintains the appearance of youth, such as face-lifting and hair transplants, are commonplace for both men and women without the secrecy of semi-stigma of two decades ago.

Within the last decade we have been forced to realize that pouring more money into the health care system will not improve people's health to any great extent. People must take the responsibility for their own bodies. As they develop lifestyles which reduce major health risks, the emerging theme of self-care will change people's conceptions of their bodies. They will value them more, listen to them more intently, relate behavior to what goes on with the body and take their own risks with their bodies. Nurses will play an important role in this change in focus and function. People will need to be motivated and taught in ways nurses have yet to develop.

In summary, the women's movement, the sexual revolution, an increase in obesity, a greater proportion of aged in the population, advances in medical technology, speed, drugs, violence and the prospect of self-care are the major changes which have affected our body image in the last 15 or 20 years.

OBESITY AND BODY IMAGE

Obesity as a health problem has increased to the point where more than one out of every three people is more than 10 percent overweight, and the number of people overweight is even higher among those over 30 because of weight increase as people get older. Most medical literature focuses on the increased risk of stroke, heart attack and some types of cancer for an overweight population, but by focusing on the body image of overweight people we can see their self-hate, self-derogation, and feelings of failure and helplessness.

We can also look at the feelings of helplessness and rage of professionals who have produced few lasting cures and no generally successful treatment for obesity in 50 years of exhortation, diet invention, dire threats, hypnosis, psychotherapy, surgery and behavior modification.

Most researchers and clinicians differentiate between overweight and obesity, though both may create the same body image problems. Some investigators use the term overweight to indicate all weight above a given standard. One common standard is the Metropolitan Life Insurance Company's table of the normal range of men and women's weights according to age and height. (Though in general use, this was developed using mostly white, middle-class people who purchase insurance.) However, overweight, according to this type of standard, may have nothing to do with fat. The extra weight might be lean muscle mass that would make an athlete weigh more than someone the same sex, age and height with a desk job. The term obesity is used by investigators to indicate all excess body fat, while some clinicians define obesity as 20 percent overweight. Thickness of skin folds is used by some to measure body fat, and there are other ways to compute it. Regardless of method of measurement, excess body fat is not in vogue in our culture. Forty years ago, causes of obesity were ascribed to overeating or to the endocrine glands. So few endocrine cases were found that this cause was almost dropped and overeating became *the* cause. Gradually, the spare or thin human figure has become popular. Fat people have become stigmatized in two ways. First, they are viewed as ugly, repulsive, and to some degree unemployable, and second, as undisciplined pigs who could stop gorging if they wanted to. Almost 100 percent of fat women and about 50 percent of fat men know they are overweight and feel some degree of self-hate. Studies indicate that members of this large group have all tried to slim down.

One of the sad commentaries on medical, self and other treatment of obesity is that most successful weight loss is quickly followed by failure—weight gain. And this situation, especially when it is repeated over and over, compounds the feelings of self-hate and helplessness. Many fat people are unable to look in a mirror; they avoid their reflections in store windows as they walk down the street; they put off shopping for clothes until they are threadbare, and when they do shop they find few attractive clothes in large sizes. Studies indicate that most obese people exaggerate their body size, particularly width.[1] This discrepancy between their actual body size and their concept of it increases the body image problem. This is what an essentially unicausal etiology and a rigid cultural value have done to a considerable portion of the population.

What is the real situation today with excess body fat? In addition to psychological causes, genetic, thermodynamic, endocrine, neuroregulatory, biochemical factors in metabolism as well as ethnic factors and family practices have been found to be related to obesity. It is also recognized that obesity occurs much more frequently among poor people who have no status or prestige in the community.

If obesity is a subconscious way to camouflage feelings of helplessness and inadequacy, then the resulting projection of a huge body makes a lot of sense as compensatory behavior. Who is going to see a large hulk of a person as vulnerable? Who is not going to think twice before taking on a person bigger than one's self? Whatever unsolvable problems excess body weight attempts to solve, if there were any other choices for coping fat people would take them. H. Bruch, after extended contact with many difficult individuals who repeatedly tried to diet and became depressed or acutely disturbed by failure, concluded that "as handicapping as overweight is, there are people who function better with extra weight. Obesity, although a faulty adaption, may serve as a protection against more severe illness; it represents an effort to stay well or be less sick."[2] Bruch goes on to indicate that difficulty in losing weight is not the problem, although this is the focus of medicine, much of the research and to a great extent weight reducing programs. If this is not the problem, reducing is not the cure. The underlying problem has to be identified and worked through.

Obese people do not receive the same kinds of messages from their bodies as other people. Most people eat when they are hungry and in response to increased gastric motility. Obese people respond more to messages from the environment, like the odor of food, time of day, availability of food or the degree of stress experienced from the environment. Obese people are also much less active than other people and feel no pleasure from activity. Obese people often say, "I don't like to do anything I can't do in a rocking chair." It may be that people with excess fat are more awkward than other people. This lack of activity and awkwardness is thought to be related to their disturbed body image. If people do not move about, do not interact and do not get feedback from their environment, how can they know about size, functions, boundaries or where self leaves off and the nonhuman environment begins? Being glued to a chair or seeming to be a part of the furniture takes on new meaning from the perspective of obese people's body image.

There is little or no explanation of why there are so many people who overeat and do not get fat if the basis of excess body fat is the intake of calories in excess of those needed for energy output. There are few data on why a person who diets and loses 20 pounds regains only 20 pounds when he or she goes off the diet, returning to the original weight. Why not gain 30 pounds or stop five pounds short of the original weight?

All obese people are not the same. Excessive weight gain is not uncommon in infants or even newborns in the first four weeks of life. Because adipocytes can increase in number, at least in the first year of life, obesity in infants is a hyperplastic process compared to obesity in adults, whose adipocytes only increase in size with the increased deposition of body fat. Adult obesity is a hypertrophic process. The problems of adult obesity built onto infant obesity, with the increased number of cells available for storage of fat, can readily be seen.

The infant at risk of obesity is usually the formula-fed infant. The breast-fed infant determines the quantity he or she gets, not the mother. The formula-fed infant is encouraged, even urged, to take a prescribed amount. The formula may be richer than breast milk in both electrolytes and nutrients, which would cause thirst and further ingestion of formula to reduce the thirst; and, also, infants on formulas often have solid foods introduced earlier. Mothers may feel guilty about not breast feeding and mix a formula richer than directions call for. Overprotective mothers (those ambivalent about the baby or motherhood) will overfeed and force feed their infants. When food is offered to solve every problem (rage, frustration, hunger, anxiety) the child cannot learn the difference between hunger and other needs. Also it is not long before the child becomes slow, ungainly, awkward and sluggish. The feedback from this kind of activity, plus disapproval from people, makes development of a normal body image impossible. When fat children draw pictures of themselves, the drawings are more global and less differentiated than normal children's. Their self-drawings are immature in form and concept; they are less detailed than the drawings of normal controls; they lack sex differentiation and contain more distortions than the drawings of normal controls.[3] There is some evidence that childhood and adolescent obesity predispose to adult obesity, but there is little agreement about the nature and scope of this relationship.

Nurses might think of preventing life-long body image problems, thus reducing great human suffering. First, nurses might want to develop skills that support breast feeding, such as working through fears of great intimacy and dependence, feelings of repulsion at breast feeding, concern about confinement required by breast feeding and fears about not having enough milk or the ability to breast feed. Nurses need to help mothers who decide not to breast feed to relax about it so they do not stuff the baby. These mothers need to feel comfortable making the formula according to directions, offering water between feedings and withholding solid food until the infant is three months old or weighs 14 pounds. Mothers may need help in differentiating between hunger and other infant communication and in developing a repertoire of appropriate responses to the needs being expressed. A feeding schedule in which the infant takes enough for a three- or four-hour period without having to be forced may take some patience. On the other hand, nurses need to be alert to mothers who, in their anxiety, keep waking the baby. Case finding of obese infants and young children should allow for early intervention. No reports were found on the treatment of obese young children.

An increasing number of adolescents are becoming obese, and it is beginning to appear that there are certain stressful periods when obesity is apt to occur as a maladaptive response. Obesity seems more likely to occur at puberty, just after marriage, after the delivery of a child and at menopause. No studies were found that looked at hormonal changes or hormonal levels in relation to the development of obesity.

Obese people live in a hostile, stigmatizing, rejecting environment. They are unable to control their own bodies or eating behavior. They are full of self-loathing and are more different from other people than the simple fact of obesity might lead one to believe. Nurses need to get the pressure off of these people. Medicine, with its high failure rate, has joined society in focusing on fat as the problem and in castigating overweight people as neurotic, unwilling to change and weak. Nurses need to alleviate guilt and reduce the stigma. They need to identify with the person's need to eat and relate the needs to antecedents, expectations or feelings in the ongoing situation. If the focus must be on eating, one could support eating five small meals a day. In cultures where the total population eats five meals a day, there is less obesity, and trying this as treatment has been suggested.

Of the thousands of articles written about obesity and its control, very few document the real feelings of people about themselves and how much these people suffer on an average day. There is no systematic documentation of the things these people say about their bodies, their activities or their relationships. There are materials in psychiatric theory indicating that grossly obese people feel helpless and have such needs to control that they try, symbolically, to incorporate people and the environment as well as food. Real documentation about the problem gets lost in the professionals' and investigators' preoccupation with overeating and overfeeding. It is a wide open area, long overdue for depth research.

THE CHANGING BODY IMAGE OF WOMEN

Women and the world in which they secure health care are different from what they were 15 years ago. Women have had to confront the medical care system, in particular, because medicine for more than a century has contributed substantially to defining women. Women were defined as incomplete in body, unwell when menstruating, sick when pregnant, nonwomen after hysterectomy, mentally disturbed during or after the menopause, often hypochondriacal and at all times slaves to the cyclical nature of their physiology. In society as a whole, beauty, good breasts, rounded buttocks and good legs were the valued components of the body.

Women have worked hard with physicians to have their complaints investigated seriously and to remove the psychogenic labels from their symptoms. As women have become more sure of themselves and more in tune with their bodies, they have become less accepting of medical and social values concerning their bodies. When unable to secure the health care they wanted they established their own health care centers. Women are learning to listen to themselves and to assess themselves and each other. They are learning and helping each other to enjoy their own bodies. At one level they are promoting heightened body awareness in social and business relationships through consciousness raising and assertiveness training. At another level they are helping each other learn sensuality to enjoy their bodies and helping each other with problems that cause women to be nonorgasmic. Women, by being better informed about contraception, can be as sexually free, or almost as free, as males. Women have done a great deal to remove the stigma and guilt from masturbation as an alternative way of enjoying their bodies. And they are working to demedicalize normal processes such as pregnancy and childbirth. There is a large group of people whose new faith in their bodies helps them resist being dependent, unintelligent, weak and invalided to conform to the expectations of those delivering medical care.

Of even greater importance is the demand that women have control of their own bodies. While it has been common practice to have husbands or parents sign for certain operations on women's reproductive organs, in most states much of the legal work has been done to clear the way for women to have abortions and sterilization surgery with only their own approval. In a civilized world it seems alien to have to demand control of one's own body, but there are strong social and political forces at work to take away the gains of the last few years.

Nurses need to think about working with two groups of women. Some older women have not changed their concept of body image or beliefs about who controls their bodies. Some younger women have consciously chosen the same value system. But many younger women who have been socialized differently have changed. For example, it is common for young women who have had mastectomies to refuse prostheses. They do not have to conform their bodies to the old norm of having all the right sexual symbols. Women over 40, on the other hand might be expected to be uncomfortable without a prosthesis to conform to their norm.

Nurses need to be knowledgeable, open and articulate about the female body, reproductive functions, female sensuality, female orgasm, and alternative sexual practices and lifestyles as well as self-examination and self-care. Like most women, nurses, have been both uncomfortable talking about and unknowledgeable about masturbation, intercourse, orgasm, homosexuality and bisexuality. They have been extremely uncomfortable when confronted with the person who masturbates, is homosexual or is bisexual. Nurses are often ill-prepared to discuss the issues involved in tubal ligation, abortion, oral contraception and intrauterine contraceptive devices. All of these practices provide for active communication from the external and internal surfaces of the body and the higher centers of the brain. All of them have some effect on the ever-changing body image, body boundaries and sense of the physical self.

Assault, rape and battery of women have been brought out in the open. Women have insisted that these practices be halted and that severe punishment be meted out to the perpetrators. Police, physicians and hospital emergency services have had to develop more humane methods of treating women victims of violence, and refuges have been developed for battered women. Subjugation of one person by another by inflicting physical pain, wounds or bruises is always considered demeaning, but in middle-class America physical assault is equated with barbarism. How one sets body boundaries and feels secure within one's body in such a milieu is not known, particularly when the victim, whether beaten, battered or raped, is often made to feel guilty of somehow instigating the violence. Many women fear battering but remain silent because they fear they will surely die from more battering. Woman-beating has been a brutal sub-rosa theme of the subjugation of women in Western society for a long time. Hopefully, legislation will outlaw beating and battering as well as rape, and refuges, financial aid and legal protection will be provided. Until they are, professional nurses' tasks with these women will be difficult to accomplish.

Nurses need to be able to deal with the state of emotional shock which traumatized women are in when seen. Battered women come for help feeling injured, dirtied, broken and vulnerable as well as guilty. Nurses need to help these women to feel rage and take action. They need to be gentle with bruised bodies as one way of affirming that the body is good.

Now there is greater emphasis than before on women's sports from school through professional ranks. Women athletes have new prestige and prominence. Women are demanding opportunities in all-male occupations, such as heavy equipment operation, truck driving, mining and heavy duty assembly line jobs. Women are beginning to view their bodies as stronger, more competent, more whole and more equal to the task of hard physical endeavor than before. We can expect some changes in the kinds of illness (increased heart disease) and injuries seen in women because of changes in occupational hazards.

THE SEXUAL REVOLUTION AND BODY IMAGE CHANGES

The subject of body image, male or female, cannot be separated from the sexual revolution of the last two decades. While there are many causes for the sexual revolution, a few that provided impetus and gave it shape are: (1) the idea that human sexual pleasure is separate from reproduction, an idea that is not generally true among other animals; (2) the women's movement; (3) the population explosion and subsequent zero population growth concept; and (4) the development of technology providing acceptable, effective contraceptive methods. Thus the sexual revolution has resulted in sexual freedom for women as well as men and vastly increased the number of sexually active teenagers, teenage and extramarital pregnancies, and the range of normality for sexual relationships and practices. Premarital casual or contractual sex lifestyles have much greater acceptance. Group and communal sexual lifestyles also have greater acceptance. Masturbation, oral sex, artificial instruments for increasing sensual experience, and sexual experimentation are all better accepted as long as the people involved are consenting. The sexual revolution has also made legalized abortion an acceptable alternative to dealing with pregnancy among a large group in the population, and several states have legalized abortion. Seven million abortions were performed in 1975, and there was an 8 percent increase in 1976. Fifty percent of all extramarital pregnancies occur in the 15-to-16-year-old group. It is estimated that more than 4 million teenage girls are sexually active.

Both men and women seek variety and greater heights in sexual experience. There is almost no end to the books published to help people toward this goal. It is common knowledge that scratching, bathing, chewing, biting, urinating, sucking and other primitive activities provide pleasure in one or more erogenous zones, and though it is not discussed in polite society, the enjoyment of these activities is enhanced in a variety of ways. Warm water, water under pressure, electrical vibration, locally applied drugs and creams, and smooth or rough textured materials are among agents that stimulate peripheral nerve endings.

As women have begun to feel whole and their bodies have become free, the ways women feel about and present their bodies have also become free. Women's clothing has become much less restrictive. Certain age groups have essentially given up girdles and brassieres. Looser, briefer clothing allows more freedom of movement and sitting positions. The many acceptable "in" styles from which women may choose allow them to enhance their body scheme with individuality. Lack of clarity about one's body, however, puts some women in conflict and creates disorganization and ambivalence in their dress. Men, too, are freer in dress. New styles drawing attention to their sexuality by emphasizing the genitalia and permitting rough estimates of size have become accepted and popular.

Despite the revolutionary increases in sexual activity, lack of knowledge about reproductive system functioning, contraception and sexual practice is still widespread, especially among teenagers. Even married women with children are often unsure about such things as when ovulation occurs in the menstrual cycle. While it is difficult to explain the degree of ignorance of one's body that exists, one might speculate that adolescents are only working through the great changes in body image and testing their attractiveness and sensory ramifications without making rapid advances toward responsible adult knowledge and behavior. Another explanation for women in general is that in the past men took responsibility for all knowledge about sex and are still determined to legislate certain aspects of sex. It may be that there is a time lag between freeing one's body and taking responsibility for it. The client/patient education role of the nurse needs to be developed so all nurses can function as experts in sex teaching.

The vast number of 13 to 16-year-old school girls who become pregnant each year needs to be a concern of nurses. Nurses who work in schools, clinics, VNAs and hospitals have these young people as clients and patients. These girls are subjected to a threefold maturational crisis. They are struggling with a large order of developmental tasks. While completing their anatomical and physical growth, they are also working out their identities as persons and as women, which includes sexual identity, heterosexual commitment, independence from parents and home, choice of vocation and commitment to work at it, learning of mature emotional skills, development of the ability to form lasting relationships, learning of love and tenderness and adoption of a personal value system and ethical guidelines. On top of this they are confronted with an unexpected pregnancy and must learn new roles as wife and mother, unwed mother and child or unwed mother alone.

Discovery of the pregnancy, often made by teachers or family members before the girl knows she is pregnant, is another crisis. Each girl's crisis is different, but fear of telling parents, embarrassment, guilt, grief for hurting family, leaving school, having nothing to do, disbelief and denial are common reactions.

Another kind of crisis is the high risk nature of teenage pregnancy. While toxemia and prematurity are the most severe of these high risks, weight gain, depression, hypochondriasis, fear of labor and delivery and suicide attempts are also common. Later, child-battering may be another kind of high risk for these girls.

The bodies of these girls become very fragile to them. They cannot talk enough about labor and delivery. They greatly fear the pain and what the whole process will do to them. They constantly pump their peers who have been through labor and delivery for information and overuse nurses who are available and accepting. While they may be distrusting of adults and ambivalent about authority, they will generally use adults who go out of their way to show acceptance. It should be obvious that the younger the pregnant girl the more severe her problems will be, including the body image one. Many girls, when the pregnancy begins to show or even before, will wear a large covering coat that they never remove or will not face people. They turn their heads or whole bodies aside. They demonstrate lack of acceptance by saying, in effect, "I cannot bear what my body is telling about me." We need to study these girls in terms of what kinds of reactions and behaviors correlate with subsequent child-beating. Nurses, providing care, need to be ego supporting, support hope, be consistent, promote satisfaction for achievements, help to identify challenges and support facing the future. These functions are in addition to fostering the emergence of tools needed to accomplish the tasks of adolescence.

Tubal Ligation and Vasectomy

In 1975 one of the partners in more than 31 percent of all married couples had been sterilized. The total number of men and women who have been sterilized is about equal, although sterilization of women is increasing rapidly. The recentness of this solution to the termination of reproductive capacity for large numbers of people prevents careful delineation of problems. But it is known that some of these people do have problems. These problems do not usually appear immediately after sterilization, but within six months to two years later women may become inorgasmic and men may become impotent. Some men and women overreact in their sex roles. Men become more aggressive, more authoritarian and dramatize their masculinity in dress, speech and action. Women may do the same in overreacting to the feminine stereotype. The rigidity of the body image probably accounts for the delayed reaction. The reaction itself is probably related to the body image change finally registering in people whose sexual identity is somewhat fragile or contains latent homosexual tendencies which remained quiescent while the intact sexual organs provided an adequate defense. Prevention of this type of outcome must rest in developing presurgical assessment tools that identify the poor risks. Actually, many surgeons doing these procedures do no in-depth interviews and do not have skills necessary to assess unconscious conflicts. Nurses who see these clients preoperatively are in a position to contribute useful data about them and can be useful to them by exploring their needs or helping them explore alternative solutions if this is indicated.

Sex Reassignment

Transsexual treatment programs, or sex reassignment as it has come to be known, are hardly ten years old in this country, and while the citizenry hardly raises eyebrows over the concept any longer there is still considerable disagreement among professionals. Those opposed do not usually differentiate between transsexuality and homosexuality. They refer to the treatment as gender transmutation, since one is born and dies the same sex. They believe that by eliminating external and internal sexual organs as well as giving intensive hormone therapy all chance of reversal is destroyed should the person have a change of heart. Some people have regretted going through with the procedures. They see professionals putting people into a course of treatment in the expectation that internal sexual conflicts and other problems will be resolved by changing the body image. Those against sex reassignment programs point out the possibility that people obsessed with having surgery and neurotics with an overwhelming desire for change could be processed into these programs, which require a considerable number of surgical procedures producing drastic change. They also point out the rigidity of body image in many people who have to integrate plastic surgery, noting that depression and even psychosis may be part of the outcome.

In 1966 the Johns Hopkins Hospital established the Gender Identity Clinic. While there are now about 40 such clinics, this was the first in this country and it did a great deal to legitimize sex reassignment. In most clinics an interdisciplinary team evaluates people for admission to the program, using a number of tests and in-depth interviews. In simplest terms, transsexuals are differentiated from other people, including homosexuals, in that they have always felt they belonged to the opposite sex and never accepted the primary or secondary sex characteristics of their sex, feeling that these parts were a mistake and inconsistent with their body schema.

After assessment and acceptance into a sex reassignment program, there is a period of intensive hormone therapy that changes the secondary sex characteristics to some extent. Then, in the male, the scrotum and penis are amputated. Some penile tissue is saved to line and make an excitable and functioning vagina. In some cases plastic surgery further enlarges the breasts, which usually have increased in size with the hormone therapy. In the female bilateral mastectomy and panhysterectomy are performed. It is not possible at this time to create a functional penis.

Nurses caring for these patients need to be aware of behaviors and verbal communications that express doubts about sexuality and conflict about the sex reassignment program. Nurses need to learn to accept this alternative for the people who select it. People who select alternative sexual lifestyles have not had good experiences in hospitals or with nurses. Effective nursing for transsexuals requires moving beyond American middle-class orientation to sex. Nurses need to be prepared for some participants in this kind of program being disappointed and be able to work with them as with anyone who has had an irretrievable loss and is grieving. They also need to be prepared for the patients who constantly press for more surgery. This need has to be explored in terms of inadequate sexual identification, masochism, interpersonal inadequacy and other problems surgery symbolically deals with. Depression, irritability, demanding and inconsistent behavior are all clues that the patient faces some kind of body-image dilemma.

One final point before leaving the subject of sex reassignment is its relationship to the generally accepted idea of penis envy by females. There are five men for every woman requesting sexual reassignment. Also, research findings show that men whose wives are pregnant draw larger and larger pictures of themselves as the pregnancy progresses. The drawings show an identification with pregnancy almost as if the men were pregnant. What is going to happen to penis envy as a concept in women's development? Are women going to be born complete at long last?

BODY IMAGE PROBLEMS CREATED BY ADVANCED MEDICAL TECHNOLOGY

"The miracles of survival are often so spectacular that no one can blame the surgeons for failing to weigh the costs of the procedure against the likelihood of a workable rehabilitation result."[4] Never in the history of medicine has there been such daring invasion, replacement and grafting of the human body as there has been within the last decade. Kidney transplants are common now. Heart valve replacements are common. We anticipate liver and more successful heart replacements and there is talk of brain replacement. Transplants involve the body image of two people, a donor and a recipient. This sounds simple enough. However, living donors are providing a gift of inestimable value. They often provide it under considerable duress. Transplant teams consciously structure their behavior to avoid pressuring potential donors, but the prospective donor knows it is a life-death situation to be resolved. The prospective donor may also be the only suitable donor available. Since suitable living donors are usually close relatives of the recipient, they may be pressured into donating an organ by the recipient or other family members. In this society one who gives a gift may expect a gift or a service of equal value in return. Sometimes donors' ambivalence and fears about giving an organ for transplant are hard to identify. Some donors never feel the same again about their bodies and speak of feeling an empty space where their kidney used to be.

Recipients are often ambivalent about accepting an organ from the suitable donor because of their existing or anticipated relationship. Recipients often feel as if they have something alien in their bodies. They have fantasies about how part of another's body will affect them, especially if the donor is of the opposite sex or a different race.

When a cadaver's organ is used for transplant, relatives of the donor must approve the gift. When they know the name of the recipient, they often feel they have an investment in him or her and may try to build a close relationship. At the symbolic level, their loved one is not dead as long as a part of him or her is alive in someone else. If the recipient rejects the donor organ or dies, they usually grieve all over again for this final death of their loved one. Occasionally a person will become angry when the recipient's body rejects the loved one's organ.

Losing an organ of one's own and gaining an alien one create complex intra- and interpersonal situations as people resymbolize their losses and gains and act them out with each other. These are major problems for nurses and others on transplant teams. They can become major problems among members of the team if they become personally involved or take sides about courses of action. Nurses need to study the dynamics of organ loss and replacement in terms of body image and interpersonal dynamics. They need to be able to help patients clarify what is going on with them and sometimes work through relations with significant others, not just because of the donor-recipient situation but also because the patient is in a critical situation and needs a great deal of support. In their relationships with potential donors and families of potential cadaver donors, nurses need to be nonpressuring and nonjudgmental while the donors struggle with the problem, especially once the compatible donor or donors have been identified. Nurses need to be alert to signs of ambivalence and resistance in both donor and recipient. They need to support and participate in problem solving as sensitively as possible. They need to have input about their findings and what they are doing so the whole transplant team can make useful decisions. Then, nurses need to be supportive as both recipient and donor work at integrating a new organ or loss of an organ into their body schema.

Patients with third-degree burns over a large portion of their bodies can be saved. However, disfigurement is appalling. Only slightly less appalling is the pain suffered from the burn and from innumerable plastic surgeries using the skin of the patient, relatives, cadavers or animals. Many of these patients give up, withdraw from all social relations and cannot even be found for follow-up. They have been called "closet people,"[5] but socially dead may be a truer description. Facial disfigurement produces the greatest crisis for a person. The face is a basic instrument of communication. Everyone learns how to read and respond behaviorally to many nonverbal facial cues. Second, facial disfigurement produces a large number of emotional responses from other people. Severe anxiety is triggered and rapidly pervades the feelings, thoughts and actions of people with normal appearing faces when they are confronted with a nonhuman face on a human body. Victims of severe facial disfigurement are treated like things. This is not a phenomenon unique to unbearable ugliness, however, and nurses need to be aware that people of great beauty are also treated like things.

Many badly burned people who have lost hair, nose, eyes, ears and chin have also lost hands and fingers or toes and feet. These people often express the wish to die. Many fight to die even to the point of insisting on a lawyer to represent them. They cannot integrate so much destruction into their body schema or face the prospect of living as a "monster" or crippled person. The trend for these people to terminate treatment and disappear raises moral questions for physicians. Should horribly maimed patients' demands to die be respected? How can a physician treat a patient as free and still look out for that patient's best interests? Is paternalism in health care practice legitimate? When is a choice free? When is allowing the patient to choose really abandonment? What are the criteria for allowing free choice in the matter of dying?

Nurses work closely with and influence both patients' and physicians' decisions whether consciously or not. What they report and how they conceptualize their observations are added to the data pool. It then becomes a nurse's responsibility to identify and study the issues and ethics involved. Only a few years ago people so badly maimed *could not* have survived, but now we must answer the question of how much of the patient's body image must be destroyed before free choice about his or her future—death or life—is allowed. How much pain in relation to ultimate outcome of appearance and function is too much? The precedent was set several years ago for renal dialysis, and people still choose to die by making the decision to go off the machine. At the same time, it is not useful to assume that gross loss, innumerable surgeries and great pain make all people wish to die. Where the self-concept is strong, the values in living have their origin internally and activity plays a lesser role in lifestyle and the management of anxiety, the drive to live may be great. People adapt and help others become comfortable with them.[6]

AGING AND BODY IMAGE

Since body image represents all of individuals impressions about their bodies as they more or less systematically move along the growth and development continuum, we would expect that each individual's body image in aging would be different. Cognitive, affective and motor input about the body boundaries, body competence, physical disability, and body worries over a lifetime require complex integration and interpretation by the cerebral cortex. We are all aware that some people's body image and consequent level of activity, work, productivity and body care is old at 60 while others at 90 perceive their bodies as effective, responsive, competent and having worth.

There are 25,000,000 people in the United States over 65 and many more between 45 and 65 who are experiencing changes due to aging, about which there is much sensitivity. In normal uneventful aging, one would expect inner psychological and intellectual components of the self-system to reduce threats presented by changes in body image. Changes in size, strength, physical efficiency and productiveness, reduction in speed as well as outward physical signs of aging are usually integrated without major crises. However, there are major social themes which put an extraordinarily high value on youth.

One social theme has an impact on the whole aged person, but since much of the data on age are communicated by the whole body the material is relevant here. The status of the aged is inversely related to the proportion of aged in the population. If aged people are few they have high value. Where there are many their value is low. Also, the aged have more prestige in a static society than in a society with a high rate of change.

Another social theme that still persists concerns America's image as a young country of young people, a beautiful country of beautiful people, and a new country full of young new ideas. This theme does not have room for the aged and aging in the job market, economy, family or even community in any natural way, such as the extended family. For more than a decade we have manufactured for the aged jobs, housing, social relationships and ways to get health care. The wish that the aging and aged would disappear is expressed in much of the housing specially designed for them, the maintenance of the proprietary support base for the operation of nursing homes (Would the society allow people to make so much money off the misfortunes of children?), the talk of voluntary euthanasia (such as living wills), and the level of care in nursing homes, which in some instances amounts to involuntary euthanasia.

The result of these and other devaluing themes is an all-out attempt among the aging, beginning even as early as age 30 or 35, to maintain the illusion of youth. This occurs even though people left to their own devices could integrate the changes of aging very well. Economic necessity and need for social acceptance force a certain amount of regression to the adolescent level of body image development. Facial reconstruction, neck reconstruction and hair implants are common today. Only a few years ago they were only for Hollywood stars and millionaires. Many business men and women and other members of the middle class feel these surgeries are important to their success. Wigs, hair dyes, skin bleaches, preparations to remove wrinkles and youth maintaining hormones are all in common use. Some products have little effect and others put skin and endocrine system in jeopardy, but people—not just women—feel desperate and take the risks. Great attention is paid to dressing to create the appearance of youth but not too youthful for one's age. Health spas have sprung up everywhere and are widely used to maintain figure and physical fitness. For some, inability to wear contact lenses is a major tragedy.

Recently, Paris dress designers have started to design glasses that provide glamour and hide circumoptic wrinkles.

When people have to build in so many props to achieve an acceptable body image, they may experience considerable emotional reaction if they are unable to maintain the props for any reason, such as illness or travel. It may be of the utmost importance for nurses, wherever they work, to make referrals or find community groups to assist such patients in maintaining a body appearance that conforms to their internalized body image. It is a shock to look in the mirror and see an inch of white hair framing the face or bushy white eyebrows instead of an arched brown line. It is even a greater shock to look in the mirror and see one's gray-haired parent looking back, especially if one's parent has died. Billions of dollars are spent each year in search of the fountain of youth and in carrying out the charade of being eternally young. The relationship between enforced youth and job failure, emotional crises and marriage failure is not known, but always having to portray the perceived values and ways of youth must accentuate these pressures for some people.

As aged people are devalued, they take on some of the stigma of untouchables. Loss of loved ones and distance from family in a mobile society may leave these people with no one to touch and no one who wants to touch them. It is not unusual, where there is freedom to tell the truth, for student nurses to admit feelings of repugnance about touching the elderly. Touching others and physical activity are both important in the development and maintenance of the body schema. If activity is limited and there is no touching of others, distortions in body image and changes in the whole self-concept can be expected. Older people use a variety of strategies to be touched, and there are a variety of interpersonal bids for touch that are almost literally pleas to be touched. Many aged people who flatter or flirt and reach out to touch are misunderstood; not that older people do not make sexual approaches, but most simply want body and skin contact with another human.

In the last decade we have come to a clearer understanding of sexual interest and activity among the aged. We now know that sexual activity is common through the seventies, when a sexual partner is available. Because of women's longer average life, masturbation has become one alternative sexual outlet for some widows. The social belief that sex life ends at 40 has existed so long that older people have not been open about their sexual interests or solutions to sexual problems. As older men and women began to live with each other out of wedlock to avoid loss of Social Security support, the society was confronted with their sexual needs. Companionship may have the higher priority in many of these living arrangements, but it is a fact that, though there is decline with age, older people are more sexually active and have greater sexual interests than was previously thought. If sex is central to body image, we can expect greater demands for freedom and understanding from this group. Nursing and retirement homes do not promote intimacy, to say nothing of sexual intimacy, but there are those who are beginning to raise questions and ask for change.

The male climacteric, with consequent impotence, is creating more interest among researchers and clinicians now. The climacteric may occur as soon as the early forties in a few men and as late as 100 in another few, but usually it occurs in the late fifties or sixties. Impotence may be increasing at earlier ages with increasing work pressures and aggressiveness, including sexual aggressiveness of women, which increase both physiological and emotional stress. The climacteric may be more critical for men than the menopause is for women. They both herald old age in a social sense, but women can still function sexually. Nurses need to keep the climacteric in mind in assessing midlife changes in men and women and post-midlife changes in men. Both men and women may be depressed, change jobs, become physically ill or even psychotic.

Nurses need to be able to accept and support alternate lifestyles for older as well as younger people. But first they may need to accept the importance of sexuality and sexual activity to the body schema and thus the self-concept of all people—young and old.

GENERAL NURSING CONCEPTS

Intrusion and Invasion

We need to look at some medical and nursing activities as potentially threatening to people. For a few patients, especially children, the thermometer may be a threat. When we say, "I am going to *take* your temperature," one wonders whether this choice of words is intentional or accidental. Other intrusive activities of nurses that might be threatening are enemas, catheterization, insertion of gastric tubes, intravenous infusion, intramuscular and subcutaneous injections, suctioning and the like.

Perhaps we should also study the threat such intrusive diagnostic procedures as gastroscopy, bronchoscopy, sigmoidectomy, cystoscopy and dilatation and curettage may represent or the other effects they may leave on body image.

Another component of the mending and revising aspect of surgery is the nature of the threat or other experience that is posed by the "knife." A. M. Sutherland has demonstrated that the experience of cancer as a threat to the patient's body image cannot be separated from threat inherent in the curative measures—surgery and radiation.[7] Some of the postoperative emotional responses to artificial heart valves need to be explored from a body image point of view as well as a physiological point of view. Such studies would help us deal with the problems of body image in the rapidly developing field of organ transplantation.

Assessing the Nature of the Threat

Because the body image provides a base for identity, almost any change in body structure or function is experienced as a threat. This occurs even in normal growth; the maturing process may be welcomed, but it still may be accompanied by the threat of new expectations and being found inadequate. This is particularly true of adolescence, in which we observe a great deal of comparing, testing, and experimenting in relation to particular changes and to the whole body.

Psychiatric theory and research in body image indicate that serious threat to body image is related to many factors and that, in order to understand a particular patient's problem, one needs to construct a pattern of adaptation through study of the variables involved. The cultural values of youth, wholeness, normality and attractiveness enter into definition of threat. Dr. Martin Steinberg tells a story that illustrates how doctors may be caught up in a cultural bias about wholeness:

> One of our specialists is a man called Buerger and a disease was named after him—Buerger's Disease . . . hundreds of patients had come to us (with this disease) with the ever-present danger that they would lose the circulation in their legs. And there was always the question of trying as much as possible to keep the amputation rate low and save these legs. This was a tough clinic with hundreds of these patients. The nurse, however, refused to accept this goal of keeping the legs. She took an awfully good look at it and finally convinced us that what we were doing was leading to the wrong goal; that just saving these legs wasn't good at all; that these people were now living without legs. They couldn't use them. They had legs and they got out of bed into chairs and had to be pushed around—but they had legs. She did the thinking and she said, "No, this is not the right thing." She got more people interested, and we began to realize that we're not talking about saving legs, we're talking about functions. It was much better to give somebody a prosthesis that he could use and get him functional than to have him stop *everything* he was doing. . . .[8]

Some cultural groups do not allow the taking of pictures because of the belief that the one who takes the picture is stealing the identity or spirit of the person being photographed. Navajo Indians will never tell you their names, because this would allow you to take their names away from them. Then they would have to look for other names. In some cultures, thieves are punished by cutting off one or more fingers. A person from such a culture who lost fingers in an accident would be especially traumatized because of the stigma attached. In our country we are committed to wholeness, beauty and health. As we learn more about disease and accident prevention, it will be interesting to study changes in public attitudes toward those who do not meet the culturally determined criteria of health.

Threat is also related to the extent to which the individual's patterns of adaptation are interrupted. Each person develops patterns of behavior that meet needs for security and does this within the framework of the requirements of his or her environment. These habits or patterns may depend heavily on certain organs of the body. If these organs become diseased or have to be removed, the threat is greater than if an organ unimportant to the patient is affected. In one study of three women who had hysterectomies, data were collected about the meaning that the uterus and its removal had for patients.[9] The range of meaning is impressive: anxiety about the effect of the operation on sexual activity; anxiety over loss of sexual desire, inability to respond to spouse; fear of loss of sexual attractiveness, inability to have intercourse;

expectation of painful intercourse and having to refuse spouse on this basis; fear that spouse would not obtain satisfaction because of damaged sexual organs; fear of loss of husband; fear of destruction of marriage; fear of loss of strength and ability to work; expectation of being an invalid for a long time ("strength comes from womanly organs"); belief that one will never be the same again; concern for loss of childbearing capacity; fear of looking older and losing beauty or youth; fear of going insane; fear of becoming unable to control husband with whom sex has been used as a bargaining point; fear of loss of independence from husband; fear of increased vulnerability; fear of development of personality changes; concern about loss of menstruation as a means of keeping body "cleaned out."

M. Ullman[10] gives recognition to the concept that one's patterns of adapting to the environment play an important role in perception of threat to the body image when he notes that if a stevedore becomes mildly aphasic he might have only minor anxiety about it, but a teacher who becomes mildly aphasic might panic. Thus, we observe that the degree to which loss of functional control creates loss of customary control of self, physical environment, time, and interpersonal field is very closely related to degree of threat. In the aging process, as well as the illness process, the prospect of still further loss mobilizes a great deal of anxiety.

The meaning that the curative procedure itself, particularly surgery, has for the patient is another variable among threats to the body image. Some patients feel that to sign a release for surgery is to sign away one's life. Others feel that to sign for general anesthetic is to sign away control of one's body and render oneself absolutely helpless. There is also the fear of being cut, being in pain and being mutilated.

The person who has limited coping abilities to deal with stress, and who is easily made to feel helpless and powerless, will experience greater threat with a change in body image.

To understand the nature of the threat, then, one needs to know the pattern of adaptation, the value of this pattern for the particular individual, and what coping capacities the individual has.

Other people in some instances influence to a considerable extent a person's response to alteration in body image. A study of 38 married colostomy patients who were from 5 to 13 years postoperative revealed that 25 of their spouses had never seen the colostomy or had seen it only initially. Only 13 of these patients (16 were women) were given body care that involved sight of the colostomy by their spouses after being discharged from the hospital. At least nine spouses had severe reactions to the colostomy, which included refusing to look at it, fainting, vomiting or expressing disgust. Some patients concealed their colostomies because they felt their spouses could not take it.[11]

One study indicates that there are great differences between the person who has had a colostomy and the one who has had an ileostomy. Some ileostomy patients feel reborn or created anew after unbearable misery (with ulcerative colitis). They are described as having positive and productive changes in personality and lifestyles. They become more aggressive, enjoy a high level of social functioning and are vocationally successful. They may be exhibitionistic, as evidenced by their willingness and requests to demonstrate their ileostomy to student groups. The question was raised about the pleasurable aspects of ileostomy in that a new connection between skin and mucous membrane may be as enjoyable as the stimulation of this type of junction in other body areas. People who have had an ileostomy also seem to enjoy the attention gained through surgery, which is often dramatic when life is in the balance.[12]

Keeping in mind the three sequential aspects of the development of the body image, one can recognize the identity threat to some extent because one knows what aspect of body image is of primary importance in each phase. For example, to a young child, a disfiguring illness would not be as threatening in itself as one that is immobilizing or takes away some aspect of self-mastery. A sixteen-year-old who suffered disfigurement would be greatly threatened, because he or she is concerned with attractiveness and normality. In adults one would expect the threat to be balanced by satisfactions that emanate from the soma and satisfactions attained in the intellectual, spiritual and social spheres of the psyche.

Other factors that influence the degree of threat include the extent or degree of change and the rate at which it occurs. One great and sudden change will be more threatening than numerous small changes over a period of time.

Supporting Adaptation to Alteration in Body Image

Adaptation to alteration in body size, function or structure, as has been noted, depends on the nature of the threat, its meaning to the individual, his or her coping ability, the response from significant others and the help available to patient and family to undergo change. If surgery is involved, adaptation really starts beforehand. In the study of colostomy patients cited earlier,[13] three patterns of family responses to the recommended surgery were identified. One type of family gave encouragement and support, hiding its own fears and anxieties to encourage the patient. Another type of family became threatening, attempting to force the patient into surgery immediately and warning of the dire consequences of delay. These families went into action at the point of emergency at which the diagnosis became known, rather than from the point at which the patient had symptoms. The third type of family became immobilized either from fright or illness of another family member and left the patient alone to make the decision and arrange for hospitalization. Also included in this group is the uninterested, rejecting family. This study provided evidence that the family's preoperative pattern of behavior toward the patient indicates how they will behave postoperatively. The groundwork is laid for postoperative healthy adaptation in the healthy preoperative patient-family relationship.

In elective surgery a preoperative adaptation task for patients is to project themselves into the experience ahead. Signs of potential maladaptation are absence of anxiety, joking about the surgery or matter-of-factness about it. A normal person is concerned and begins dealing with it. The serene patient who communicates that the surgery will bring an end to all difficulties, or that the part to be removed will never be missed, is anxious to such a degree that the anxiety is repressed, only to come to the fore later as panic or in some way to alter the postoperative course.

Accidents account for over 1,800,000 traumatic injuries per year. Thus, almost 2 million people experience some alteration in body image which cannot be prepared for in advance. One might expect that after the shock of trauma wears off, these patients would experience the attacks on their body images more sharply and acutely than would the person who elects surgery.

Patients often initiate the adaptive process by requesting to see the changed body part. They may not ask, but instead peek a little more each time dressings are done; they study the area, using a mirror. Being able to look at what has happened to the self is one step in coping with it. Victims of accidents or emergencies may have more difficulty at this point because of the lack of opportunity to "prepare." However, if patients are still in a state of shock or have a concussion, they may accept change calmly, only to panic when they again have full use of faculties.

Testing and experimenting with those persons significant to them may be the next steps for most patients in coping with change. Nurses, as persons significant in the patients' recovery, are often the first ones tested. Many nurses find this a difficult task and some misunderstand the patients' need to show "my operation." Patients may give the nurse a choice and ask, "Have you seen my operation?" or "Would you like to see my operation?", or complain of pulling, itching or local pain, hoping to coerce the nurse into an examination. Other patients will raise their gowns and demand, "Look at my operation!" This even happens in social situations. There are probably two related problems operating in these patients. The afflicted part is a source of both fascination and revulsion. The patients can hardly tolerate the thought, sight or idea of the change in body image, but cannot stop looking and exploring the significance of the change. Another explanation for these patients' behavior might be that they are really saying, "I don't know whether I'm as attractive or worth as much as I was. What do you think?" Hopefully, these patients will be able to take the next step up to testing with family and friends. This does not mean that showing is the only way of testing. Discussion and observation of the behavior of others is testing, too. The patients' expectation of rejection or their feelings of guilt over what happened to them may cause errors in perceiving the behavior of others, so that pessimistic expectations seemingly are confirmed. Another patient problem in the early verbal-testing phase is questioning that pleads and beguiles the respondent into giving a positive or hopeful answer. It is important that any conversation about change in body image go well. As soon as emotionally laden material can be talked about, one step in acceptance has occurred; the subject is no longer too painful to mention.

If the body image change has been highly threatening, the patient may rage and grieve. This is a very normal reaction which may be necessary before hope and positive action can supplant it. Prolonged grief and rage, such as one may see in the adult paraplegic victim, may be very difficult to interrupt.

Denial is a common response also. It has been noted that this can occur preoperatively as a maladaptive response in surgical patients. The denying patient is headed for further such responses, some of which are reworked into a way of living. Feelings of emptiness, vague symptoms of illness such as weakness and fatigue, feelings of fragility and vulnerability, intractable pain, hypochondrical problems, psychosomatic conditions involving organ or system pathology, nervousness, obsession, or phobias are some of the conditions that may develop and persist as ways of coping with trauma, including trauma to the body image. Denial is often the result of repressed anxiety, but it may be related to altered perception. Ullman describes this kind of problem in patients after stroke, in which they are unaware of their illness.[14] Their thinking goes "If I can't feel it, if it feels like it's missing, if I can't find it, then, indeed, it isn't mine, but must belong to somebody else."

In patients who have lost control of complex, coordinated neuromuscular activity, denial may be the only alternative to psychosocial death, psychosis, or succumbing to apathy and resignation. Shame is nearly always a response to threat in which control of self or one's immediate space—such as the ability to manipulate a urinal, bed pan, meal tray—is lost.

Time, as has been noted, is a factor in adaptation. It takes time to cope adequately with threats. However, if anxiety is high and support is low, pathological coping mechanisms go into operation early and are more difficult to alter than to prevent.

Nursing Process

The content of other disciplines provides a general theoretical framework for understanding the development of body image, its dynamic nature, its importance to self-actualization, its socially and culturally determined facets, the variety of psychotic traumata that occur when the body is attacked, and the variety of coping and succumbing responses of which humans are capable.

The nursing process that makes this content become meaningful and operational may be called nursing assessment, nursing examination or nursing history. Whatever we call it, the basic problem of this process is how to structure the nursing history, assessment or examination so that we elicit the information needed to make a nursing diagnosis.

The conceptual frame of reference for this examination has many dimensions. Cultural values and prejudices concerning wholeness, independence and attractiveness can be used to determine whether patients feel isolated, excluded, stigmatized, helpless or ashamed. Knowledge about the patients' occupation, social group membership and habitual ways of interacting can be used to decide to what extent their lives are disrupted. Knowledge about persons' needs for inclusion, affection and control helps the nurse look at them in light of the attack on their body image. Knowledge about patients' feelings of self-esteem and security, as well as operation of their methods of coping, is helpful in identifying actual and potential problems. Knowledge of family dynamics helps the nurse assess family solidarity—whether the family provides sustained support or, at the other extreme, is emotionally impoverished and cannot rise to any crisis. Knowledge of useful or nonuseful human coping activity helps the nurse to identify avoidance, compensation and problem solving. Nurses should be able to recognize the grief that accompanies final permanent and irrevocable loss, which may elicit rage or oppositely, succumbing behavior. They will be helped greatly also if they recognize that body image attack involves problems of altered appearance, discomfort, dependence, stigma, social isolation, action and movement limitation, vocational threat, deformity, and loss of control. Age is always a consideration, and nurses also need to be aware of the vast discrepancy between psychological, physiological and chronological age. It should not surprise them that some middle-aged spinsters grieve more deeply over a hysterectomy than do some young and newly married women. In all aspects of assessment nurses should be aware of the patients' definition of the situation—their perception of what is to happen, or what has happened to them. Actually, casual or laconic patients are the easiest to describe and diagnose, but most difficult to work with because of the effectiveness of their denial. The stroke patient, mentioned previously, who denies because of disordered perception and sensation is even more difficult to approach.

In the history-taking process, usually the most useful attitude for the nurse to assume is to regard the patient as a person coping, in however inadequate a way, with what is an overwhelming experience. If the nurse labels the patient "disoriented" or "crazy," it may be difficult to identify coping mechanisms.

In relation to patients' body image, the nurse should look for indications that life roles are challenged, threatened or are meaningless; that the patients are questioning who they are; that they are experiencing strange bodily sensations, loss of feeling or contact, detachment or depersonalization, as if observing what is happening to themselves instead of experiencing it. Intellectualizing in which patients are both very reasonable and logical is related to this observation. Nurses need to ask about what they see. If they feel threatened by this, they will be unable to explore its meaning with the patients. The nursing diagnosis needs to include an appraisal of the families' ability to support the patients, to tolerate stress, and to deal with all the realities of the situation. It needs to include the patients' reality orientation to their experience, the problems with which they are trying to cope and how they are trying to cope with them. The nursing diagnosis should include predictions insofar as possible, since this alerts others and sets up expectations.

The nursing care plan needs to include means of supporting family members and helping them develop the strengths needed to cope with the patient's problem. It also needs to include support of positive moves the patient makes and ways of dealing with inadequate coping mechanisms. The need to express grief and rage to an accepting person cannot be ignored for the period immediately following an abrupt change in the body image. This period may be a long one if the loss is very great. Following this period, reinforcing hope and suggesting moves to compensate for the problem must be considered within the total plan.

The nursing therapy aspect of intervention in matters involving the body image is limited at present because of the need for more nursing research in this area. Valid nursing theory requires more adequate descriptions of patient response to body image threats. It must look for ways to characterize patients and their response to threat into some kind of typology, identifying the variables that provide for prediction, and then test situations in which nurses prevent or intervene in these problems.

REFERENCES

1. Garner, D. M., Garfinkel, P. E., Stancer, H. C., and Molofsky, H.: Body image disturbances in anorexia, nervosa and obesity. Psychosomatic Med. 38:327-36, September-October 1976.
2. Bruch, H.: Eating Disorders. New York, Basic Books, 1973, p. 4.
3. Nathan, S.: Body image in chronically obese children as reflected in figure drawings. J. Personality Assessment. 37:456-63, October 1973.
4. Hackett, T. P. (guest ed.): Problems created by advanced medical technology. Psychiatric Annals. 6:9-13, October 1976, p. 13.
5. McGregor, F. C.: Facial Deformities and Plastic Surgery. Springfield, Ill., Williams, 1953.
6. Tierney, E. A.: Accepting disfigurement when death is the alternative. Am. J. Nurs. 75:149-50, December 1975.
7. Sutherland, A. M.: Psychological impact of cancer and its therapy. Med. Clin. North Am. 40:705-72, 1965.
8. Conference on Preparation for Leadership in Psychiatric Nursing Service: Teachers College, Columbia University, New York, Columbia University Press, 1963, p. 74.
9. Drellich, M. G., Bieber, I., and Sutherland, A. M.: The psychological impact of cancer and cancer surgery. Cancer. 9:1120-26, 1956.
10. Ullman, M.: Disorders of body image after stroke. Am. J. Nurs. 64:89-91, October 1964.
11. Dyk, R. B., and Sutherland, A. M.: Adaptation of the spouse and other family members to the colostomy patient. Cancer. 9:123-38, 1956.
12. Druss, R. G., O'Connor, J. F., Stern, L. O.: Changes in body image following ileostomy. Psychoanalytic Q. 41:195-206, 1972.
13. Dyk and Sutherland, Adaptation of the spouse and other family members to the colostomy patient.
14. Ullman, Disorders of body image after stroke.

ADDITIONAL READINGS

Andreasen, N. J. C. et al.: Management of emotional reactions in seriously burned patients. New Eng. J. Med. 286:65-69, January 13, 1972.

Bernard, J.: Sex as a regenerative force. *In* Otto, H. (ed.): The New Sexuality. Palo Alto, Science and Behavior Books, 1971.

Bernstein, N. R.: Emotional Care of the Facially Burned and Disfigured. Boston, Little Brown, 1976.

———: Medical tragedies in facial burn disfigurement. Psychiatric Annals. 6:31-49, October 1976.

———: Psychological changes caused by aging of the face: aging and the facial body image. *In* Höhler, H. Plastische und Weiderherstellungs-Chirurgie. New York, Schattauer Verlag, 1975.

Blessing, S.: The development of body image in the child. Nurs. Clin. North Am. 7:579-607, December 1972.

Boston Women's Collective: Our Bodies Ourselves. New York, Simon and Schuster, 1976.
Bray, G. A.: The Obese Patient. Philadelphia, Saunders, 1976.
Burland, W. L., Samuel, P. D., Yudkin, J. (eds.): Obesity Symposium: Servier Research Institute Symposium. New York, Churchill Livingstone, 1974.
Burnside, I. M.: Accoutrements of aging. Nurs. Clin. North Am. 291-301, December 1972.
Busse, E. W., Pfeiffer, E.: Behavior and Adaptation in Late Life. 2nd ed. Boston, Little Brown, 1977.
Clausen, J., Fisher, S.: Effects of amphetamine and barbiturates in body experience. Psychosomatic Med. 35:390-405, September-October 1973.
Cleveland, S. E.: Personality characteristics, body image and social attitudes of organ transplant donors versus nondonors. Psychosomatic Med. 37:313-19, July-August 1975.
Craft, C. A.: Body image and obesity. Nurs. Clin. North Am. 7:677-85, December 1972.
Davis, R. H.: Aging: Prospects and Issues. Los Angeles, University of Southern California Press, 1976.
Dynneson, L.: Sexual self concept in elderly women. Tucson, University of Arizona, School of Nursing, Masters Thesis, 1975.
Engelhardt, H. T., Jr.: A demand to die. Case Studies in Bioethics. Hastings on Hudson, New York, Institute of Society, Ethics and Life Sciences, June 1975.
Fisher, S.: The Female Orgasm: Psychology, Physiology, Fantasy. New York, Basic Books, 1973.
Foster, T. A.: Why patients decide to discontinue renal dialysis. J. Am. Women's Med. Assoc. 31:234, June 1976.
Fox, R. C., Swazey, J. P.: The Courage to Fail: A Social View of Organ Transplants. Chicago, University of Chicago Press, 1974.
Goldman, G. D., Milman, D.S. (comp. and eds.): Modern Woman: Her Psychology and Sexuality. Springfield, Ill., Thomas, 1969.
Hackett, T. P.: The psychiatrist's view of the ICU: vital signs stable but outlook guarded. Psychiatric Annals. 6:14-27, October 1976.
Howard, A. (ed.): Recent Advances in Obesity Research. Westport, Conn., Techonomic, 1974.
Jennings, L. G.: The changing health care needs of women: clinical specialists take heed. JOGN Nurs. 6:44-46, May-June 1977.
Kaufman, R. V.; Body image changes in physically ill teenagers. J. Am. Acad. Child Psychiatry. 11:157-70, January 1972.
Kubie, L. S., Mackie, J. B.: Critical issues raised by operations for gender transmutation. J. Nervous & Mental Diseases. 147:431-43, 1968.
La Barre, M.: Emotional crises of school age girls during pregnancy and early motherhood. J. Am. Acad. Child Psychiatry. 11:537-57, July 1972.
Laron, Z. (ed.): The Adipose Child: Medical and Psychological Aspects. Basel, Karger, 1976.
Leon, G. R.: Personality, body image and eating pattern changes in overweight persons after weight loss. J. Clin. Psychol. 3:618-23, October 1975.
Lindgren, T. W., Pauly, I. B.: A body image scale for evaluating transsexuals. Arch. Sexual Behavior. 4:639-56, November 1975.
Malo-Juvera, D.: What pregnant teenagers know about sex. *In* Browning, M. H., Lewis, E. P. (comps.). Human Sexuality: Nursing Implications. New York, Am. J. Nurs., 1973.
Muslim, H. L.: The emotional response to kidney transplant: the process of internalization. Canad. Psychiatric Assoc. J. 17, Suppl. 2:3S3, 1972.
Pluchik, R., Weiner, M. B., Conte, H.: Studies of body image. I. body worries and body discomforts. J. Gerontol. 26:344-50, July 1971.
Roberts, A. R. (comp. and ed.): Self Destructive Behavior. Springfield, Ill., Thomas, 1975.
Slvan, S. H., Wahl, C. W.:The eye and I. *In* Perlman, J. T., Adam, G. L., Slvan, S. H. (eds.): Psychiatric Problems in Ophthalmology. Springfield, Ill., Thomas, 1977.
Vann, D.: Psychological aspects of vasectomy. Med. J. Australia. 1:959-60, May 12, 1973.
von Uexküll, T.: The problem of psychosomatic theory and the mind-body unity model. Psychotherapy and psychosomatics. 18:103-16, 1970.
Weininger, O., Rotenberg, G., Henry, A.: Body image of handicapped children. J. Personality Assessment. 36:248-53, June 1972.
Zelnick, M., Kantor, J. F.: Sexual and contraceptive experience of young unmarried women in the United States, 1976 and 1971. Family Plann. Perspect. 9:55-71, March-April 1977.

2 STIGMA

Betty Blackwell

This chapter is addressed to the discussion of the concept of stigma, using sociological literature on the management of spoiled social identity, labeling theory and the study of deviance. A primary assumption is that illness, particularly when certified by medical authority, elicits attempts by both the ill person and cointeractants to provide meaning to the changes in his or her condition. The meanings provided frequently involve a decrease in the ill individual's feelings of self-worth, as well as in the cointeractants' estimation of his or her social worth.

According to Erving Goffman,[1] persons are stigmatized when expectation based on a value judgment of what persons of a certain social identity should be differs from what they actually present to others. The judgment of persons' social worth as less than anticipated is inherent to the assignment of stigma. If their stigmatizing aspects are visually obvious or personal histories available, they are termed discredited. If their disabilities are not obtrusive, either by sensory or cognitive means, they are defined as discreditable.

For instance, the skid row alcoholic is discredited; the middle-class alcoholic who continues to meet role obligations is discreditable. The student who is caught cheating is discredited; the successful cheater is discreditable. Although recently changed attitudes toward women's rights and abortion have decreased the stigma for some, the pregnant unwed woman who maintains her primary and secondary relationships may be discredited; the pregnant unwed woman who interrupts the pregnancy before it becomes visible or severs primary and secondary relationships before delivery to control information about the pregnancy may be discreditable.

Goffman declares the major assumption made in the normal person's response to the stigmatized is that they are not human or less than fully human. From this assumption, normal individuals develop a stigma theory to explain the stigmatized's inferiority and to account for their dangerousness to the social structure. This process permits the use of words with negative emotional connotations, such as "bastard," "cripple," "sot," and "looney." Gradually, a mythology evolves imputing a "wide range of imperfections on the basis of the original one, and . . . some desirable but undesired attributes, often of a supernatural cast, such as 'sixth sense' or 'understanding.'"[2]

Beatrice Wright suggests that, when normal individuals encounter the disabled, they are apt to experience dissonance between their expectations and actual perceptions of the disabled. She calls this phenomenon expectation discrepancy. She states that reconciling the discrepancies in expectation "may be accomplished by such cognitive changes as *expectation revision, altering the apparent reality* and *anormalizing the person.*"[3] In anormalizing the person, the laws that apply to normal persons are transcended.

> Anormalization that reconciles a discrepancy in which expectations are lower than apparent reality leads to sanctification, but where the expectations surpass the apparent reality, anormalization leads to vilification.[4]

Anormalization through sanctification occurs when normals ascribe exquisite aural and tactile sensitivity to the blind, high tolerance for tedious and boring tasks to the mentally retarded or business acumen to those with gastrointestinal ulcers. Anormalization through vilification is demonstrated by viewing those with cerebral palsy as mentally retarded or those with ethnic or physical differences as inferior in morals or character. This process is further elaborated in the following discussion of essences as moral identifiers.

Jack Katz,[5] in discussing the verifiability and responsibility in imputations of deviance and charisma, explicates essences as moral identifiers. He defines essences as "inherent qualities which may be manifested, reflected, indicated, or represented by, but do not exist in, conduct."[6] He comments on the use of nouns and present tense to refer to what the other is. "Nouns purport to locate qualities as general states in individuals; they gloss the situational limits of the identity and ignore the responsibilities of others for the identity's interactive existence."[7] He further notes that there are two related themes in moral identifications: (1) "persons conceive of essences as personal qualities which exist independently of, and cannot be verified in, observed conduct"; and (2) "persons give moral significance to the essences they impute."[8]

Katz distinguishes between two kinds of moral identities, the deviant and the charismatic. The former includes those who, in comparing themselves with others in an interaction, believe themselves to be "of inferior capacity, ability, competence, etc. The charismatic is someone of relatively superior capacity."[9]

John Hepburn[10] suggests that there are three deviant identities in interactions between audience and an actor. These are public deviant identity, consensual deviant identity and private deviant identity. In the first of these, the audience identifies the behavior as deviant but the actor does not. In nursing such interactions include behaviors which the nurse defines as health risking and the patient does not—a client's failure to follow prescribed medical regimen—or behaviors which the client defines as appropriate for the nurse and the nurse does not—the nurse's failure to give a bed bath when the patient deems it a perquisite.

The consensual deviant identity arises when both actor and audience agree the behavior is deviant. This category corresponds most closely to Goffman's discredited and suggests similar examples. The final category, private deviant identity, applies when the actor defines him or herself as deviant and the audience does not. Similarities to Goffman's discreditable and examples of it are obvious.

Hepburn notes that the above categories are "based on subjective criteria of deviance"[11] and

> ... the identity of the actor is allowed to (1) emerge through active negotiation; (2) change in the negotiation process as one party is successful in its attempt to structure reality and thus alter the other's definition of the situation; (3) adjust to the different audiences encountered, in some of which a public deviant identity may prevail, in others of which a different identity may prevail; (4) respond to situational rules and definitions of deviant behavior; such that "being a deviant" may be nondeviant in a deviant group.[12]

Hepburn's terminology suggests the interactive and dramaturgical significance of the interpretive work accomplished between the deviant actor and the audience. The following discussion of features of the deviant role concentrates on the analysis of deviance in role theory.

Ralph Turner[13] lists five features of deviance as a role: linkage of diverse action, role and meaning of action, role cues, economy of roles and role and self. Linkage of diverse actions is the repetition of a deviant act in conjunction with other acts, which leads to assigning these other acts to the deviant role. This feature is similar to Wright's anormalization and to Katz's essences. The role and meaning of action stresses the need to impute meaning to the action for the deviant role to be so labeled. The process is similar to that suggested by Katz in the use of essences as moral identifiers. Recognition of role cues precedes labeling the individual as deviant and corresponds to Wright's process of expectation discrepancy. Economy of roles emphasizes that the recognition of role cues leads to a clumping of the signals and hence to a lack of discrimination between different types of deviant roles. Role and self capsulizes the idea that deviant role behavior is more likely to be ascribed to the person than to the actor of a role. That is, an individual's mental or physical illness may lead cointeractants to interpret behavior (symptoms) as properties of the person, his or her previous actions or both rather than as features of the performance of the sick role.

The following features of stigma have been suggested by the foregoing discussion.

1. Deviation from the expectations for one with that particular social identity.
2. Recognition of the deviance by the actor, the audience, or both.
3. Development of a stigma theory utilizing essences as moral identifiers.
4. Spread of moral valuations to other characteristics of the actor.
5. Devaluation of the individual's self and social worth.
6. Pervasiveness of the stigmatization to the individual which is temporally, spatially and interactively related.

RESPONSES TO STIGMATIZATION

Wright and Goffman both note that every human being experiences increased tension in perceptually unclear, unstructured or ambiguous situations. Both writers also hypothesize that disabled persons encounter such situations more frequently and any of their social interactions may involve undertones of ambiguity or unanticipated behavioral responses.

Wright uses the term *spread* to characterize the process in which the audience sees physical disabilities as cues to interpret and understand the actor's total personality. In discussing spread, she emphasizes the significance of physique in determining expectations regarding one's own and others' personalities. Physique is the central feature in assessing the individual. The viewer may impute to the disabled a sensitivity to the needs of others, especially if he or she considers physical perfection important—and few Americans are not imbued with the cult of youth, health and beauty. This sensitivity is presumed to result from suffering. A vocational capability may be assumed to grow out of a handicap. Intelligence, or the lack of it, may be seen as stemming from an atypical physical behavior, and so on. In short, the viewer may attribute all the disabled person's interpersonal difficulties or successes to the disability.

Disabled persons' acceptance of such imputations may make them uncertain of whether they are being treated stereotypically in recurring social situations. It also may put into play all the dynamics of the self-fulfilling prophecy.

The mythology surrounding stigma places stigmatized persons in the position of expecting to be treated like anyone else of the same social position while recognizing that such expectations may not be realistic because of their disability. Goffman says that disabled persons, in the presence of normal people, may feel their privacy is being invaded "most pointedly perhaps when children simply stare . . . [at them]."[14] They join other not-quite-people, such as policemen and children, in being considered approachable to strangers. They are asked personal questions about their condition. Goffman states that this is considered proper by the questioner, provided the questioning is "sympathetic to the plight of persons of [their] kind."[15]

Wright summarizes the effects of being disabled in this way:

> The disabled . . . rarely has the kind of group sanction and personal valuation that endorse behavior reflecting the disability. Rather, the typical advice is to appear as much like a nondisabled person as possible, and his adjustment is often measured in terms of his skill as an actor. Even where there is a high degree of acceptance of the disability, there is resistance against behavior that unnecessarily spotlights the handicap.[16]

After describing the trying psychological states of shame, self-pity and inferiority, their effects on the disabled person, and the tendency to hide or weaken one's identification with a devalued group, Wright notes that "the vigilance required for covering up leads to strain, not only physically but also in interpersonal relations, for one must maintain a certain distance in order to fend off the frightening topic of the disability."[17]

Discussing the acting that the disabled must do in attempting to emulate the able-bodied person, Wright says:

> Even should the person with a disability achieve or surpass the standards of normal performance, this by no means guarantees a success experience, for as long as he views his disability as a stigma, he can have only the feeling that at best he is an imperfect facsimile of a nondisabled person.[18]

Internalizing culturally derived standards of behavior, even about such matters as the proper way to walk or talk, can produce feelings of shame and guilt—shame at being inferior and guilt for violating a moral code. "Thus, the means of extricating oneself from more shame becomes the means of submerging oneself further."[19]

The desire to escape identification as a member of a devalued group often leads to avoidance of labeled members of that group. This avoidance protects the disabled from reminders of his or her implicit membership in the group. Furthermore, avoidance removes the threat of discovery "for by the mere fact of contiguity, he fears that likeness will be exposed; he may also sense that a person like himself will see through his mask."[20] In avoiding others similarly afflicted, individuals implicitly concede the correctness of society's assignment of stigma, and its accompanying shame, to them. In addition, they may be deprived of others who more intimately understand their conditions.

One obstacle that the disabled faces in establishing understanding human relationships is the pretense by both participants that the disability does not exist. This pretense leads to "the feeling that the person with a disability is only seemingly accepted, i.e., that he is not really accepted at all."[21]

Wright describes the techniques used by the disabled to manage the curiosity of others:

> 1. Attacking the offender with either biting sarcasm or dramatic prevarication.
> 2. Excluding the disability from the situation by an ostrich reaction or by redirecting the course of the interaction.
> 3. Minimizing the disability and preserving the relationship by goodnatured levity and superficial discourse.[22]

Joseph Rogers and M. D. Buffalo[23] suggest additional modes of adapting to being labeled deviant. These modes might also describe adaptations to stigmatization. The first of these is acquiescence, which includes the following four subtypes.

1. The "true believer" is one who accepts the definition developed by the interactants.
   Example: The patient with an acute myocardial infarction who is admitted to a CCU.
2. The adopter of a "compliance facade congruent with stereotypical expectations."[24]
   Example: The clinic patient who, during visits to the clinic, reports compliance with the medical regimen but may not follow it rigorously outside the clinic.

3. The user of acquiescence as a weapon.
   Example: The new father who accepts duties for infant care, thinking them unmanly, in exchange for greater freedom in recreational activities.
4. The acceptor of shame and accompanying self-hatred.
   Example: The burned patient who sees him or herself as a monster.

Other modes suggested are repudiation, flight, channeling, evasion, modification, reinterpretation, redefinition and alteration. Repudiation involves a process in which the person denies the imputation of deviance and the efforts of audiences to affix the label to him or her. The most obvious example in nursing is the patient denying an illness or its symptoms.

Flight may be accomplished either physically or socially. Patients may sign out against medical advice. They may withdraw from discussion of the symptoms they consider stigmatizing. Other examples include former mental patients or addicts who move to other parts of the country and attempt to establish new social identities.

In channeling, "The person not only assents to the label but utilizes the label as a fulfilling means of self expression, personal identity and social effectiveness."[25] Included among those using this mode of adaptation are spokesmen for voluntary organizations such as Alcoholics Anonymous, Lost Chords or the Gay Liberation Front, and children with various corrective prosthetic devices, such as glasses, dental braces or hearing aids.

Evasion and modification may be seen as related phenomena. In the first, the actor relies on verbal mechanisms to escape the imputation of deviance. Through modification, the label is exchanged for one with less stigma attached. Thus, the patient with mobility problems may attribute them to weakness, age or temporary incapacity.

One of the major distinctions between reinterpretation and redefinition is that the label is accepted by the actor in the former but not in the latter. In reinterpretation, the interactants agree that the actor is stigmatized at first glance but further interaction indicates that the label is not appropriate to his or her moral or social identity. Redefinition is more dependent on ongoing and changing legal and social definitions of deviance. For instance, changes have occurred over time in attitudes toward seeking and accepting psychiatric care, particularly for certain classes of people. One can also note recent changes in beliefs because of social and legal recognition given to working women, the handicapped and other formerly stigmatized groups.

Alteration is the process of rehabilitating the deviate. In the health setting, the patients are cured or learn to control the information about their stigma to prevent its intrusion into their interactions. In Goffman's terms, they are no longer discredited but may be discreditable.

Goffman describes two categories of persons who significantly affect not only the stigmatized individuals, but also public opinion about them. These classifications are the own and the wise.[26] The own are those who suffer from the same affliction. The wise are nonsufferers who have become or are considered knowledgeable and understanding of the sufferer's plight. Goffman distinguishes between two types of wise. The first are persons such as doctors, nurses, and social workers, with whom the individual relates because of his or her condition. For the purposes of this chapter, these may be called the professional wise. Goffman's second type includes those who participate in primary group relationships with the individual. These shall be called the intimate wise.

Wright's description of the inside position corresponds to Goffman's wise and own. The outside position is maintained by strangers. Because of the interactive significance of stigma to the discredited/discreditable and their cointeractants and the fuzziness of Goffman's term normals or Wright's strangers, nonafflicted audience might more clearly designate those who are neither own nor professional or intimate wise. This would be particularly helpful when discussing the effects of face-to-face encounters on both actor and audience.

A survey of recent nursing literature discloses a rather standard approach to the nursing care of the disabled. The usual paper is either a personal case history of the disabled or an attempt by a knowing nurse author to communicate the status of the disabled, his or her response to attitudes and feelings expressed by others and suggestions about treatment. Most of the literature deals with the individual in a specific disease category, such as the blind, those with cerebral palsy or muscular dystrophy, the burned, and so on.

Generalizations applying to the conclusions and recommendations of most articles reviewed are: (1) nurses interact with the discredited in the same manner as the general public; (2) the discredited are worthwhile, thinking, feeling beings who should be treated like anyone else, except that one should do specified things for them; (3) the nurse should use purposeful interviewing techniques to determine the meaning of the disability to the patient; and (4) the nurse should use the information gathered to provide additional data, support, reassurance, and so on.

Notable exceptions to the articles mentioned above are those by Beatrice Kalisch[27] and Susan Jones.[28] Kalisch discusses in considerable detail the nursing care implications of the obesity stigma. Jones's discussion of illness as deviance focuses specifically on orthopedic injuries. Both papers are excellent examples of the application of sociological theory to the understanding of patient behavior and consequent implications for nursing practice.

Goffman stresses that the main task for both discredited and normal (nonafflicted audience) in a mixed interaction is the management of tension. As noted earlier, for those with visible or widely known stigmata, each encounter brings into question continued acceptance of the individual's personal and social worth. In encounters between nonstigmatized individuals, an assumption is made that both will be and act in a manner consistent with past encounters. In mixed encounters trust in this assumption is frequently lessened, which leads to increased surveillance by both interactants.

Recognition of this increased surveillance within and between the interactants leads to a decrease in spontaneity and an increase in tension.

In interactions between the discreditable and the nonafflicted audience, the principal task is the control of information about his or her defect. In health-illness situations, the means for controlling the spread of information about a possible stigma are available to the individual through commonsense knowledge of everyday life and acceptance of instruction from the own and professional wise.

Both tasks, the management of tension and the control of information, are of prime importance here and will be discussed in the following sections on implications for nursing the discredited and the discreditable. As suggested earlier, Hepburn's consensual and private deviant identities are similar to what Goffman has labeled the discredited and discreditable, respectively. Hepburn's category of public deviant identity will be discussed separately because it not only shares features of the Goffman labeling but is also significant for both the interpretation of health-illness behavior and the implication for nursing practice.

IMPLICATION FOR NURSING—THE DISCREDITED

Two aspects of nursing practice relate to the discredited individual. The first is how the nurse assists the patient to manage tension during the nurse-patient interactions. The second is how the nurse helps the patient manage tension with others.

In nurse-patient situations, both parties ordinarily will anticipate that the disability is a topic of mutual concern. Depending on such variables as length of time discredited and previous experience with nurses, the patient may expect that the nurse knows the medical implications of his or her condition, is willing to assist in regaining the best health possible, sympathizes with the patient's suffering and knows about others who have the same condition.

Tension management in nurse-patient interactions has been discussed at length in nursing literature. Still one of the most helpful articles is Dorothy Gregg's "Reassurance."[29] She describes fully the rationale, techniques and anticipated outcomes of nursing practice aimed at tension management. (Also see Chapter 3 on Shame and Chapter 12 on Humor.)

The second nursing aspect, helping the patient manage tension with others, has been explored less but is critically important. If one regards many of the teaching and rehabilitative tasks of nurses as assisting patients to manage tension with others, it follows that nurses aid them to develop a circle of own and intimate wise who will support them and decrease their tension. This process is illustrated by the following examples:

1. After a patient has had a leg amputated, the primary objective of teaching and rehabilitation is to restore mobility. A secondary objective is to provide a lifelike prosthesis and thereby enable the patient to share information about the disability only with those he or she chooses.

2. For the patient with a colostomy, the primary objectives of the nurse are maintenance of nutrition, elimination and skin integrity. Of equal importance are measures that permit the patient to maintain privacy.

3. When a woman has had a mastectomy, the teaching relating to a prosthesis is done solely to give her control of the information about her disfigurement.

IMPLICATIONS FOR NURSING—THE DISCREDITABLE

Despite wide publicity given to the ills suffered by prominent figures today, a person's value in this culture usually depreciates when information about his or her poor health is available to cointeractants. Increasingly, the individual is held responsible for becoming sick, probably because of modern medical knowledge and mass communication of preventive measures.

In this society, in which more and more previously private information is becoming public, it appears that professional nurses must make a philosophical decision about the issue of privacy. If nurses believe that patients have the right to control the spread of information about their health status, then they must devise techniques and skills to help prepare patients for this task.

Two factors that make nurses potential discreditors of individuals with whom they work are the growing emphasis on community participation and the need for adequate information to plan personalized nursing care plans. For example, certain types of behavior, lifestyles and socioeconomic ills once were considered outside the purview of nursing. Now these are regarded, with an attendant increase of involvement, as legitimate nursing concerns. There is increasing expectation that nurses understand and work with the so-called culturally deprived or different.

When hospitals had one routine for all patients—time for bathing, eating, visiting—there was less reason for the nurse to secure information which might discredit the patient. With the present trend to personalize care, the nurse often obtains such information. Personal information is needed in order to personalize care. The hospital patient may be asked for minute data concerning sleeping, elimination, dietary, sexual and exercise practices. Answering such questions may seem to be discrediting to him or herself.

Besides facing requests for potentially discrediting information, the patients encounter an army of personnel. They cannot be certain which workers have access to the information gathered about them; but if they know anything about the team approach to health care practice, they can be sure that the information supplied will have wide circulation.

Four conclusions for nursing practice are that the nurse (1) must be able to justify the seeking of information, for both short- and long-term goals; (2) must anticipate receiving some inaccurate information if the patient is cognizant of his or her own deviations from cultural norms; (3) is responsible to the patient for controlling the spread of information; and (4) must assist the patient to learn methods for managing information about his or her condition.

While the first three conclusions are important, this chapter will concentrate on the fourth because it states a nursing responsibility less emphasized than the others and it promises to help determine nursing action.

The three previously cited examples of nursing and medical actions which helped patients control information about their health status also demonstrated how the patients' status was changed from discredited to discreditable. A logical next step is to discuss measures to assist the individual to control information about the stigma which may lead to being discredited.

In a utopian world, deviations form the norm in health status undoubtedly would not be labeled stigmata. Since we are far from Utopia, it would seem defensible to help patients develop techniques for protection from attacks on self-image. Patients should not be encouraged to deny their illness but rather to identify those aspects of their behavior which cause them trouble in relationships with others. Following are examples from everyday practice that illustrate this sort of help.

1. Teaching the blind to "look at" those speaking to them eases the tension in the interaction and at times prevents awareness that the blind persons cannot see.
2. Suggesting that the expatient who has been hospitalized for mental illness supply this information only when asked by appropriate persons protects him or her from stigmatization.
3. Diet teaching for the individual with diabetes not only assists in the maintenance of health, but also gives control over the spread of information about his or her illness.
4. Instruction in caring for the newborn not only safeguards the infant's health, but also helps the mother achieve the status of a good parent.

In each of these examples, the instruction given to the patient also provided help in information control. Conscious application of the instruction in information control would enhance the total nursing care plan for those who are discreditable.

All of us worry about our behavior in untried situations in which we wish to maintain self-control, poise and face. Within the nurse-patient interactional system, there are several factors that limit patients' ability to control information about themselves. Among these constraints are the stress ordinarily connected with health-illness matters, cultural expectations of the sick role and the health care institution as a social system.

Applying the concept of stigma to some relatively simple but often stressful situations provides new insights for nursing practice. For example:

1. When an adult is waiting to be immunized or to give blood, one concern is pain. Another, and perhaps the major concern, is whether one's behavior will meet adult norms. Crying or fainting might discredit the individual.
2. The person awaiting general anesthesia worries about pain, outcome of

the procedure and death. An equally important concern is unintended disclosure of information, including unruly behavior.

3. An individual who knows but does not practice dental hygiene fears that a dental examination may provide information that will discredit him or her.

Active participation in the treatment program is a major responsibility of the sick person in this society. Examples of individuals who must provide discrediting information in order to enter the treatment process are numerous and obvious: the person with diabetes who does not follow the treatment regimen; the individual who attempts suicide; the alcoholic who drinks; the person with emphysema who smokes; and many others.

IMPLICATIONS FOR NURSING—PUBLIC DEVIANT IDENTITY

Application of Hepburn's category of public deviant identity to the health-illness continuum suggests that people in this category share the tasks of tension management and information control mentioned previously. Because their behavior is publicly labeled deviant while they categorize it as normal, an additional and probably primary task is information manipulation.

Perhaps the most dramatic examples of public deviant identity which nurses encounter are those medically defined as risk-taking. Risk-taking may be divided into activities with high probability of physical injury, such as Evel Knievel-type exploits; dietary lapses; addiction; and sedentary lifestyle.

Some of the modes of adaptation to deviance suggested by Rogers and Buffalo are helpful in discovering implications for nursing practice. Among these modes are repudiation, evasion and modification. Each is a frequently used tool for manipulating information between the individual with a public deviant identity and the nonafflicted audience.

The sociological interpretation of repudiation is like the psychological concept of denial. In repudiation, the physical injury risk-taker negates cointeractants' allegations that his or her activities are suicidal or at least health endangering. Those whose eating practices lead to obesity refute accusations that they are risking their health. The addicted deny that their activities are unhealthy, as do those who ignore suggestions that their bodies need exercise.

As noted previously, evasion and modification are somewhat related modes of adaptation to deviance. In their verbal behavior those whose risk-taking involves the probability of physical injury evade discussions of this type of risk-taking and subsequently modify definitions of the situation. They refer to the economically beneficial and emotionally stimulating aspects of the endeavor rather than its health-risking features.

In mixed encounters, individuals whose dietary practices are health threatening evade discussions of those practices or note the sensual and esthetic values of their dietary habits. Modifications in the definitions of health-risking may also be seen in variations in categorizations of healthiness and beauty among different ethnic and cultural groups. Examples of this are the idea that fat babies are the healthiest babies and the recent formation of voluntary groups designating fat as beautiful.

Other examples of individuals using evasion and modification are users of drugs, alcohol and cigarettes who evade discussions of their practice and modify the labels of drug addict, alcoholic and smoker to the more acceptable ones of users of mind-expanding, relaxing or socially expediting materials. Similarly, discussions of sedentary lifestyles are evaded and modifications of the label are made.

The functions of the nurse in interacting with individuals manipulating information are prevention of risk-taking, treatment of the consequences and rehabilitation. In prevention, consideration of the assumption that behavior is goal-directed raises the question of what the individual's priority of goals is. Through purposeful interviewing, the nurse may find that consideration of the risk of physical injury or illness is secondary to economic, stimulative, sensual or esthetic goals. Through education, confrontation and reality testing, the reordering of goal priorities may be achieved. The same procedures may be utilized to decrease the risks by altering the environment to minimize hazards.

Treatment of the consequences of risk-taking involves the recognition by the risk-takers that the assertions of their audience have been correct. Their behavior has resulted in injury or illness. The modes of adaptation they have been using—repudiation, evasion and modification—are no longer defensible or useful. The risk-takers are discredited.

In rehabilitation, the goals discussed previously under implications for nursing the discredited and discreditable are applicable. Assistance in the management of tension and information control are the appropriate nursing objectives.

IMPLICATIONS FOR NURSING EDUCATION

There are three principal implications in the concept of stigma for nursing education. The first implication relates to the special burdens borne by the stigmatized group refered to by many contemporary authorities as alienated from society. The concept of alienation is presented in many nursing curricula. So, too, the concept of stigma should be a common theme in the nursing major. Nurses are in daily contact with most persons labeled inferior by this society—the mentally and physically disabled, minority group members and lower socioeconomic group members. By utilizing the concept of stigma in nursing curricula, it is possible to identify the major social problems faced by individuals with a wide range of disease conditions. Such action would decrease the amount of time spent in teaching what appears to students as repetitive material about specific diseases. Early identification of the need for techniques of tension management, information control or recognition of information manipulation can lead to more individualized nursing care planning.

The second implication is that nurse educators should consider the education of the nursing student as the preparation of the professional wise. Although nurses may become one of the wise with many and varied groups, it is doubtful that they are at present. Notable exceptions may be nurses in some rehabilitation, psychiatric and other special care units. Possibly, educating nurses to be the professional wise to many persons is not a feasible objective of an undergraduate program.

Integrating the stigma concept into nursing education dramatizes what seems to have been a latent purpose of clinical experience. Like the family of the discredited patient, the student nurse must achieve a drastic revision in values. This revision involves not only the individual with a particular stigmatized condition, but also large numbers of people with a multitude of conditions who are devalued by the larger society. Nursing educators, perhaps intentionally, have tried to hasten this change in students' values by diversifying patient assignments and emphasizing patients' strengths instead of weaknesses.

The third implication relates to the student nurse as discreditable. Applying the concept of stigma raises troubling questions. Do some stresses students encounter arise from expectation that they perform as fully accredited practitioners? It seems that the student, instructor and patient collaborate to prevent the student's lack of full accreditation from spoiling the student-patient interaction. What is the effect of this "as if" performance when the patient and student cooperate to keep the instructor from learning that the student's performance has not been satisfactory? And how much stress does the student experience when the information everyone has been trying to hide finally obtrudes and the student is discredited?

REFERENCES

1. Goffman, E.: Stigma: Notes on the Management of Spoiled Identity. Englewood Cliffs, N.J., Prentice-Hall, 1963.
2. Ibid., p. 5.
3. Wright, B.: Physical Disability—A Psychological Approach. New York, Harper, 1960, p. 72.
4. Ibid., p. 73.
5. Katz, J.: Essences as moral identities: verifiability and responsibility in imputations of deviance and charisma. Am. J. Soc. 80:1369-90, May 1975. Quoted by permission.
6. Ibid., p. 1371.
7. Ibid., p. 1372.
8. Ibid., p. 1370.
9. Ibid., p. 1375.
10. Hepburn, J. R.: The role of the audience in deviant behavior and deviant identity. Soc. Sociological Res. 59:387-405, July 1975. Quoted by permission.
11. Ibid., p. 397.
12. Ibid.
13. Turner, R. H.: Deviance disavowal as neutralization of commitment. Social Problems. 19:308-21, Winter 1972. Used by permission.
14. Goffman, Stigma, p. 16.

15. Ibid., p. 16.
16. Wright, Physical Disability, p. 19.
17. Ibid., p. 24.
18. Ibid., p. 25.
19. Ibid., p. 27.
20. Ibid., p. 40.
21. Ibid., p. 211.
22. Ibid., pp. 212-16.
23. Rogers, J. W., and Buffalo, M. D.: Fighting back: nine modes of adaptation to a deviant model. Social Problems. 22:101-18, October 1974. Quoted by permission.
24. Ibid., p. 106.
25. Ibid., p. 109.
26. Goffman, Stigma, p. 30.
27. Kalisch, B. J.: The stigma of obesity. Am. J. Nurs. 72, 6:1124-27, June 1972.
28. Jones, S. L.: Orthopedic injuries: illness as deviance. Am. J. Nurs. 75, 11:2030-33, November 1975.
29. Gregg, D.: Reassurance. Am. J. Nurs. 55:171-74, February 1955.

3 SHAME

Silvia Prodan Lange

The following are everyday situations in nursing settings. Their common denominator is the emotion of shame.

A teenage girl with downcast eyes tells the school nurse that she is ashamed to tell her parents that she is pregnant.

A woman delays examination of a lump in her breast because of her horror that a possible mastectomy would lessen her sense of femininity.

A high school athlete, quadriplegic from a diving accident, flushes crimson as the nurse tends to his bowel and bladder needs.

The parents of a child with symptoms of mental retardation keep him hidden away in a back room from friends, other children and family.

A nursing student holds back tears of humiliation when the anxious surgeon snaps at her awkwardness.

A woman, severely beaten by her husband, asks him not to visit her so that he will not be embarrassed by the hospital staff.

A man returns to the hospital with DTs after repeatedly promising himself and the staff that he would never drink again.

"Can't *you* do anything *else* to stop my pain, nurse?"

A meeting is held on the psychiatric ward in which the staff members share their feelings of inadequacy, failure, guilt, and shame after a patient on pass has committed suicide.

A four-year-old on the pediatric unit wails in despair after soiling his bed in the night.

A man berates himself for crying with pain.

A nursing instructor feels that she has failed when her students do poorly on a nationwide, standardized test.

For many people the experience of illness is in itself shameful. The diagnosis, medical treatment, body changes, reactions of family and friends, hospitalization, and many contacts during nursing care all may precipitate feelings that range from social discomfort to embarrassment to abject humiliation. Sick persons are suffering persons and very vulnerable. Their whole lives have been changed, at least temporarily, and they struggle with the resurgence of past experiences as they attempt to cope with present realities and plan for the future.

Nurses are central figures in their immediate lives. Through sensitive and compassionate understanding and actions they can provide multiple opportunities for the patients to maintain self-esteem and to share and explore with them the threatening aspects of their illness. Nurses can develop awareness of what shame means to individuals in all sorts of situations. In order to do so, they must be aware of their own feelings of shame in both their professional and personal lives. Shame leaves no one alone. Experience in observing illness, and daily contact with any group of patients, gives the nurse many opportunities to observe, analyze, and intervene therapeutically in the reactions of people being shamed and shaming others.

DEFINITION OF SHAME

Shame is only one emotion or affect among many, although it is central, complex, and interrelated with the others. Its importance in any person's life depends to a large extent on its intensity, duration and frequency. Other emotions are often mixed with and experienced with shame. One can be afraid and feel ashamed of cowardice; one can feel humiliated and cover it up with anger; one can feel jealous and be ashamed of one's pettiness. Shame, guilt and feelings of inferiority are often present together.

Shame and its synonyms are used frequently but without precise definition. Webster defines shame as "Painful emotion excited by a consciousness of guilt, shortcoming, or impropriety."[1] Disgrace, humiliation, embarrassment, tragedy and guilt can all be expressed by "It's a shame." Other popular expressions include, "Shame on you!"; "I was too embarrassed for words"; "A shameless hussy"; "I could have sunk through the floor." Children sing a mocking chant, "Shame, shame, double shame, everybody knows your name." A social blunder may be erased by the jingle, "It's better to burp and bear the shame, than squelch the belch and bear the pain." (Not everyone would agree.)

S. S. Tomkins, who wrote extensively on shame, stated:

> . . . shame is the affect of indignity, of defeat, of transgression and of alienation . . . shame strikes deepest into the heart of man . . . shame is felt as an inner torment, a sickness of soul. It does not matter whether the humiliated one has been shamed by derisive laughter or whether he mocks himself. In either event he feels himself naked, defeated, alienated, lacking in dignity or worth.[2]

The early psychoanalytic definition indicated that shame is a defense against exhibitionism and voyeurism: "I feel ashamed" means "I do not want to be seen."[3]

Threat of exposure is part of shame. Erik Erikson stated:

> Shame supposes that one is completely exposed and conscious of being looked at—in a word, self-conscious. One is visible and not ready to be visible. That is why we dream of shame as a situation in which we are being stared at in a condition of incomplete dress, in night attire, "with one's pants down" . . . the destructiveness of shaming is balanced in some civilizations by devices for "saving face." Shaming exploits an increasing sense of

being small, which paradoxically develops as the child stands up and as his awareness permits him to note the relative measure of size and power.[4]

H. M. Lynd regarded shame as being closely associated with self and therefore a clue to a broader understanding of identity:

Experiences of shame . . . are experiences of exposure, exposure of peculiarly sensitive, intimate, vulnerable aspects of the self. The exposure may be to others but, whether others are or are not involved, it is always . . . exposure to one's own eyes.[5]

The relation of physical exposure—nakedness—to shame is shown in the account of Adam and Eve, who felt shame after eating of the fruit of the tree of the knowledge of good and evil and subsequently covered themselves from the sight of each other and God. The German word from which our word "shame" is derived is part of a compound word relating to the genitals. However, experiences of shame involve much more than sexual exposure. The uncovering of weakness, failure, physical defect, passivity, misplaced confidence, and lack of recognition are all shameful experiences.

When urged to participate in a therapeutic speech group by reading a poem, a 28-year-old woman rushed out of the room cursing and slamming the door. Later, she told the nurse she was very ashamed of not knowing how to read and that she usually covered this up by bluffing or getting angry. The nurse conveyed her impression that the patient was an intelligent person, and later was able to help make arrangements for special tutoring.

A teenage girl received severe burns on her breasts as the result of sunbathing in the nude. She delayed medical treatment because of her embarrassment about the location of the burn and her feelings of shame that she had been so stupid.

One cause of shame for a girl seeking a therapeutic abortion was that she had put her trust in a man who turned out to be the local Casanova. She was ashamed because she had been seduced by an unworthy man and felt so guilty that she could only consider abortion or suicide, and she was ashamed that she must ask other people for help. She was embarrassed by her tears and her dependence.

A 77-year-old woman was restless and anxious after emergency surgery until she confided that her chief concern was that the black from her recently-dyed hair was rubbing off on the pillowcase. The nurses were surprised that she had so much pride in her appearance at her age.

Hair, dentures, make-up, privacy, and toilet rituals are taken for granted until a person is plunged into the often bewildering, impersonal, and embarrassing hospital environment. In the home, a sudden visit by the public health nurse may precipitate feelings of exposure and shame regarding children who will not behave, an alcoholic husband, or even dishes piled in the sink.

Shameful experiences are characteristically sudden and unavoidable. The incident may appear trivial or inconsequential to others, but it can precipitate intense feelings of self-consciousness and personal failure. Another aspect of shame involves admitting to oneself parts of the self that have been unrecognized or unacceptable. Shame may occur when one deceives others into believing something about oneself that is not true. Feelings of shame for others may be acute. Children may be painfully ashamed of, and for, their parents, and parents may experience helpless feelings of shame for their children, whose behavior may reflect their own parental failures. Parents of hippies often demonstrate this.

The feelings and reactions that have been labeled shame are often complex and difficult to distinguish from other feelings, such as anxiety, guilt, and inferiority. Shame and guilt are often linked as if they were synonymous. However, closer study has differentiated between them. Although they may be operating in the same individual at the same time, they are considered to be overlapping, rather than identical, emotions. For instance, a girl may feel guilty about her promiscuity, ashamed of her frigidity, and inferior to other girls. The young child who has difficulty with anal control feels bad, ashamed and inferior.

The following identify some of the differences between shame and guilt.

1. Shame is generated when a goal or ideal is not being reached; guilt is more tied to transgression of a specific code or law.
2. Shame concerns the more basic, unalterable aspects of the self (appearance, intelligence, race) as compared to the ideal—the should-be's and ought-to-be's; guilt concerns violations of social codes of behavior, cleanliness, politeness and rules—the do's and don'ts.
3. The unconscious, irrational threat in shame is abandonment; in guilt it is retaliation, mutilation and castration.
4. Shame may involve the feeling of having loved the wrong person or being inadequate for the person one loves; guilt involves a feeling of wrongdoing toward a love object. Unconscious hostility is often a part of guilt.
5. Shame results from tension between the ego and ego ideal; guilt stems from conflict between ego and superego.
6. Shame pertains to what one is—weak, inadequate. Guilt pertains to what one has done—bad things.
7. To be shameless is to be brazen, unblushing, insensitive to self and others—"bad"; to be guiltless is to be exonerated, innocent—"good."
8. Shame refers more to visual exposure; guilt occurs predominantly in reaction to verbal demands, prohibitions and criticisms.

Is there a feeling opposite to the feeling of shame? If this reaction stems from experiences of failure or as a defense against exposure, can self-confidence and pride be regarded as the other end of the continuum? G. L. Engel supports this view:

> Pride is the affect specially indicating success in living up to standards of the ego ideal. It pronounces satisfaction with the self, which feels correspondingly strengthened, loved, admired, and invulnerable. The person feeling pride is eager to display himself and to be seen . . . [Pride] is particularly related to all varieties of achievement, the various ways in which mastery is achieved in relation to the environment and to objects. The earliest expressions of pride are particularly related to the development and mastery of the body.[6]

In writing about the effort to maintain social poise, Erving Goffman stated that individuals who sense that they are "in face" will typically respond with feelings of confidence and reassurance.[7] They can hold their heads up high and openly present themselves to others. According to Goffman, poise is the capacity to suppress and conceal any tendency to become shamefaced during encounters with others.

Pride is as complex an emotion as shame, and its consideration cannot be oversimplified. It ranges from compensatory measures for feelings of inadequacy and inferiority to genuine feelings of self-respect and accomplishment.

DESCRIPTION OF SHAME REACTIONS

Who needs to be told what it feels like to experience shame? Ranging from mild embarrassment to excruciating humiliation, the subjective feeling involves a sudden awareness of anxiety, a sense of painful self-consciousness, and the wish to hide or escape. Statements of self-blame and self-derogation may be made, along with other verbal reports that the person feels embarrassed, ashamed, or humiliated. The more intense the feeling, the less likely one is to report it or mention it.

Shame can be recognized by some characteristic body reactions which may be observed in oneself or others. These are the general signs of anxiety, with specific relevance to the state of being observed. Some signs are:

1. Complete or partial withdrawal from visual contact—lowering of the eyes, blinking, bowing the head, turning the back, avoiding eye contact, glancing up furtively, covering face with hands.
2. Sudden changes in skin color—blushing, blanching, flushing.
3. Nervous physical gestures or manifestations—twisting of the fingers, nervously playing with hair or clothes, inspecting hands carefully, scuffing the feet, tremors, hesitating or vacillating manner, weak knees, tense muscles.
4. Difficulty with speech—stuttering, very soft voice, voice pitched very high or very low (or breaking), dryness of mouth, inability to speak, incoherence.

Modification and control of the reaction to shame are seen in the adult who abbreviates the response by a quick raising of the eyes and head. The frozen face of chronic shame may look continually humble and bowed down. A person may assume an anti-shame posture, in which the head is tilted back with the chin jutted out to help in obeying the command against admitting shame: "Keep your chin up." The embarrassed laugh is an attempt to cover up the discomfort, as is the burst of anger.

The mixture of shame with other emotions may produce such facial expressions as the following: with fear—humble and terrified; with distress—sad and defeated; with excitement—eyes glancing around, although the head is bowed; with anger—tight jaw, lowered head, a frown.

Blushing is a reaction to the experience of shame that has been mentioned repeatedly in both classical and psychiatric literature. Usually related to sexual feelings, the sudden, involuntary flushing of the face is a common symptom. This reaction is generally not regarded as pathologic, although as erthyrophobia it may reach such proportions as to keep a person from social situations that are stimulating and shaming. Because blushing is an open signal of inner discomfort, the shaming situation may be compounded. There comes the wish to cover one's face, sink into the floor, or become invisible. Young male patients, especially those on orthopedic wards, exploit this phenomenon to the nth degree with young female nursing students by means of a barrage of suggestive remarks, dirty jokes and excessive compliments. Learning how to cope with this situation is a special kind of learning experience.

> A man frequently shifted attention away from himself in group therapy by observing correctly that the therapist was blushing. The therapist would then blush even deeper, but handled this matter-of-factly by saying, "Yes, and you know how to make it worse," and refocusing on the patient.

Another specific way of expressing and handling shame reactions is the use of hand-to-mouth movements, which restore social and psychic equilibrium.[8] Such things as playing with the mouth, biting on a pencil, thumb sucking, lip biting, and covering of the lower face serve to hide a quivering lip. Gum chewing, the cocktail glass, cigarette smoking, excessive cosmetics, and moustaches help to accomplish the same purpose. L. Rangel developed the following sequence of security operations:

1. Infant with its mouth and snout buried in the breast.
2. 1½-year-old in its mother's arms, when approached by a stranger, turning away and burrowing into its mother's shoulder.
3. Older child turning its face into a corner so as not to be seen.
4. Adult, unpoised, blushing, and wanting to cover or hide his or her face.[9]

THE DEVELOPMENT OF SHAME

Shame results from tension between the ego and the ego ideal. The ego ideal refers to standards, aspirations, and goals which are internalized through identification with the culture—specifically, with the parents. Parents can either be loving and reassuring or trying to impose their own ideals (often unachieved). In their ego ideal children also include qualities they wish the parents possessed—such as beauty, wisdom, strength—as well as qualities of their own. Keys to the ego ideal include the answers to such questions as: What did you want to be when you grew up? What did your parents want you to be? Who was your childhood hero? Why? What is the ideal—whether girl, woman, wife, mother, or boy, man, husband, father—like? What is the ideal nurse like? If you had a magic wand, what about yourself would you change?

Shame, according to Engel, involves a discrepancy between the idealized self and the self as actually perceived.[10] The failure to achieve one's standards stimulates a fear of abandonment as expressed by the reaction "I am not worthy." The susceptibility to shame is increased when the internal standards are too high or too perfectionist. If parental figures demand too high a performance as the price for love, the "failing" person may feel unlovable and, therefore, not deserving of attention and love. The feeling of utter worthlessness and being held in contempt with the threat of abandonment is the most extreme shame reaction. Lesser degrees involve less harsh and final judgments and therefore greater chance of making good, regaining pride, and reestablishing a favorable opinion of oneself. Success in meeting the ego ideal results in pride.

S. Kaplan and R. Whitman developed a way of looking at shame as stemming from two origins—the positive and the negative ego ideals.[11] The negative ego ideal includes the qualities that have been ridiculed, disparaged and held in contempt. For instance, if courage in the face of physical pain is part of the positive ego ideal, then cowardice is part of the negative ego ideal. Therefore, shame can result when one falls short of interalized aspirations, and also when one behaves or feels about oneself in a way that approximates the negative ego ideal.

Beginning nursing students frequently experience embarrassment, humiliation, and a sense of personal failure because they set unrealistic goals for themselves as expert practitioners. They compare themselves unfavorably with more experienced students and RNs and are mortified when they have to admit to a patient that they do not yet know how to do a simple procedure.

At times hospital staff members and instructors may add to this stress by shaming the student, either consciously or unwittingly, for ineptitude and lack of knowledge. Nursing instructors can help students to deal with the situation more adequately, assisting them in sorting out their educational goals, discussing their assets and limitations, and talking about their ideals and the steps needed to reach these goals.

Engel also considered disgust to be linked to the development of shame.[12] Disgust is the affect that is a reaction against the oral and anal drives which are primarily involved in tasting, swallowing and smelling. Disgust contributes to the standards that are part of the ego ideal and the superego and that inculcate a special kind of guilt and shame. To be disgusted with oneself involves judging oneself as being dirty (fecally or sexually) and malodorous, therefore deserving only to be pushed away, segregated and isolated. To feel disgusted with others is to see them as unclean, unacceptable, unpleasant, and to wish to be rid of them.

Nurses need to come to grips with the reaction of disgust and learn to understand it in order to give nursing care to patients whose condition is repulsive. Sometimes disgust is an automatic response of some persons to such things as feces, vomit or foul-smelling drainage. Other people are disgusted by obesity, disfigurement, emaciation, congenital anomalies, sexual deviations, lice and body odor. Before patients can be helped with their conditions, nurses must understand the basis of their own reactions and deal with them appropriately.

Shame is generally considered to be first experienced in regard to body function and image. The child feels ashamed of weakness, smallness, nakedness, and lack of control, especially when compared with parents. A derivative of this is feeling shame because of a deformity or disfigurement.

Shame for adults involves abstract concepts such as the values of physical and mental health; intellectual performance; beauty; strength; sexual, vocational and monetary success and power; racial identification; national prestige; and socioeconomic status. In any society there may be moral and ethical codes that conflict with these concepts, and the child may be presented with standards different from those of parents, educators, peers, and the broader society. The ego ideal changes as new and different identifications are made; however, under stress, the individual generally returns to original constructs.

J. Ruesch identified some of the overall American values as being related to our pioneer and Puritan heritage, with the virtues of toughness, resourcefulness, purpose, purity, equality, sociality and change.[13] He recognized the powerful influence of the cultural group on the individual's feelings and behavior, with the degree of conformity being a common consideration. Competition and the need to win are stimulated at an early age, when American parents covertly require and demand of their babies that they be larger, healthier, and more precocious than other children. Love is given conditionally to reward these achievements, which can be demonstrated in quantitative terms—number of hits in the Little League, Girl Scout cookies sold, A's on the report card, and dates a week. As a social group hippies challenged many of these values; they are interesting to study in relation to shame because of their questioning attitudes toward many traditional values. Ethnic groups that have not been assimilated may have different values.

In the development of the personality, some experiences are of special significance in relation to shame; one such is muscular control. According to Erikson, the child struggles with the problems of muscular control during the second stage of personality development—roughly, from the second to the fourth year. Achievement of self-control results in the feelings of autonomy, pride and self-esteem. Failure to do so results in shame, doubt and diffuse anxiety.

Later, illness may reactivate conflict about bodily control and thereby impose stress, which complicates complete recovery. Such conflict is particularly characteristic of illnesses or treatments that radically change the body image and functioning. For instance, a colostomy is generally regarded by the patient as disgusting, ugly and unnatural, despite preparation before surgery, and the task of regaining bowel control is closely linked with shame, humiliation, pride and self-esteem.

Child-rearing practices often involve shaming, particularly in relation to toilet training and the inculcation of appropriate social behavior. The control of bed-wetting is often handled (or mishandled) through shaming techniques.

If shaming is used extensively in the socialization of the expression of emotions, the individual may later experience shame in many situations in which a display of emotion takes place.[14] For instance, if a child is made to feel shame for noisy excitement and laughter, the child may later feel shame over any source of enjoyment and excitement, sexual or otherwise. If he or she is shamed because of crying in distress, the child may later feel shame whenever distressed by hunger, pain, fatigue and frustration. This may pose particular problems during illness. The child may be shamed for expressing anger, contempt, fear, surprise, curiosity and shame itself.

Tomkins emphasized the importance of child-rearing practices that are based on an "anti-shame" ideology.[15] Through attitude, word and deed, parents can convey an attitude of respect and caring. They nurture the child with sympathy and understanding, to help him or her cope with discouragement and failure and learn ways to avoid defeat. Good socialization of shame experiences may: attenuate shame; allow the child to express, deal with, and reduce shame; increase trust; increase willingness and ability to offer sympathy and help to others and self; potentiate progress; develop physical courage; increase tolerance in problem solving; and aid in the achievement of identity. The nurse, especially in maternal-child and public health nursing, has many opportunities to help parents develop these attitudes toward their children.

As the child enters the latency or juvenile period, he or she shifts to peers for recognition and for hope of inclusion in a peer group. Differences in background, abilities, maturation, and social standing help to create in-groups and out-groups. Ostracism becomes a powerful weapon, which the child seeks to avoid. Disparagement and ridicule of others may develop at this time. Learned from parents who teach the child to notice the shortcomings of others, it can be a means of maintaining a shaky self-esteem by attacking and depreciating others. If used extensively, disparagement can interfere with correct appraisal of one's personal worth—everyone is "bad," including me.

Adolescence is also a crucial period in which shame is operative. Physical appearance, masculine and feminine identity, emancipation from dependence on parents, achievement in school and work, and comparisons with both the younger people's and older people's worlds—all may be shame-provoking. Loss of face, embarrassment, humiliation, exquisite sensitivity make this period a trial for many. Adolescents who become ill bring all their pride and shame to the treatment situation. This is one reason that nursing students find it particularly difficult and challenging to work with someone in this age bracket.

During the years of middle and old age, individuals may experience painful and devastating feelings of shame for what they have not accomplished, for becoming socially useless, and for failure of their physical and mental capacities. At their extreme, these feelings may lead to suicide.

THE FUNCTION AND VALUE OF SHAME

Although it is generally considered a "negative" emotion, shame has both function and value. It can be regarded as an important message to oneself and can provide opportunities for further self-development.

Engel has divided emotions into two main categories—the drive-discharge affects (anger, love, tenderness, sexual excitement) and the signal-scanning affects (shame, guilt, sadness, hopelessness, contentment, joy and pride).[16] The latter fulfills a warning function—an evaluation of one's performance—a "how am I doing?" The judgment of "good," "bad," "pleasant," "unpleasant," "success" or "failure" is sent back as part of ego function, either to maintain present behavior or to make a shift.

The drive-discharge affect reaches a peak and is either discharged or blocked. In either case the emotion is then replaced by one of the signal-scanning affects, pleasurable or unpleasurable, depending on the ego's evaluation of the consequences. A teacher might shout at a student in anger and feel ashamed for losing his or her temper and not "understanding" the student. A nursing student may reach out in great tenderness and compassion to hold a sick toddler and then feel embarrassed and bewildered when the child screams.

Shame provides a warning to the ego that some impulse, thought, fantasy, or act has failed or will fail to meet the standards of the ego ideal. When the signal is effective, psychic processes or behavior, or both, maintain the standards. A twinge of shame at the dean's reception might prevent one from acting inappropriately and making a fool of oneself. Ego defense mechanisms that prevent expression of the impulse may be used as well as activity directed toward accomplishment, creativity, and achievement.

If the signal is ineffective, the unpleasant affect of shame is felt with increasing intensity. Secondary psychic and behavior processes occur. An overwhelming sense of total personality failure may result in labeling oneself a "slob," "fink," "jerk," "sucker," "weakling" or "square." In this way, shame may be reduced by lowered aspirations or expectations of self. Self-deprecation is one of the most destructive results of discrimination and ridicule, in that one becomes deeply ashamed, seeing oneself through the eyes of the prejudiced, and accepts their evaluation as true.

Although shame-provoking experiences are characteristically painful, they may throw an unexpected light on who one really is and thus may point the way to a more complete understanding of who one might become. Such experiences may lead to a greater understanding of all people and how they live their lives.

In the trusting relationship, there is a paradox regarding shame experiences. If you reveal yourself to someone you care about and who accepts you, there is a strengthening of the bond and a boost of self-esteem. However, rejection by one who is important is much more humiliating and shameful than rejection by a mere acquaintance.

The act of sharing a "shameful" experience may in itself alleviate the fear of rejection, abandonment and disgust. After all, everyone is human—and what is shameful about that? However, one of the most difficult aspects of dealing with shame is the private nature of the things one feels ashamed about. They are the very things one *wants* to hide and *not* talk about. Yet, when one is able to talk about it, there is a sense of relief and universality. People are just not so very different from one another in their dreams, fears, hopes, hates, lusts and loves.

F. S. Perls has labeled shame and embarrassment as "quisling" emotions because, like the Norwegian collaborator who turned against his own country, these emotions tend to obstruct and restrict the individual's expression.[17] On the other hand, endurance, acceptance and expression of the shame will enable the person to bring the repressed material out, establish contact with and confidence in another, and discover with amazing relief that the facts behind the embarrassment were not so incriminating after all. Such liberation makes it possible for a person to experience the basic feelings of love, fear, hurt, anger and trust.

> Hank had repeatedly referred to things that he "couldn't talk about" in group therapy. The nurse received a phone call from a former friend of his, asking about his progress and inquiring if he was still getting cobalt treatments. This was new information. She decided to ask Hank about this in the group, knowing it would provide both support and pressure. He became very angry and refused to talk except to threaten to leave treatment. When he talked with the nurse privately, he maintained that the group wouldn't understand him. She expressed her concern for him whether or not he had cancer or had had treatment and encouraged him to take a chance.
>
> Two days later Hank took a deep breath, asked the group to listen to him first and condemn him later, and confessed that to his deep shame he was a pathological liar. He had made an elaborate web of lies of which the cancer and treatment were only a small part. Instead of condemnation, the group applauded him for his courage and helped him to sort out his present problems. "I feel like a thousand-pound weight has been lifted," he said with relief.

Shame can either be a spur to accomplishment—an incentive that helps a person reach a higher level of achievement and self-esteem—or it can be an overwhelming reaction that results in progressive self-derogation, withdrawal and hopelessness, and may lead to suicide.

Shame in the Interpersonal Context

The cause and feelings of shame may be known only to the person with a secret shame, but generally other people are part of the experience of being exposed and shamed. In relating poise to shame, Rangell stated that these reactions occur only in the presence of others, for although anxiety may be present when one is alone, social threat and fear of ridicule are not. He stated:

> When one is alone, one can let oneself go, assume a posture of which one is not proud, examine in the mirror a skin blemish of which one might be ashamed, let one's stomach stick out, grimace at oneself, or squeeze a blackhead; unless, that is, one fantasies other persons as still present; in the absence of this, even the most unpoised and vulnerable can achieve a relaxed state when alone. In company and in a social setting such is not the case; a stiffening-up takes place and a certain armour, no matter how subtle, is assumed.[18]

Lack of privacy in most hospital settings forces the patient to deal constantly with the threat of social disapproval when poorly equipped to do so. Interaction with others raises the questions, "How will I do?" "Will I be accepted?" "Will my needs be met?" "Will I be welcomed, respected, noticed and listened to?" In early clinical experiences, nursing students are preoccupied with these questions pertaining to themselves, and then they gradually shift the focus to concentrate on the patients' needs. One student reported:

> I was to care for a two-year-old boy who was in traction with synovitis of the hip. When I went in to become acquainted, I noticed that his father was there with the child. When I approached the youngster, I found that he did not wish to cooperate with me. He fought me and yelled for his father every step of the way. I usually get along very well with children, and I began to get embarrassed and to completely lose confidence in myself. . . . I lost my effectiveness altogether, and I became so "still" and unnatural that I never could communicate effectively with the child after that.[19]

Like anxiety, shame and embarrassment may be contagious. Therefore, considerable efforts are often exerted to protect oneself and others from recognizing these reactions.

Goffman stressed the importance of interpersonal situations in the precipitation of the sense of shame. Regarding all encounters as situations in which "face" is established, maintained, threatened, and recovered, he said:

> Should he sense that he is in wrong face or out of face, he is likely to feel ashamed and inferior because of what has happened to the activity on his account and because of what may happen to his reputation as a participant. Further, he may feel bad because he has relied on the encounter to support an image of self to which he has become emotionally attached and which he now feels threatened. Felt lack of judgmental support from the encounter may take him aback, confuse him, and momentarily incapacitate him as an interactant. His manner and bearing may falter, collapse, and crumble. He may become embarrassed and chagrined; he may become shamefaced.[20]

An incident reported by a nursing student illustrates this point:

> I had to do an abdominal perineal prep on this woman who was scheduled for surgery. She made many comments about how embarrassing it must be for me to do this procedure. When I said I wasn't she replied that a nurse would get used to doing it and would become hardened about doing things like this so it would not bother her. I wasn't embarrassed at first, but as she continued to make comments of that sort, I became embarrassed and fumbled in my work.[21]

Tomkins has identified five different positions in relation to feeling shame and being shamed.[22]

1. I may feel shame for many things for which no one has shamed me (failure to achieve my own goals or violation of my own standards).
2. I may not feel shame although another has tried to shame me. (If the person expressed contempt of me, I may just get angry or contemptuous of him or her.)
3. I may be shamed by another person even though it was not intentional. (The other person is so busy or preoccupied that he or she ignores me. Closely identified person—spouse, child—may produce shame by behavior which would shame you if you did it.)
4. I may feel ashamed because another expresses negative feelings toward me even though it was not intended to shame me as such. (If the person is

angry at me or distressed by me or frightened by me, I may feel shame for my behavior.)

5. I may feel shame because the other person is trying to shame me. (If I am doing the best I can and am satisfied but another claims to be disgusted with me, I could feel shame.)

The last position was elaborated on by A. Leveton in discussing reproach and "shamesmanship."[23] Shaming can be a powerful interpersonal weapon, ranging all the way from tears to suicide on the part of the patient, and counterattack on the part of the therapist, by means of abandonment or inappropriate treatment.

The hypochondriacal patient, the depressed patient, and many families of schizophrenic patients use shame to an extensive degree. Hospital staffs may be demoralized by the master of reproach, who has the skill to elicit expectations and shame someone into trying to fulfill them unsuccessfully. Shaming tactics between staff members, nursing and medical, are also usually destructive.

Nonverbal aspects of the act of shaming another person include the derisive laugh, staring a person down, and using the shaming gesture—one forefinger stroking downward on the extended forefinger of the opposite hand.

Disparagement, when expressed openly and verbally, is called ridicule. Particularly vulnerable are people who deviate visibly from the norms of appearance or behavior. Wright, using many first-hand accounts of shame and humiliation, points out the devastating effects that taunting and ridicule can have on the child with a physical defect and suggests that such a child be given special preparation to avoid lasting damage to self-esteem.[24] Ridicule from adults is generally more covert, though it may be expressed through curiosity, pity, ostracism, and oversolicitude.

> A 13-year-old boy who was extremely sensitive about his crippled legs from polio had always been overprotected. For the first time in his life he went downtown alone to a movie. As he was standing in front of the theater with a half-empty box of popcorn and his crutches, a passerby solicitously dropped a quarter in the box. On return to the hospital, the boy told the nurse about his humiliation and his fury. She listened with the feeling, "It *would* have to happen to *him*." After agreeing with him that it had been a thoughtless but perhaps well-meaning gesture, she helped him cope with the situation by saying, "Well, at least it will pay for the popcorn the next time." He did go out alone again.

Two basic methods of handling shame situations are avoidance and correction. The person who seeks to avoid being shamed will conceal parts of the self he or she thinks are unacceptable, use cautious and ritualized behavior, conform socially, and keep away from "loaded" topics. Corrective efforts include acknowledging and challenging the shamer, seeking special achievement through acts that restore pride and self-confidence, maintaining a façade, denying that one has been shamed, and reacting with anger or joking.

To avoid shaming another person, an individual may provide physical and psychological privacy, keep away from touchy areas, explain why the other person need not be upset, utilize face-saving etiquette, overlook shortcomings and deviations, and use humor.

Once the situation has been precipitated, the shamer can attempt to correct it by helping the victim to restore face, apologizing and making amends, stating that the comment was a joke or was meaningless or unintentional ("just my way"), stating that he or she was acting under the influence of another, and purposely ignoring shame reaction.

People are shamed by different things at different stages in their lives. An experience that was humiliating at the time may be funny in retrospect.

> When I was a beginning student, I was very anxious to be a good nurse and give "complete" nursing care. I was giving morning care to an elderly man who had had a stroke which left him somewhat disoriented as well as hemiplegic. He was in a six-bed ward with only curtains drawn to separate us from the other men. When it came time to "finish the bath," I realized that he didn't grasp what I meant. I lifted up the bath blanket and began diligently scrubbing away. He began to moan and groan so that the whole room could hear him. "What's the matter?" I asked, afraid that I was hurting him. "Oh, lordy, oh, *lordy*," he shouted, "Does that feel good!" To make matters worse, he reached up and pinched my cheek saying, "You delightful little devil, you!" I was very, very embarrassed—not wanting to stay with him and not wanting to leave the sanctuary of the curtained bed and face the other men. Later that night, I told my classmates in the dorm and they roared. I am still telling the story and can now laugh about it, too.

APPLICATION OF THE CONCEPT OF SHAME IN NURSING

Nurses must develop a sensitivity in relation to shame. Their knowledge of general sociocultural values that affect patients must be used with an awareness of individual differences to minimize stereotyping. They need to be alert to their own cultural background and biases so they do not impose them on the patient or misinterpret behavior. Some situations that would precipitate shame in the nurse might not in the patient, and the patient may be embarrassed by actions that are commonplace to the nurse, such as questions about elimination. Many nurses and other health team members come from a white, middle-class background. The common values that form their ego ideals might differ considerably from those of the patient who comes from another background.

This point is illustrated by I. D. Cahill in the description of the misunderstandings by nurses of the attitudes of Negro and Puerto Rican lower-class women toward illegitimacy.[25] The assumption that all unmarried mothers feel shame was often found to be a reflection of the nurse's value system but not that of the patient. Strenuous efforts to "protect" all such patients may be unwarranted and possibly even destructive.

General nursing actions related to shame are:

1. Avoid causing shame.
2. Give anticipatory help in situations in which shame is likely to occur.
3. Encourage the patient and family to share shame feelings and to deal with these constructively.
4. Minimize the need for shame in the nursing situation.

An example of this last approach:

> A woman, severely injured in a hurricane, was having her clothes cut off in the emergency room. Increasingly anxious, she blushed and blurted out, "I wear falsies." "That's o.k.," the nurse replied, "I wear them, too." The patient was visibly relieved.

Nurses have the responsibility, opportunity, and privilege of helping people in crisis situations. Many times these situations involve radical shifts in ways of thinking, acting, and feeling because of the impact of illness and the necessity of altering patterns of living. Shame can be precipitated by almost any situation.

A person's perception of self and situation determine whether shame is precipitated. Some common nursing situations in which shame can be anticipated and dealt with are:

1. Modesty situations
   a. Lack of privacy and exposure of the body during physical nursing procedures (enemas, catheterization, bathing)
   b. Elimination and reactions to loss of bowel and bladder control
   c. The obstetrical situation, with exposure of the genitals and discussion of the reproductive cycle
2. Regressive behavior under stress
   a. Anger
   b. Crying
   c. Loss of control during anesthesia, toxic reactions or alcohol intoxication
3. Reactions of the patient and family to critical situations such as:
   a. Loss of limbs and/or other disfigurement, especially of the face
   b. Mental retardation, mental illness
   c. Adjustment to physical disability, immobility and/or enforced dependence (such as being in traction)
   d. Suicide or unsuccessful suicide attempt of a family member
   e. Venereal disease and genitourinary conditions
   f. Congenital defects
4. Body changes
   a. In adolescence
   b. In the aging process

Many more could be added. Therapeutic failures and disturbed staff relations may be shame-producing for the nurse.

The following examples illustrate the application of the concept of shame in three major clinical areas—medical-surgical, maternal-child, and psychiatric nursing. Shame is viewed from three different perspectives: shame that comes from changes in body functioning, shame that comes from failure to meet social values, and shame that results from another's behavior.

Shame that results from changes in body functioning: For example paralysis, whether from a cerebrovascular accident or an external injury to the spinal cord, presents complex problems. Along with grief, fear, bewilderment, anger, and denial, the patient may experience shame. This is often related to extreme dependence, interruption of ability to care for bowel and bladder needs, lack of ability to control muscles of locomotion and speech, loss of sexual function, and impaired control over emotional expression. The nurse needs to consider the impact of illness in order to help the person utilize rehabilitation opportunities to the fullest.

Application of the concept of shame would include the following:

1. Nurses explore their own experiences, backgrounds, and feelings in regard to radical changes in body functioning and dependency.
2. The patient may be experiencing many emotional reactions, some of which may be shame, embarrassment, and disgust in relation to changes in body image and lack of control over functioning and temporary dependency. The intensity depends on the patient's unique personality and plans for the future.
3. Anger, denial, and withdrawal may be used to reduce feelings of shame, inadequacy and despair.
4. Regaining personal control over body functions increases self-esteem and descreases shame. The nurse helps the patient by giving expert physical care, by encouraging maximal decision-making by the patient, and by teaching self-help skills.
5. Shame can be felt for another and can be precipitated in interpersonal contacts. The family and members of the nursing team are included in the nurse's understanding of the dynamics of shame for this patient.
6. Mastery of a shameful experience may lead to further personal development and a sense of pride. The nurse helps the patient to cope with limitations and to develop alternate ways to maintain self-esteem, and may provide contact with other patients who have made a good adjustment to their condition. This helps both persons.

Shame that comes from failure to meet social values: A typical situation calling for an understanding of shame in relation to social values is that of the premature infant. Viewing the birth of a premature infant as an acute emotional crisis in a family, D. M. Kaplan and E. A. Mason expressed that the mother often experiences a deep sense of failure because she has a small, weak, often ugly baby, who barely holds on to life.[26] Such babies rarely inspire pride; congratulations, if any, are cautious. The mother feels useless, helpless and undeserving of even being in the hospital. In her shame she avoids the nursery and the baby.

From this research it was determined that a definite pattern of psychological tasks must be accomplished in order for the mother to master the situation, so that in the future she can provide a healthy mother-child relationship. One task for the mother is to face and acknowledge the fact of her failure to deliver a normal, full-term baby. If she is not able to do so, it is all the harder for her to use the time with her baby in a psychologically productive way. A possible lifetime of misery and emotional disturbance for the family may result.

The nurse can help the mother of the premature (or birth-injured) infant admit, express, and come to grips with her feelings of failure and shame. Awareness of the following may be useful:

1. Part of the positive ego ideal of most women is that they will be able to deliver healthy, normal babies of which they can be proud. Part of the negative ego ideal would be inability to do so, this inability being a reflection on them as women, wives and mothers.
2. Along with feelings of inadequacy and shame, the mother may experience anger, distress, fear and guilt, which she directs at others, including her family and the medical and nursing staff, in an effort to reduce anxiety.
3. Because shame may be lessened by recognition and sharing, the nurse provides opportunities for the mother and father to talk about the baby and to express disappointment and grief without further shaming. Both privacy and companionship should be provided for.
4. Shaming can be decreased, and self-esteem increased by opportunities for achievement that will relate to the shameful experience. The nurse may provide appropriate opportunities for the mother to participate in the care of the baby.
5. Feelings of shame can be reactivated—the nurse should be alert to this possibility in subsequent pregnancies of this mother. Also, the mother may attempt to compensate for her initial failure by overprotection, and she may need help in allowing the child to grow up as a normal person with normal needs.
6. If the premature infant has other congenital anomalies or is brain damaged, the nurse should recognize the long-term needs in regard to helping the family and child make an optimal adjustment in terms of self-esteem and accomplishment without shame.

Shame as the result of another's behavior or condition: In examining the effects of the husband's mental illness upon the family, M. R. Yarrow et al. reported that wives of hospitalized mentally ill men expect the illness to be stigmatized.[27] Wives are quoted as saying, "I'm not ashamed, but people who don't know the hospital would take the wrong attitude toward it." "I live in a horror—a perfect horror—that some people will make a crack about it to Jim (child) and suppose after George gets out everything is going well and somebody throws it up in his face. That would ruin everything." "At first I was a little ashamed, but now I'm getting to understand it better. . . . Of course, I have cut out seeing all but a couple of our friends . . . in fact, Joe asked me not to tell his friends . . ." This study presented much fascinating data about this difficult situation and indicated in summary that the wives are generally subject to conflicting emotions as to whether they can communicate with others about the husband's illness—they need help and understanding, but are generally unwilling to reveal the nature of the illness and the anxieties associated with it.

Nurses could help the members of the family as well as the designated patient with feelings of shame, failure and stigma. Some ideas are:

1. Mental illness is still a stigmatized condition in this country which often produces a feeling of shame in the individual and family. This may result in a delay of treatment.
2. Part of the ego ideal is that one will marry a happy, stable, productive mate. Mental illness in a spouse may produce feelings of failure, guilt and shame.
3. It is difficult and painful to talk about shameful experiences, even with professional people who are offering help.
4. Nurses should look at their own feelings, background and experiences in relation to mental illness and determine if they view it as shameful, embarrassing, or frightening. They must discover whether they tend to blame or shame the family members for the patient's condition.
5. Family members of hospitalized psychiatric patients may express feelings of shame, resentment, anger, and inadequacy to the patient and toward the staff. The nurse can refrain from retaliating and can help them to develop more realistic expectations of themselves, of others and of treatment.
6. Loss of self-esteem and feelings of inadequacy, shame, and guilt are common among patients with mental illness. Their feelings are particularly related to depression and may precipitate suicide attempts. The nurse interacts with the patient and family in such a way as to mobilize ego assets, restore and maintain self-esteem, and regain confidence. She or he creates a therapeutic environment to foster this.

Application of the concept of shame is useful in examining the educational process—from how nursing students move from being flustered and embarrassed by their first bed bath to being experienced nurses coping with the complex reactions in which the feelings of patient-nurse-physician are intimately entwined. Nurses should develop their own ego ideal for nursing, which will help them to achieve maximal satisfaction under the common stressful situations in which shame, inadequacy, guilt and helplessness play a part.

Basic Assumptions Regarding the Application of the Concept of Shame in Nursing

General Application:

1. Shame is a complex, common reaction which occurs in a wide variety of situations throughout life. Many people seeking medical attention may expe-

rience feelings of shame because of the illness, the necessary treatment and the changes in patterns of living.

2. The experiences of shame one has had in the process of growing up play a significant part in behavior regarding self-esteem, self-confidence, guilt, doubt, disgust, poise, ability to persevere, and ability to cope with failure.

3. Shame reactions can be identified by subjective feelings, verbal descriptions and nonverbal behavior, with varying degrees of intensity and significance.

4. Shame occurs in an interpersonal context—it can be precipitated, intensified, relieved, or resolved through communication. Nurse-patient-physician relationships may be influenced by shame.

5. The professional nurse is expected to be able to cope with feelings of shame, guilt, disgust and inadequacy in order to be able to anticipate, recognize and intervene in shame reactions with patients and families when it is deemed appropriate.

Specific Nursing Intervention:

1. General nursing action related to shame involves maintaining the dignity and self-esteem of the individual through both obvious and subtle means—verbally and nonverbally. Basic to such action is an attitude of not blaming and not shaming the patients for being who they are and helping them to be more like they want to be. It includes common courtesies, such as knocking on the door, providing privacy, calling a person by name, and encouraging individuality.

2. Specific verbal intervention includes the nurse helping patients under the appropriate circumstances in the following sequence:

   a. The nurse, recognizing that patients are experiencing shame, encourages them to acknowledge it to at least one other person.
   b. The nurse helps the patients to determine the reason for the shame—in what way do the patients feel inadequate, humiliated and a failure?
   c. The nurse draws the patients' attention to the relationship between the reason and their ego ideal—in what ways did they fall short of this ideal or come close to the negative ego ideal? How did they acquire this expectation? Is it still appropriate? Was it ever appropriate? What do they want to do?
   d. If the patients decide that the goal is still desirable and worth working toward, the nurse helps them to determine what steps can be taken to approximate the goal more closely.
   e. If they decide that their previous ego ideal was inappropriate, skewed or incomplete, the nurse helps them to determine what they do want for themselves and what is possible.
   f. If it is determined that the patients were shamed through the behavior of the nurse, other staff members of institutional practices, the

nurse will act to make amends and avoid such behavior in the future. She or he will also try to evaluate accurately when it enhances the patient's self-esteem more not to discuss the situation.

3. Nurses can apply the concept of shame to themselves in order to increase their own understanding of self, so that they can be happier and more productive, professionally and personally.

REFERENCES

1. Webster's New Collegiate Dictionary. Springfield, Mass., G. & C. Merriam, 1958, p. 777.
2. Tomkins, S. S.: Affect, Imagery, Consciousness. Vol. 2. New York, Springer, 1963, pp. 6-118.
3. Hinsie, L. E., and Campbell, R. J.: Psychiatric Dictionary. New York, Oxford University Press, 1960, p. 677.
4. Erikson, E., Kluckhohn, C., Murray, H. A., and Schneider, D. M.: Personality, in Nature, Society, and Culture. New York, Knopf, 1959, p. 200.
5. Lynd, H. M.: On Shame and the Search for Identity. New York, Science Editions, 1962, pp. 27-28.
6. Engel, G. L.: Psychological Development in Health and Disease. Philadelphia, Saunders, 1962, pp. 177-78.
7. Goffman, E.: On facework. Psychiatry. 18:213-31, 1955.
8. Rangell, L.: The psychology of poise. Int. J. Psychoanal. 35:317, 1954.
9. Ibid., p. 325.
10. Engel, Psychological Development in Health and Disease, p. 170.
11. Kaplan, S., and Whitman, R.: The negative ego-ideal. Int. J. Psychoanal. 5:183-87, 1965.
12. Engel, Psychological Development in Health and Disease, pp. 172-73.
13. Ruesch, J., and Bateson, G.: Communication: The Social Matrix of Psychiatry. New York, Norton, 1951, pp. 97-98.
14. Tomkins, Affect, Imagery, Consciousness, pp. 227-28.
15. Ibid., pp. 305-17.
16. Engel, Psychological Development in Health and Disease, p. 128.
17. Perls, F. S.: Ego, Hunger and Aggression. San Francisco, Orbit Graphic Arts, 1966, p. 178.
18. Rangell, The psychology of poise, p. 315.
19. Seman, M. A.: A survey of stressful and satisfying incidents of nursing students during pediatric clinical experience. Master's Thesis, University of Washington, 1964, p. 83.
20. Goffman, On facework, p. 215.
21. Yasuda, P. M.: Some factors contributing to interpersonal relationship problems experienced by first-year nursing students with medical and surgical patients in a selected general hospital. Master's Thesis, University of Washington, 1958, p. 42.
22. Tomkins, Affect, Imagery, Consciousness, pp. 154-55.
23. Leveton, A.: Reproach: the art of shamesmanship. Br. J. Med. Psychol. 35:101-11, 1962.
24. Wright, B. A.: Physical Disability—A Psychological Approach. New York, Harper, 1960, pp. 242-50.
25. Cahill, I. D.: Facts and fallacies about illegitimacy. Nurs. Forum. 4, 1:39-55, 1965.
26. Kaplan, D. M., and Mason, E. A.: Maternal reactions to premature birth viewed as an acute emotional disorder. *In* Parad, H. J. (ed.): Crisis Intervention: Selected Readings. New York, Family Association of America, 1965, p. 122.
27. Yarrow, M. R., Clausen, J., and Robbins, P.: Personality and family-community. *In* Smelser, J., and Smelser, S. (eds.): Personality and Social Systems. New York, John Wiley, 1963, p. 397.

ADDITIONAL READINGS

Appleton, W. S.: The blame of dying young. Am. J. Psychoanal. 35, 4:377-81, Winter 1975.

Bermosk, L. S., and Corsini, R. J.: The price of sarcasm. *In*: Critical Incidents in Nursing. Philadelphia, Saunders, 1973, pp. 45-53.

English, F.: Shame and social control. Trans. Analysis J. 5, 1:24, January 1975.
Heller, E.: Man guilty and man ashamed. II. Man ashamed. Psychiatry. 37:99-108, May 1974.
Lewis, H. B.: Shame and Guilt in Neurosis. New York, International Universities Press, 1971.
Lowenfeld, H.: Notes on shamelessness. Psychoanalytic Q. 45:63-72, January 1976.
Nakushian, J. M.: Restoring parents' equilibrium after sudden infant death. Am. J. Nurs. 76:1600-04, October 1976.
Piers, G., and Singer, M.: Shame and Guilt, A Psychoanalytic and a Cultural Study. Springfield, Ill., Thomas, 1953.
Roberts, S.: Depersonalization of the critically ill (Chap. 3). Body image and self concept (Chap. 4). *In:* Behavioral Concepts and the Critically Ill Patient. Englewood Cliffs, N.J., Prentice-Hall, 1976, pp. 57-96.
Stierlin, H.: Shame and guilt in family relations. Theoretical and clinical aspects. Arch. Gen. Psychiatry. 30:381-89, March 1974.
Ward, H.: Shame—a necessity for growth in therapy. Am. J. Psychotherapy. 26:232-43, 1972.
Woods, N. F.: Aftermath of sexual assault: rape (Chap. 6). Sexual adaptation to hospitalization and illness (Chap. 7). Alteration of body image and sexual adaptation; enterostomy, mastectomy, and hysterectomy (Chap. 9). *In:* Human Sexuality in Health and Illness. Saint Louis, C. V. Mosby, 1975, pp. 95-123, 140-59.

4 LOSS

Carolyn E. Carlson

Loss is probably one of a very few events that is experienced by everyone regardless of personality, economic status or culture. Losses may be of body parts and functions, valued persons or possessions, abilities, and even more abstract things, such as certainty or predictability in life. In this chapter loss is defined in relation to changes in goal accessibility brought about by life events. Goal differences, objective and subjective definitions of loss, and many types of loss are described. Nursing implications include the importance of assessing actual and potential losses and understanding their meaning to the individual, and methods of preventing or lessening the impact of loss.

Various aspects of loss have been of interest to this writer for many years, beginning with recognition of individual differences in responding to the death of a loved one and broadening to concern about reactions to losses of such things as body parts or functions. Generalizations about phenomena are important and essential aspects of developing knowledge; however, they lose their usefulness in professional practice when individual differences are overlooked.

THE RELATIONSHIP OF LOSS TO GOALS

Although everyone can think of examples of having lost things or an important person, defining a loss and understanding its significance to the individual are not simple. It is not uncommon to hear people say such things as "I couldn't live if I lost my husband" or "I would never get used to losing a breast." Most people agree that such statements refer to major losses. On the other hand, there are other losses that may be equally devastating which are not always met with the same recognition or compassion. Some examples are the death of a pet, the paralysis of a hand or the appearance of wrinkles on a previously unmarked face.

What constitutes a loss? Are there commonalities in the myriad events or experiences that people call losses? When we speak of losing something we are referring to a type change we have noticed. Something once present or available is now absent or inaccessible. The fact that the change is noticed is evidence that the object had some significance to the individual.

Definition of Loss

Thwarting of desires, hopes or goal achievement seems to be inherent in most events or experiences involving losses. A person, object, body part or body function may be missed because certain desires or outcomes are no longer attainable rather than because the object itself is gone. For example, the pianist with a paralyzed hand may no longer have a means of self-support, of gaining recognition, or of relieving tension. A spouse who has died may have been so centrally involved in the bereaved person's methods of meeting goals that the latter feels absolutely desolate. In such an instance all goals may be viewed as inaccessible.

Since the individual's goals are important to the perception of something missing, they are included in the definition of loss. Loss is defined as any change in the individual's situation that reduces the probability of achieving implicit or explicit goals. It is assumed that a person's goals, ends, or hopes exist to satisfy the person's needs. Severity of loss is related to the salience of goals that have become less accessible or inaccessible and the extent of the goal disruption, displacement or extinction.

Goal Characteristics

Since loss is defined within the context of goal achievement, it is useful to understand ways in which personal goals may differ. First, goals may differ in clarity or explicitness. Some persons are very capable of stating clearly what their goals are while others say they have none or are unable to be definite about them. It is assumed that most behavior has direction and to that extent is goal-oriented, but the direction may not always be recognized by the person. Second, goals have different levels of concreteness or abstractness. For example, the goal of being a productive human being is more abstract than a goal of completing the writing of a book. Third, goals differ in the number of actual or potential paths or methods available to reach them. This is closely related to the concreteness-abstractness dimension, with fewer paths likely to be available for the more concrete goals. A fourth type of difference is in the nature of the relationships of goals to each other in a hierarchical structure. Goals may be broken down in such a way that lower-level goals are seen as steppingstones, that is, as methods or pathways to reach higher goals. Goals vary in centrality within one's goal structure. Some individuals may be dominated by one all-pervasive goal. All other goals may be subordinate to it or part of it. For example, the individual striving to become president of a company or country might direct all goals and activities to be in line with that primary goal. Other individuals may have many goals of equal importance, some of which can even be substituted for another. For example, an individual may strive to be a "good" teacher, athlete and musician rather than outstanding in any one role, or achievement of excellence in any one category might substitute for lack of excellence in another.

Goals may be interrelated in such a way that progress toward the achievement of one enhances, impedes or has no effect on the achievement of a goal parallel to or superordinate to it. For example, completion of a college degree may facilitate getting wanted recognition as well as reaching a career goal. Achievement of a second goal is obstructed when paths to the goals conflict. The case of conflicting paths is similar to the antagonistic or conflictual psychological situations described by L. Meyerson.[1] Here, progress in achieving one goal prevents progress in achieving another. Achievement of the goal of health, for example, may require the amputation of a leg, which blocks achievement of goals requiring an intact body. In the case of independent goals, different methods are required to achieve each. This seems more likely to occur when goals are stated in very concrete terms.

Nurses who know these characteristics of their patients' implicit or explicit goals are in a much better position to understand and sometimes prevent loss experiences than those who lack this knowledge.

Goals have physical, psychological and social components. Work toward most goals requires specific physical processes and abilities. Attainment or lack of success has numerous psychological consequences. Finally, few goals can be reached without at least some reliance on social resources external to the self.

In summary, there are many ways in which people's goals vary. There is variation in aspects of specific goals (clarity, concreteness, numbers of paths available) and in the relationships between goals (hierarchical, parallel arrangement, centrality) and in the effects on goal achievement (facilitation, obstruction, no effect).

Goal characteristics are influenced by such factors as education, development level, intelligence, personality, culture, past experience and environment. Many of these factors also influence the loss experience.

FACTORS INFLUENCING THE LOSS EXPERIENCE

Although the primary determinant of how a loss will be experienced is the extent to which it interferes with goal achievement, this is not the only influencing factor. There are objective characteristics of changes or losses, person characteristics, and external resources that affect the extent to which changes disrupt goal attainment.

Objective Factors

Objective factors include characteristics of events uninfluenced by the subjective meaning attached to them. The most obvious example of such characteristics is the objective description of facts concerning a change that everyone aware of the change agrees on. "Her husband died," "all four limbs are paralyzed," "the left leg was amputated below the knee," "he has total loss of vision in both eyes," "the child's dog was killed," "the patient's personal belongings were removed from the bedside" are statements that qualify as objective descriptions because they include facts without qualification. They do not include the meaning these facts have for individual goals and goal achievement.

Major objective characteristics of an event that influence goal achievement potential are visibility; duration; abruptness; extent of change in physical structure or function; time required for treatment, relearning and reconstruction; and financial requirements.

Visibility: Visibility of a change can have various consequences. As described in Chapter 2, a visible deformity or defect usually has negative social consequences. Thus visibility tends to add social losses to the already existing physical limitations. On the other hand, the visibility of a destroyed home may stimulate others to help out by providing housing, contributing money or giving time. Thus the potential expansion as well as the duration of losses is limited.

Duration: The duration of a change or a loss refers to the extent to which it is temporary or permanent. In the case of death, severance of the spinal cord or loss of limb, the physical changes are permanent. On the other hand, immobility caused by paralysis or a body cast may be temporary, at least in part. Obviously duration can influence the number and type of goals that become less accessible. For example, family and friends may get tired of helping and drift away if demands persist for a long time.

Abruptness: Abruptness concerns how quickly changes occur. A death can occur without warning or after years of struggle with a progressive illness. Likewise paralysis can happen instantly from a dive into shallow water or after years of living with multiple sclerosis. Long-term gradual change may lessen goal disruption by allowing time to develop alternate methods to achieve important goals.

Extent of Loss: Extent of loss or change can be defined objectively (such as loss of home, spouse, spouse and children, function of lower extremities) or subjectively (extent relative to goal disruption). The extent of objective loss does not necessarily correspond to extent of loss actually experienced, however, since individual goals are so variable.

Time Required: Time required for treatment, rebuilding or relearning can be critical to success or failure in achieving goals. This variable is similar in some ways to duration of change but needs to be singled out for emphasis. Frequently time that must be spent reestablishing one's physical, psychological, or social equilibrium is time taken away from other goal-directed activities. Education and work are often delayed because of physical illness or disability, making attainment of goals related to these activities less accessible.

Financial Requirements: Little needs to be said about this variable. Most persons are painfully aware of the financial drain that occurs with illness and disability. Many other changes in life are accompanied by financial requirements also. As noted previously, one's financial status is often instrumental in the pursuit of numerous goals.

Although there are other objective characteristics of life changes that might affect goal accessibility, those noted are some of the prominent ones. This writer hopes that the discussion will alert the reader to others.

Person Characteristics

Previous discussion has already included some person-related variables: clarity of goals; number of goals relevant to the person; centrality; number of pathways available to achieve goals; compatibility of goals; and the like. Openness, coping mechanisms, flexibility and motivation are other important person characteristics. Although little research has been done on these variables, there are some influences that can be deduced logically.

Clarity of Goals: The more certain people are about what goals they are striving to achieve, the more successful they should be in reaching them. Clarity of direction allows the individual to search for and put energies into methods rather than into aimless activity. Clarity, however, would have a negative influence if goals were extremely unrealistic. In such a case, much energy could be wasted.

Openness: Openness refers to the individual's willingness and ability to take in available information with minimal or no distortion. It is hypothesized that the more information that is available to a person the more alternatives for goal achievement that person can generate. Information often can increase opportunities or suggest which opportunities are blind or unproductive.

Coping Mechanisms: Coping mechanisms are defined simply as the methods of handling actual or potential disruptions in one's purposeful, goal-directed activity. Some individuals flee into a fantasy world at the first sign of difficulty, while others try to define logically and precisely the nature and extent of disruption and find methods of removing whatever is problematic. Individuals have many ways of trying to deal with changes in life that go beyond pleasant novelties. Anticipation, within limits, may be a helpful aspect of an individual's coping style, by giving a person time to prevent a loss or lessen its impact.

Flexibility: Flexibility refers to the ability to change set or substitute methods for achieving a given goal. For example there are many ways that the goal of recognition might be achieved. Flexible people are more likely to succeed since more pathways are open to them. Also, if one pathway is taken away the availability of others makes the goal still accessible. The person who is fixed on one method to achieve a given goal is much more vulnerable to loss.

Motivation: Motivation generally means some movement on the part of the motivated person and usually implies a goal or direction. J. R. Barry[2] insists that all persons are motivated and that the person who is described as "unmotivated" is simply not motivated to achieve the "right" goals from the describer's perspective. J. W. McDaniel[3] has suggested that motivation to achieve a goal and subsequent effort toward that end are a result of three subjective estimates: the probability estimate of a positive outcome; estimate of costs; and utility or value. All three of these variables may be significant in influencing a person's perception of loss. For example, the person who is sure of success, estimates few costs and great utility in accomplishing a goal is expected to be more devastated than one who is more tentative about success and utility and perceives numerous potential costs.

Summary: Only a few person variables that are considered important in the perception of loss have been described here. Many others, such as age, education, past experience with loss, attitudes, and internal-external control orientation, may exert their effects. Until research is sufficient to determine the critical variables in the perception of loss, health workers need to determine logical relationships between person variables, goals and goal achievement pathways and to share hunches about them based on observations.

External Resources

Goal achievement usually requires persons or things external to the individual. Certain supplies manufactured and sold by others are needed. Jobs may be needed from others. Feedback is needed to develop one's body image, self-concept and roles and to learn of progress in working toward goals. Although a few insist that they are independent from others, most agree that they are very dependent on and interdependent with others. Opportunities for success diminish in a hostile environment and tend to increase in a supportive one.

There are many ways to view the influences of external resources on one's perceptions of and vulnerability to loss. The availability of resources during development influences attitudes, coping styles, modes of perceiving and thinking about events, self-esteem, body image, self-concept, goals and methods of goal achievement possible. Also, alternative methods of goal achievement available when one method is blocked depend on the individual's external resources. The greater the number of acceptable methods to achieve a threatened goal, the more likely that loss will be averted or diminished.

Availability is an important word to keep in mind when considering external resources. For a resource to be available, the individual needs to know about it, have access to it and know how to use it. Lack of any one of these factors increases vulnerability to loss. A physical event that diminishes the ease of locomoting may decrease the availability of numerous resources. Brain damage, on the other hand, may reduce the number of resources that are usable.

External variables with the potential to influence loss are many. Past and present resources such as people, physical aspects of the environment, agencies, and job and educational opportunities are but a few of the important external factors.

Little research has been done on the effects of any of the objective, person and external variables on loss as perceived by the person experiencing the change event. Identification of the critical variables and the nature of their effects should improve nursing assessment, planning and intervention.

THE NATURE OF LOSSES

Since loss is defined as any change in the person's situation that reduces the probability of achieving implicit or explicit goals, it is a very subjective event. An observer may be able to define some of the objective characteristics of a change; however, only the individual experiencing it can know its full meaning. The subjective description of a loss may be very similar to or very different from its objective description. There is a tendency to assign generalized meanings to objective descriptions of changes. Loss of parent or spouse is generally thought of as a negative event, whereas, a promotion is considered to be a positive one. In actual fact the experiencing person might define the events quite differently.

Consider the situation of a daughter caring for a demanding, helpless mother who is in constant pain. The daughter is unable to work and consider marriage and having children. She cannot even have friends over, since her mother becomes very angry and combative. Death of the mother in such a situation might very well be experienced as a liberation rather than a disruption in goal achievement.

A promotion may mean more responsibility, more demands, inability to live up to expectations, loss of self-esteem, loss of security and less time to meet family goals. In such a situation the promotion and the accompanying circumstances may well be perceived as losses rather than gains.

The importance of determining the meaning or subjective definition of a change in one's life cannot be overemphasized. Accurate assessment is critical to planning any nursing intervention. Objective events, however, frequently are signals to be alert to actual or potential losses to the individual involved. Some such objective events involve changes in the people in one's environment while others are alterations in body parts or functions. Another type of objective event that may cause subjective perception of loss is change in inanimate objects in the environment.

Changes in People

The most written about change in the people in one's environment with respect to loss is the death of a significant person. Many goals may become less accessible or even unreachable after a significant person has died. The degree of inaccessibility depends to a great extent on how much the bereaved person relied on the deceased to achieve important goals. For example, some marriages exist in name only and partners are involved minimally in each other's goals or pathways to goals. In such a situation, the loss of one or the other through death or separation may cause minimal disruption. On the other hand, in situations where many goals and pathways to them are shared and intertwined or when a dominant goal is unattainable without a specific person, the absence of that person can have devastating consequences. Financial security, emotional security, sexual fulfillment, belonging, companionship, rest and comfort are only a few goals or states that may be at least temporarily inaccessible following the loss of a significant person.

It is important to note that these consequences may not occur all at once. As mentioned earlier, losses may be experienced over a long period of time if the individual who dies had a condition that gradually limited his or her participation in mutual goal-directed activities. Suddenness of loss may be a critical variable influencing the grief experience, which is described in the next chapter.

Interpersonal changes that frequently accompany perception of loss do not always involve death, nor are they limited to absence of persons. Long-term separations due to illness, injury, military service, business, moving or divorce may have devastating effects on goal achievement. Additions of people to the environment or changes in relationships that are usually viewed as positive are sometimes perceived as equally disruptive. Marriage, for example, may be perceived as a loss of freedom, independence and career opportunities. The birth of a child and child-rearing may be viewed as taking time away from work necessary to achieve other goals, as disrupting financial security or as taking love and attention away from the parents.

Changes in Body Parts or Functions

A large percentage of persons who require nursing care have experienced or are anticipating losses of body parts or functions. Physical changes or limitations can be very disturbing since the body with its parts and functions is inextricably tied to objects in the environment, social interaction and one's psychological self. There is potential for physical impairment to spread and to be experienced as psychological and social losses; therefore, it is important that nurses actively assess the total meaning of the physical change for the person.

F. C. Shontz[4] has identified seven functions of body experience that affect the individual psychologically. The body functions as: (1) a sensory register; (2) an instrument for action; (3) a source of drives; (4) a stimulus to self; (5) a stimulus to others; (6) a private world; and (7) an expressive instrument. These are normal ways in which the body functions that few persons think about until they are disrupted through illness or disability. Disruption can have many consequences especially for the achievement of social and psychological goals. Although all of the seven functions are relevant, three of the most salient are discussed here.

An Instrument for Action: Shontz[5] notes that essentially every action, whether it be thinking, talking or walking, involves performance of several body parts. The body is involved in complex ways in the simplest activities of daily living, such as getting out of bed, dressing, eating and getting necessary supplies. When the body is unimpaired, these activities are seldom thought about. Also, certain limitations in strength, agility, speed and thought processes are generally accepted without major difficulty. Sudden limitations may be much more disruptive and very difficult to ignore or accept, since goal attainment may depend on an intact instrument.

It is difficult to conceive of a goal that does not require at least some physical functioning. Since illness and accidents can affect virtually every aspect of the body, the types of possible defects in the instrument used for goal-directed action are numerous. The limits on what one can do because of an illness or disability are probably felt more acutely than the objective changes. The loss may be experienced as a change in efficiency at doing things, also. Prior methods to achieve goals may still be available but may require a greater expenditure of energy. A change in the efficiency of the instrument may result in a decrease in the number of goals toward which one can work.

A Stimulus to Self: The body provides the person much information about itself, its location in space, its integrity and its general condition. Needs and drives reach the level of awareness through body stimuli.[6] The interpretation of stimuli from the body is influenced a great deal by past experience and interaction with others. Since individuals generally share the values of their society and culture their reactions to information from and about their bodies will generally reflect those values and influence identity and self-concept.

An individual's goals include living up to expectations of him or herself. These expectations include preservation or enhancement of physical characteristics and abilities as well as other attributes. Stimuli that suggest a negative change in ability to meet these expectations has occurred indicate that something has been lost.

A Stimulus to Others: Physical aspects of the individual influence greatly how other persons will respond to him or her. In fact, physical appearance is usually the initial point of contact between two people.[7] One's appearance sends many messages that others interpret according to their own past experience, values and prejudices. An attractive, strong, intact body is very highly valued in Western culture. Evidence supporting this proposition can be seen in advertisements, the amount of money spent on wigs, cosmetics and the like. The strength and centrality of values of the physique in our culture frequently has negative consequences for the person whose body differs from the type valued. If the difference is obvious, the person tends to be discredited by others (see Chapter 2).

Potential losses to the person with a perceivable physical or mental illness or disability add up quickly when social aspects of the body are taken into account. Losses may include friends or opportunities to interact long enough to make friends, employment or educational opportunities, thus making it more difficult to gain esteem of others, companionship, love and intimacy, a sense of belonging and the like. These losses then influence feelings and attitudes about the self and psychological losses mount.

The aim of this rather brief discussion of three psychological functions of body experience was to show some of the numerous ways that physical factors can influence goal achievement. Such qualities as physical strength, attractiveness and locomotive skills facilitate or are essential to attaining many goals. Getting information from the self and others is also critical. In addition, most persons would agree that people need other people to gain satisfaction or be successful in most areas of life.

It needs to be pointed out that subjective losses can occur even when physical changes are objectively defined as gains. For example, pregnancy may be seen as a positive physical change, but it may represent losses of mobility, a perfect figure, a job and usual sexual activity to name only a few. Similarly, normal physical growth and development are often accompanied by changes in roles, statuses and expectations, all of which may be defined subjectively as losses.

Perhaps the most difficult subjective reports of losses are those that follow the return to a healthier state with a change in physical limitations. A. Meleis[8] describes the phenomenon of role insufficiency that occurs when a person experiences role transitions. There can be many causes of such transitions, including becoming well. Suddenly former roles or role behaviors are inappropriate and the individual does not know the behaviors for new roles. Subjective losses may include loss of esteem of others, self-confidence, predictability, dependency or the right to be dependent. Changes of any kind are frequently accompanied by some disruption in goal achievement. Failure to recognize this can intensify the misery of the person going through the changes.

Change in Availability of Inanimate Objects

Just as people and body parts and functions are taken for granted, so are many nonliving things on which goal achievement depends. The body was described earlier as an instrument for action. There are many articles, tools, machines, trinkets and the like that are relied upon to accomplish everyday as well as long-term goals. The significance to goal achievement of sudden absence of a car is painfully real to many. It may be surprising to some that the inaccessibility of screwdriver, wrench, saw, toothbrush, slippers, robe, shoes, jewelry, lamps, typewriter and other inanimate objects can also be very disruptive to the achievement of goals. Losses may relate to employment opportunities, grooming, maintenance of a secure home, living up to self-expectations and the like. Evidence supporting the importance of such changes is probably abundant in the reader's experience. Patients in the hospital can provide additional evidence of the significance of personal inanimate objects and security, feelings of well-being and comfort.

Losses that follow the absence of inanimate objects are frequently overlooked. It is, therefore, very important for the nurse to assess the effects of the absence and meaning of such items as family pictures, a clock, watch, toothbrush, makeup and clothes, on which people frequently depend to carry out daily activities and feel good about themselves and their appearance. Absence of such objects is extremely common.

Other Losses

Virtually any kind of change can be perceived by the individual as a loss. Most of the changes that have been described up to this point have been quite straightforward and specific. Often the losses perceived by the person experiencing the change are more abstract, such as loss of freedom, happiness, hope, dreams, certainty or predictability. These may be goals, but they can also be viewed as necessities for goal achievements. For example, patients with cancer who still have hope may continue to work toward achieving their goals while those without hope view all goals as beyond reach.

P. Marris[9] suggests that the impulse to defend the predictability of life is a fundamental and universal principle of psychology. There is a need for predictability and continuity. Thus an individual strives to maintain continuity and predictability within tolerable limits. If this is true, many of the subjective losses that people report following small and big, long-term and short-term, gradual and sudden changes are more understandable. Many catastrophic events involve concrete losses as well as more abstract ones. J. L. Titchener[10] describes the Buffalo Creek disaster in which a dam gave way and destroyed everyone and everything in its path. One hundred and twenty-five persons were killed and 4,000 lost their homes. In addition to these losses, the survivors lost security, continuity and especially predictability. Two years after the disaster 90 percent of the survivors who were interviewed had disabling psychiatric symptoms, changes in character and changes in lifestyle.

The great range of events that individuals define as personal losses is shown in an exercise carried out with nursing students. The writer, when teaching a course in the nursing care of adults with long-tern and chronic illnesses and disabilities, has asked students to describe and discuss changes or losses that they have experienced or witnessed in others. They are asked to discuss these in small groups to the extent that they wish to. The primary aims of this exercise are to learn the variety of actual and potential losses that people experience; to compare and contrast the experiences; and to learn more about things that people found helpful or disruptive in adjusting to loss.

Among the losses identified by students are being drafted, losing self-esteem and freedom, going away to college, losing the sense of smell, getting divorced, moving after establishing close relationships, losing loved ones through death, being placed in Japanese internment camps during World War II, breaking up with boyfriends, getting married, losing loved pets, being in an accident, quitting work, and starting school. Such a variety of losses points to the universality of the experience of loss events and to the importance of understanding the meaning or consequences that an event has for the individual (subjective definition) rather than relying solely on objective characteristics.

In summary, the types of potential interferences in an individual's progress toward goals are limitless. Even a seemingly small or favorable change in one's life can be accompanied by losses or lessening of the ability to achieve one or many goals. The individual's goal characteristics are important in determining loss experiences; however, as noted earlier, many other variables also exert their influence. Nurses need to be knowledgeable about goals, types of loss, changes that tend to produce loss and influencing variables.

NURSING INTERVENTION

Whether in the role of staff nurse, head nurse, clinical specialist, nurse practitioner or nurse educator, knowledge about loss and the factors influencing its perception and severity is essential in performing the role well. In any of these roles the nurse's effectiveness can be increased through recognizing potential and actual losses to self, patients and staff. Some can be prevented and others can perhaps be kept from spreading or minimized. In either case, accurate assessment is a key to success.

Assessment of Loss and Potential for Loss

The fact that loss can take many forms has already been established. Loss can occur from a change of a physical, psychological or social nature. Careful assessment of the individual's goal structure, patterns of working toward goals and level of success are necessary to discover actual or potential losses. Such assessment can be facilitated if the nurse has a framework for guidance. Many goals involve meeting basic needs essential for survival. Secondary goals often develop through the association of the pleasurable tension relief, with stimulation of body parts; certain behavior; presence of other persons; and use of objects involved in the original goal achievement. An assessment framework, therefore, should include both types of goals.

J. R. Auger[11] describes a detailed assessment tool that is used to gather information about eight integrated subsystems of behavior. This tool is an outgrowth of Dorothy Johnson's application of system theory to nursing. Each of the eight subsystems has a specific goal and other structural components (set, choice, action and sustenal imperatives). The eight subsystems are: ingestion, elimination, dependency, sexual, affiliation, aggression (protection), achievement, and restoration. The assessment tool is designed to elicit information about specific behavior patterns (methods) developed to meet each goal, the success of the patterns, the interrelationships of systems, and general regulators of behavior (objective, person and external variables).

If one uses these eight subsystems to guide assessment, a great deal of worthwhile information emerges. For example, the eight subsystems can be used to assess changes brought about by hospitalization and treatment. Anyone who has experienced hospitalization, diagnostic tests and treatment would probably agree that they are quite disruptive to the achievement of goals. Even basic needs for rest, comfort, food, activity, elimination and relief of sexual tension are often made more difficult to meet (Table 1). Privacy in the hospital is practically nonexistent. This has implications for the possibility of having quiet meditation, intimate interactions, restful sleep and other activities that are important to the attainment of many goals.

Treatment is often prescribed and carried out without consultation with the patient or family. This practice may fit into the need and goal achievement patterns of some; however, it interferes greatly with some patterns of dependency (goals of independence, freedom of choice or control over one's life).

The patient in the hospital is often stripped of all possessions except a name bracelet and few personal belongings. Few persons address the patient by name and there is little personal space. These factors tend to devalue the individual and reduce feelings of worth and self-esteem. This can interfere with many subsystem patterns.

The impact of the changes that hospitalization and treatment produce are many and varied. Some of the common changes are shown in Table 1 using the behavioral subsystem framework.

Table 1
Changes in Usual Patterns of Behavior during Hospitalization

Subsystems	Usual Pattern	Changes in Hospital
Affiliation	Variable but there is generally considerable freedom in affiliating with others	Patterns are very limited by visiting hours, opportunities to meet people, energy, and treatment requirements
Achievement	Variable specific goals, methods and opportunities	Opportunities to pursue own achievement goals are usually very limited by lack of supplies, energy, etc.
Aggression (protection)	Variable methods of protecting self	Opportunities are limited. Verbal and physical means are often prohibited
Dependency	Variable patterns of dependence, independence and interdependence	Dependency often is increased due to illness and lack of information
Elimination	Done in privacy with or without aids such as particular foods, laxatives	Often have little privacy, lack of usual eliminative aids
Ingestion	Patterns usually involve other people. Usually have choices	Usually eat alone. Minimal choices of foods, environment, etc.
Restoration	Individualized pattern of rest and activity	Rest is limited severely. Minimal privacy, many disruptions, must fit hospital routine
Sexual	Variable patterns of relating to others as sexual being	Greatly modified and curtailed

The behavioral subsystem approach is one framework. There are many others. Regardless of the framework, the information gathered should point to: (1) potential losses, (2) actual losses, (3) ways to prevent loss, and (4) ways to help the person recover from loss. The first two emerge from information about goals, pathways and achievement outcomes. Information affecting methods of prevention of and recovery from loss more often comes from the assessment of other factors, such as objective and person characteristics and external resources that influence the loss experience. As mentioned before, little conclusive research has been done on the relationship of these variables to goal and method of achievement variables and loss experiences.

It seems safe to assume that losses can be prevented or minimized by interventions that help to maintain effective methods of goal achievement. For example, a nurse may help plan a patient's day to allow for usual restorative patterns, or call a friend or relative to visit in order to maintain some aspects of affiliation behavior. Facilitating the development of functional skills such as dressing, feeding oneself, and moving about can influence the achievement of numerous goals.

Preventive interventions can be directed to helping the patient develop new methods when old ones will soon be unavailable. Similar interventions may also be successful when losses have already occurred. Goals either have to be modified or new methods must be developed to achieve them once the achievement has been disrupted. Intervention after a loss has occurred will be discussed in the next chapter.

RESEARCH

The need for research in all areas of nursing intervention is great. Just about every relationship suggested in this chapter needs to be tested empirically.

The definition of loss presented earlier is a logical one. Much can be gained by studying various goal hierarchies and how goal characteristics and other personal, objective and environmental characteristics affect loss perception. Such study may lead to the determination of specific variables predictive of perception of loss and its intensity. Methods of prevention of loss perception may be found also. It may be possible to determine the characteristics of persons who readily accept and learn new methods to achieve goals and of those who reject such learning. The exploration of loss-related variables may also help the clinician determine the intervention techniques that are most effective for particular people under certain circumstances. Such research should eventually lead to more efficient and more effective nursing assessment, planning and intervention.

SUMMARY

The writer has attempted to make several points in this chapter. First, it is imperative to distinguish between objective characteristics of events that may be loss-producing and the subjective perception of loss. It has been argued that events take on meaning according to how and how much they affect an individual's actual and potential goal achievement; therefore, loss is defined in goal achievement terms.

Second, there is an infinite number of events that can have loss consequences. Death of a loved one, change in body parts and functions, absence of important inanimate objects include many but certainly not all such events. These losses are seen in all areas where nursing is practiced. Even events that may have many positive consequences (restoration of health, birth of a wanted child) can be perceived by the experiencing person as loss events because they are disruptive to goal achievement.

Third, knowledge of types of goal hierarchies, types of loss events and other variables that influence the perception of loss should direct the nurse to find or develop a framework for assessment of actual and potential loss situations. Once such situations are recognized, attempts can be made to prevent the loss or reduce its intensity.

Finally, most of the material presented has been developed logically. This fact supports the need for empirical exploration of loss events and the numerous variables that influence the perception of them. Research on loss, as in other areas of nursing, will help make nursing care outcomes more predictable.

REFERENCES

1. Meyerson, L.: Somatopsychology of physical disability. *In* Cruickshank, W. M. (ed.): Psychology of Exceptional Children and Youth. Englewood Cliffs, N.J., Prentice-Hall, 1971.
2. Barry, J. R.: Motivation of the disadvantaged. Rehabil. Res. & Practice Rev. 3:21-28, 1971.
3. McDaniel, J. W.: Physical Disability and Human Behavior. New York, Pergamon, 1976, p. 128.
4. Shontz, F. C.: The Psychological Aspects of Physical Illness and Disability. New York, Macmillan, 1975, pp. 72-79.
5. Ibid., p. 74.
6. Ibid., p. 76.
7. Ibid., p. 77.
8. Meleis, A.: Role insufficiency and role supplementation: a conceptual framework. Nurs. Res. 24:264-71, 1975.
9. Marris, P.: Loss and Change. New York, Pantheon, 1974.
10. Titchener, J. L., and Kapp, F. T.: Family and character change at Buffalo Creek. Am. J. Psychiatry. 133, 3:295-99, 1976.
11. Auger, J. R.: Behavioral Systems and Nursing. Englewood Cliffs, N. J., Prentice-Hall, 1976.

5 GRIEF

Carolyn E. Carlson

ST. PETER'S HOSPITALS,
TEACHING DIVISION,
THE SHAFTESBURY HOSPITAL,
LONDON, W.C.2.

The last chapter presented a framework for determining the meaning of loss to people and stressed the importance of assessing loss experience. Frequently, behaviors associated with grief are the first observable signs of loss.

This chapter is addressed to the exploration of the grief that generally follows a major loss and the process of recovering from these negative feelings. The aim of the writer is to provide a knowledge base that will help the nurse: (1) understand behavior associated with grief; (2) recognize normal and abnormal variations in grieving behavior; (3) select effective ways of facilitating healthy grief work and; (4) identify areas for research.

DEFINITIONS AND THEORY

Definitions

There is much variability in the use of grief and related terms in the literature. Grief and mourning are often used interchangeably, or grief work is viewed as the same as mourning. D. K. Switzer[1] has noted that the term grief is used to apply to reactions to loss in two specific ways. First, it is viewed as a separate emotion with unique characteristics, though the unique aspects are not clearly defined. Second, grief is seen as a complex combination of numerous emotions felt at the time of loss. The second definition is the one used here. The complex emotions include anxiety, indifference, guilt, hope, hopelessness, helplessness, despair, ambivalence, anger and possibly many more. Grieving or grief work is often described as the phychological sequence or process required to adjust to loss. The process is evoked when abilities are threatened.[2] More specifically, A. W. Reed has described grief work as the inner process of working through, managing, growing through, acknowledging and making peace with a major loss or bereavement.[3] Bereavement is defined as the loss of a person, thing, body part, ideal, model or a relationship in which dependency plays a critical role. This definition is consistent with the definition of loss in the last chapter, since loss of something on which one is dependent implies a change in the ability to achieve particular goals.

The terms bereavement, grief and grief work are most often used to describe phenomena that occur when a significant person has died. These terms are used here to describe feelings and adjustment processes that commonly follow any major disruption in a person's actual or potential goal achievement.

Grief in Response to Various Losses

Although most research on grief has considered adjustment to the death of a loved person, there is evidence to suggest similarities in the recovery process following numerous types of major losses. C. M. Parkes[4] reported common features in response to lost functions due to loss of limb, home and spouse. Likewise similarities in reactions have been noted in response to loss through death and other forms of separation.[5]

The reader is reminded that the evidence supporting or negating the notion of common reaction to death of a loved one and other major life-changing losses is meager. Most likely there are both similarities and differences just as there are individual similarities and differences in reactions to the death of a significant person. Generalizations about personal experience and behavior are useful only when one maintains a commitment to the understanding and acceptance of individual variations. Attempts to force persons to fit the general rule frequently lead to unfortunate outcomes. Such attempts reflect inadequate assessment, insensitivity to individual needs and misuse of knowledge.

Theoretical Orientations to Grief

A number of theories trying to explain the painfulness of grief and the tasks that must be accomplished for successful adjustment have been offered. Freud suggested that grief work includes the painful task of removing libido from the object that reality testing has shown no longer exists and investing it in a new object or situation.[6] There is a struggle against this removal because people do not willingly remove libido from an object. The basic aim of grief work is separation from the object.

J. Bowlby's biological theory explains grief in the following way.[7] First, the brain has built up a "working model of the world" based on and modified by experience. Behavior is signaled by external events that direct attention. Previous experience and internal biochemical and neurophysiological changes determine priorities in perception and action. High priority is given to events involving persons with whom the individual desires to maintain closeness. Separation leads to behavior patterns aimed at restoring proximity.

Parkes describes grief work as the process of establishing congruence of internal and external realities.[8] Repeated discrepancies between inside and outside experiences lead to frustration and extinction of the discrepancies.

C. R. Smith[9] has suggested that all of the above theories fail to take into account the significance of interactions between the individual experiencing the loss and the social situation. Interaction with significant others is essential to validation of one's world, which includes one's own identity and legitimate place. Loss of a significant person, therefore, is compounded by loss of ways to validate identity and place in the social world.

Regardless of the specific theoretical orientation, it seems that the grieving person is trying to reestablish a satisfying life situation after events have seriously disrupted the achievement of important goals. Grief begins with the awareness of the loss.

NURSING AND GRIEF

It seems unnecessary in some ways to explain why and how nurses should be interested in and knowledgeable about grief. The nurse is continuously caring for persons who have potential or actual disruptions in achievement of significant goals.

Potential and Actual Grief Situations

The potential and actual losses that may trigger grief reactions are many and varied. A number of these were mentioned in Chapter 4. Nurses work with persons facing uncertain diagnoses and prognoses, those with confirmed terminal illnesses, those with permanent physical disabilities such as paraplegia, quadriplegia and hemiplegia, parents with dying or deformed children and others close to those experiencing physical or emotional problems. Nurses working in the emergency room observe numerous grief reactions in response to death or injury. All of these situations involve potential or actual disruptions in the achievement of important goals. Nurses therefore need to understand grief, the process of recovery from it (grieving process) and nursing's role in it.

The Role of the Nurse

Nurses have many opportunities to help persons anticipating or already experiencing loss. Helping requires an understanding of needs that change throughout the grief process. For example, a person in a state of shock requires a different kind of help from the individual at the point of trying to find ways to go on without the person or things lost.

Professional nurses are responsible for prevention of illness and maintenance and restoration of health for individuals and groups. Whenever possible, potential losses are identified and either prevented or ameliorated as described in the last chapter. When losses are unavoidable, nursing is directed toward adaptation and containment of the loss (keeping it from spreading).

Containing the Loss: Containing the loss might be viewed as similar to secondary prevention. In secondary prevention the underlying problem is identified early enough for action to be taken to prevent a greater problem. For example, hypertension may be detected early. Treatment may require giving up a few goals (losses) such as those involving anxiety-producing activities; however, a stroke resulting in greater losses may be prevented. Thus losses are contained at the treatment level.

Adaptation: Facilitation of adaptation or restoration of equilibrium following a loss great enough to disrupt equilibrium involves determining ways to help the individual find new methods to reach goals and new goals that, when attained, will be approximately as satisfying as prior goals. Such facilitation is usually enhanced when the helper knows what the prior goals were, the extent and nature of disruption, resources available to the individual, coping style, and the point in the adaptation process at which the person is. As is shown in the next section, the phases that persons commonly (but not always) go through following a major loss or crisis differ in many respects. Although the phases are not discrete and are not experienced universally by grievers, understanding of common phases of grief provides a framework for understanding the feelings, behavior and progress in overcoming the grief.

Nursing activities that are appropriate to facilitate adaptation vary according to the phase the individual is in or that is dominant at a given moment. Understanding of the feelings and behavior common to the phases and the relationships between them, therefore, should help the nurse select the most effective nursing actions. For example, in phases where anxiety is extremely high, teaching is seldom effective.

PHASES OF GRIEF

Several writers have described stages or phases that follow a major life-changing of life-threatening event. Elisabeth Kübler-Ross has identified five stages that follow a terminal diagnosis: denial, anger, bargaining, depression, and acceptance[10]; and G. L. Engel has described four stages in adaptation to a major loss: shock and disbelief, developing awareness, restitution, and resolution of loss.[11] S. L. Fink has described four stages following a crisis: shock, defensive retreat, acknowledgment, and adaptation[12]; while Bowlby has identified protest, despair, and denial.[13] Parkes has described components of grief as: alarm, searching, mitigation, anger and guilt, and gaining new identity.[14] Although there are theoretical and descriptive differences between the various approaches, the similarities seem to dominate, as shown in Table 2. F. C. Shontz has suggested that all of the stages can be described in terms of the frequency and intensity of approach-avoidance cycles.[15] Approach involves awareness and encountering of loss, while avoidance includes mechanisms and behavior that remove the individual from the problem either physically or emotionally. He has identified pre-impact, impact and post-impact phases.

The phases are described here as a guide to facilitate understanding of behavior. An individual who is grieving will seldom exhibit behavior that matches perfectly the behavior described below. Neither will the person necessarily go through the phases in the sequence presented. The phases are not clearly demarcated. There is a great deal of overlap and change from one to another.

Precrisis Phase

A significant precrisis phase does not always exist, however, sometimes there are warnings or preliminary signs of impending losses. For example, a woman in the hospital for a breast biopsy usually experiences a warning of a

Table 2
Comparison of Stages of Adaptation to Crisis or Loss

Approach-Avoidance Behavior	Shontz	Engel	Fink	Ross	Bowlby
Approach-Avoidance Starts Slowly	*Pre-Impact* Prelude Warning				
Initial Avoidance	*Impact* Shock (Initial Avoidance)	Shock & Disbelief	Shock	(Shocking news) Denial	
High Approach	Encounter	Developing Awareness		Anger	Protest Despair
High Avoidance	*Post-Impact* Retreat	Restitution	Defensive Retreat	Bargaining	Denial
Repetitive Approach-Avoidance Cycles	Acknowledgment	Resolution of Loss	Acknowledgment Adaptation	Depression Acceptance	

See text for discussion of the stages.

possible major loss. Family members who have been told that a loved one has a terminal illness also have warning of losses to come. Sometimes the precrisis or preloss phase may include signs and symptoms that are misinterpreted for a time. For example, many serious illnesses begin with symptoms very similar to those of a cold, which are often seen as very minor or insignificant.

Feelings and behavior during this phase are likely to reflect the perceived seriousness of events. F. Davis, for example, has described parents' precrisis reactions to symptoms in their children who were eventually found to have poliomyelitis.[16] Initially symptoms were interpreted as common and familiar. As they persisted, there were at least temporary moments of awareness of the possibility that something serious was happening. Actual grieving did not begin until parents were fully aware of the seriousness of the symptoms.

Nursing intervention includes helping those receiving warning signs to use their resources to interpret and cope with them as best they can. For example, if a man is reporting symptoms of dizziness, momentary losses of memory and headaches, the nurse, recognizing that these may be symptoms of hypertension and other potentially serious conditions, may intervene to facilitate his getting medical attention.

Impact and Shock Phase

Shock generally follows the perception of an event that seriously disrupts a person's actual or potential goal achievement, whether or not there was a warning. In an instant a spinal cord injury and resultant paralysis can wipe out countless dreams, hopes and alternatives in life, or the death of a loved one can shatter one's security to the core. The reality of any catastrophic, grief-producing loss is generally too overwhelming to perceive accurately and integrate fully. That which has occurred is incongruent with the reality known to the individual. The full reality of what has happened just does not penetrate consciousness at first. The individual may be aware of the facts and report "my wife just died" or "I'm paralyzed" following the tragic events, but these statements are usually devoid of feeling at this time. A 27-year-old man, for example, reported the following:

> A bunch of us were out playing around, drinking beer and swimming. I dove into the shallow water, hit my head on a rock and felt my neck snap. My friends put me on the floor of the van and took me to the hospital. I couldn't move my arms and legs, but we were all just laughing about it. It hadn't hit home.

He was not yet aware of the gravity of his injury although he was aware of the objective facts. His behavior seemed to reflect feelings of indifference or euphoria which are reported as common during the period of shock. Perception is also narrowed.

Behaviorally, unless physically injured, the person experiencing the loss event may seem unimpaired. He or she functions automatically and often very efficiently. It is useful for nurses to be able to recognize behavior that is common to shock phase. The behavior may seem cold and calculating to those who do not understand the dynamics of grief.

Nursing intervention during the shock phase is frequently directed toward protecting the bereaved individual from harm and mobilizing available supports in preparation for the phase that follows. During shock the individual may need direction in what needs to be done. The nurse is often in a position to provide this direction. Families may need to be guided and directed following the death of a loved one. They may need help making funeral arrangements and notifying family, friends and business associates. A person who has just been given a poor prognosis may also need guidance through routine activities or treatments.

Realization or Initial Awareness

Generally the shock phase does not last very long and the loss and its implications penetrate awareness at least briefly. A loss of sufficient magnitude to produce a grief reaction generally causes anxiety of panic proportions when awareness comes. It is not difficult to understand the helplessness, devastation and panic that are experienced when someone or something that is vital to the achievement of one's goals is gone—often forever.

Although there are likely to be differences, there are also similarities in the devastation accompanying the awareness of goal disruption whether it be due to death of a loved one, separation, or loss of body part or function. At this time, reality is perceived as overwhelming and the individual is usually unable to reason, plan or fully understand the situation. Sensations of somatic distress, weakness and despair are common to most who grieve.

Behaviorally, the person who is in this stage of grieving may cry, tremble, fight, flee, scream, attack, moan, sigh and move about restlessly. Parkes describes searching behavior that follows the death of a loved one.[17] This behavior is an attempt to recover the lost person. Attention is directed to parts of the environment in which the person is likely to be. A perceptual set is developed for the lost person, and the bereaved is preoccupied with thoughts of that person. Attention to personal appearance may be abandoned at this time. Parkes reported a pining for the lost functions by persons who had lost a limb. This pining is comparable to the searching behavior previously described.

The early phase of realization is a period in which the approach tendency is dominant. The reality of the situation, however, is so overwhelming that there is a move toward avoidance for protection from pain.

Nursing care during this stage of overwhelming anxiety is largely directed toward anxiety reduction. As anxiety increases, the perceptual field narrows and only a limited amount of information can be processed. The nurse can limit the amount impinging on the person by monitoring the number of people around or decreasing noise and light intensity. In addition, the nurse may facilitate information processing and anxiety reduction by giving instructions rather than requiring decision making at this time and by arranging for a comforting family member, friend or professional to stay with the person during this period of intense distress.

Many find it difficult to be around an individual in such great distress. Perhaps this is part of the reason for the tendency to give psychopharmacologic agents at this time. Dr. Kübler-Ross has noted that consulting psychiatric residents who are uncomfortable in working with terminally ill patients would rather order Stelazine or Librium than spend extra time facilitating their expression of the complex emotions of grief.[18] She has found minimal need for drugs when the terminally ill person has someone around who will listen, allow but not force the expression of feelings and tolerate the emotional expressions. Reassurance that the feelings are normal is often helpful, since such intense emotional distress may be very frightening.

Retreat

The initial awareness of the significance of a major loss is generally so overwhelming that it is intolerable. How can a wife go on without her husband on whom she depended so completely or how can the athlete with aspirations for a career in professional sports tolerate permanent paralysis of all four extremities? Fortunately, most persons have unconscious psychological mechanisms that allow at least partial retreat from the distressing realities of the situation. Avoidance tendencies are dominant at this time.

Parkes described ways by which bereaved spouses came to feel more secure in the early stages of their grief.[19] Some mechanisms served to maintain the impression that the dead partner was near, such as dreams, illusions and hallucinations. Other methods of lessening or avoiding pain are staying away from people who remind one of the loss, selective forgetting and involvement in many activities to avoid thinking. Denial is perhaps the most common defense mechanism employed.

It is important to remember that defense mechanisms are normal unless they become overused. They serve to regulate the amount of potentially disabling information that an individual has to process at once. Aspects of reality can be let into awareness as they can be tolerated.

If defenses are effective, emotions are likely to include indifference and euphoria. On the other hand, if the person's distorted reality perception is challenged by others, anxiety and anger may result as the person is not yet ready to face undistorted reality.

Behavior exhibited may include intense activity, avoidance of discussion of anything related to the loss or refusal of treatments because complete recovery from illness or disability is expected. Behavior should be observed carefully to indicate readiness to accept more aspects of reality. Anxiety levels are likely to change along with approach-avoidance cycles. Likewise, types of nursing intervention that are effective change with these cycles.

Retreat behavior should alert the nurse to the fact that the individual is too uncomfortable with reality to face it directly. Usually attempts to force reality on the person are not helpful. Allow the person to deny the loss to the extent needed; however, try not to reinforce the denial. If denial is interferring with proper treatment, the health team needs to determine the most appropriate course of action to take. Treatments and procedures should be explained in clear, concise terms, and teaching directed toward the future should be avoided at this time. If a person is denying the reality of a loss, teaching related to adaptation to that loss is likely to be threatening, anxiety producing and, therefore, ineffective.

The length of time spent in any of the above phases is quite variable and depends on many individual and situational factors. For example, it may be very difficult to persist in denying the reality of a death or loss of limb while being bombarded with cues indicating that these losses have in fact occurred. Parkes suggests that the reality of a death often hits at the time of a funeral.[20] Denial may persist in the person with paralysis due to spinal cord injury. The limbs are still present, some return of function since the injury may have been noted, or spasms may be misinterpreted as signs of improvement. The extent of permanent damage may be unknown. In such a case, failure to accept the current state of impairment is realistic and does not necessarily signify the use of defense mechanisms.

Retreat from the reality of a loss is probably seldom complete. Generally only certain aspects are denied or kept from awareness. Gradually more and more facets of the situation are confronted realistically and the individual enters the phase of acknowledgment.

Acknowledgment

The acknowledgment phase includes numerous approach-avoidance cycles. I. Glick, R. S. Weiss and C. M. Parkes describe this as the grieving phase.[21] During this phase the bereaved is confronted with the daily realities of the loss. There is often an obsessional review of events leading up to the loss. This review, conducted either alone or with others, seems to be necessary for the person to be able to integrate the loss event both emotionally and cognitively. Some may feel guilt or self-reproach because they feel they should have done something to prevent the death. Others are angry and blame other people for what happened. Profound sadness and depression are dominant during this phase. If suicide is contemplated, it is most likely to occur during this period.

This phase of grief is generally of longer duration than the previous ones. It may last several months or more. At this time the full impact of the loss is felt at least some of the time. Often the initial loss expands to include numerous secondary losses. For example, the loss of a husband may be followed by a loss of financial security or gratification of sexual needs.

The acknowledgment phase also occurs following illness and disability. It commonly comes when a physical plateau has been reached or symptoms persist and become more and more difficult to avoid. Needless to say, this is a very painful time. The individual may be very angry, depressed, bitter, or may vascillate between these states. Pre-injury or pre-illness circumstances are usually relived countless times along with "what ifs" or "if onlys . . ."

Bargaining may occur at this time, too. The person may think, "If I'm really good and promise to go to church every Sunday God will cure me," and then make such a promise. Thinking must be reorganized to be consistent with the new reality.

Nursing intervention may change a great deal during the acknowledgment phase, since emotions may change frequently and abruptly. It is not easy for the nurse to cope with some of the feelings expressed and behavior exhibited at this time. It may be of use to the helpers to explore their own feelings about death, dependency, helplessness and the like. Such exploration may facilitate the development of understanding, as well as the exercise of patience. It may be difficult for nurses or physicians to be bombarded with anger or blamed for things for which they were not responsible. Their inclination may be to retaliate or ignore the person expressing the feelings. Hopefully, understanding that anger is a normal part of the grieving process will make listening to the expressions of anger or bitterness without argument more tolerable. As noted earlier, an understanding listener will usually be far more effective than drugs.

Nursing intervention for helping individuals get through periods of depression also needs to be planned. At times when the implications of a loss are fully acknowledged, sadness and depression may be beyond measure. The affected person may be unable to see any way out of the current painful situation. Suicide may be viewed as the desirable solution. Alert nurses can pick up clues that a person is thinking of suicide, such as withdrawal, loss of interest in anything or verbal references to giving up or planning suicide. Clues may be very subtle, so it is important that members of the health team share observations in order to get a complete and accurate assessment of the patient's situation. The percentage of persons who have had at least momentary thoughts of suicide is much greater than the percentage that actually attempts it; however, it is important for members of the health team to be alert to the few who do go through with attempts. Parkes states that people should not be afraid to ask direct questions about suicide. Generally those who have thought about it will give a direct answer.[22]

The time at which depression occurs and its duration varies, therefore, nursing intervention should vary also. P. J. Clayton, M. Herjanie, G. E. Murphy and R. Woodruff, Jr., studied 109 men and women 1 month, 4 months and 13 months after the death of their spouses.[23] Forty-five percent of the widows expressed depression at some point during the 13 months and 13 percent reported being depressed all year. There was a gradual decrease in depression reported over time (35 percent at 1 month, 25 percent at 4 months, and 17 percent at 12 months).

As with anger, the person grieving usually profits from expressing feelings of depression to a caring listener. Those grieving need others even though they may not be able to respond readily to them at the time. The nurse can often be helpful by spending consistent periods of time with the person who is feeling sad and depressed even without verbal interaction. Such contacts can serve to develop or maintain the trust of the patient in the nurse or other care givers.

There are some primary things for nurses to remember at this time. First, anger, depression, bitterness, guilt and many other emotions are normal during this phase. Second, a comfortable listener who allows but does not push for expression of feelings and who does not argue with the person about how she or he feels can make a difficult period less painful. This person should not show pity because this puts the grieving person in an inferior position. Anger directed at the helping persons is usually not personal. Also, it takes considerable time for the unpleasant feelings to subside. As in earlier phases, any teaching that is done should be limited to what is needed and happening now. It is much too threatening, for example, for a woman who is just acknowledging the reality of having multiple sclerosis to be faced with the facts she will need to know when she goes home and must care for herself from a wheelchair. She may be able to learn facts about how to care for herself *now,* however. Future-oriented teaching only directs attention to the permanence of a loss.

Sometimes strangers can be more helpful than family and friends. It may be easier to talk to people not directly or closely involved with the loss. The nurse is often in the position to assess needs and call on the appropriate people (family, friends, clergy, etc.) to help the grieving individual at optimal times.

Acceptance and Adaptation

Fortunately, most individuals move beyond the painful phase of acknowledgment and go on to reorganize their lives taking into account the new realities. There is usually not an abrupt move from one phase to the next but a gradual change, with anxiety decreasing and hope slowly taking the place of hopelessness. Instead of being focused on what has been lost, attention is redirected to the present and future. An individual may never completely "get over" a major loss but does "pick up the pieces" and try to make the best of the situation. A young man who was quadriplegic following an automobile accident and is now able to ambulate with crutches said:

> I've been lucky. I've had so much return of function. I'm able to walk and do a lot of things but I'll never get over my injury. I'm brokenhearted that it happened.

This young man's comments serve to remind helpers of the meaning of events to the individual. The outsider may tend to overestimate the significance of return of function and minimize the difficulties still encountered.

During the adaptation phase, there are more approach than avoidance cycles as the person goes on to organize life to integrate the realities of loss. New, meaningful goals may be sought or energy may be directed to finding new methods to achieve goals that were important prior to the loss event. Some reorganization may begin quite early as children make demands and the like.

Glick, Weiss and Parkes found that widows were reassured by their ability to continue to perform.[24] They became more certain that they would eventually become stable again. Eight weeks following the death of their spouses, 61 percent agreed that they were beginning to feel like themselves once more. P. Marris reports that adaptation to loss of a husband takes about two years,[25] although there is, no doubt, considerable variation.

All of the phases of grief are part of the adaptation process; however, success or failure in the adaptation are more obvious after considerable time has passed. Adaptation requires "accommodation of environment and subjective experience."[26] Understanding people in the environment can contribute greatly to successful adaptation; however, the person who has experienced the loss must also be sensitive to the environment. Shontz reports three factors that contribute to this sensitivity: mental state, cognitive state and the interpersonal factor.[27] The first factor, mental state, refers to the amount of contact the individual has with the environment. The cognitive factor includes how much knowledge a person has about assistance available and what is expected of him or her. Mourning rituals help provide some of this information for the bereaved; however, persons suffering from other losses may have no such guidelines. The interpersonal factor that Shontz notes is considered very influential. It includes the feelings that the person being helped and the helpers have for each other. Too often there is failure to capitalize on this factor. Nurses are frequently admonished to keep from "getting involved" with their patients. Certainly there can be unhealthy and unhelpful interpersonal involvement with patients. However, mature, controlled interpersonal attachments between patient and nurse, doctor or others can be healthy and helpful to adjustment.[28] Openness among staff members can facilitate the maintenance of the healthy, helpful relationships and prevent the development of unhealthy, nonproductive interpersonal situations.

Anxiety generally decreases gradually as the individual adjusts to loss. Otherwise emotions during this time are likely to be determined to a great extent by situational factors that influence anyone.

Nursing intervention, of course, is aimed at facilitating adaptation. Many methods may be employed, including teaching, operant conditioning, role playing and encouraging problem solving. Selection of goals and methods of intervention should be based on the needs of the individual, resources available, the nature of the person's usual environment, the effectiveness of particular techniques and the length of time the nurse will have to work with him or her. The methods noted above are not mutually exclusive. Teaching the patient particular behaviors, for example, may involve teaching of facts, reward for the desired behavior (operant conditioning), role playing to try out behavior in a particular situation as well as other methods.

Teaching is likely to be most effective during this phase since less energy is expended in avoiding the realities and more emphasis is generally placed on the present and future. The patient with multiple sclerosis, metastatic cancer and other progressive diseases may be interested in learning ways to preserve function or control pain as long as possible. The person with a visible deformity may be anxious to learn behaviors to manage tension in social situations, as described in Chapter 2. Although there are numerous similarities in problems and needs at this stage, there are also a number of differences depending on the number and types of goals that have been disrupted, the type of life one wants to maintain or establish and other variables that will be described later. Differences are as important to notice as similarities.

It was noted earlier that common phases of grief provide a framework for assessing and understanding behavior common to them. The reader is cautioned against trying to force a person to behave according to generalities. Remember that, despite the commonalities that might be observed, each person is unique and there may be many normal patterns of grief. There are patterns of response to loss, however, that have been found to be pathological or ineffective in adaptation to the loss.

PATHOLOGICAL PATTERNS OF GRIEF

Although most individuals who grieve recover and reconstruct a relatively satisfying life, some fail to recover or do so with great difficulty. S. N. Pradhan[29] has described five types of pathological mourning:

1. affect block which is characterized by tension, inability to relax and mourn because one might break down;
2. agitated depression characterized by tension, insomnia, agitation, excessive feelings of guilt and need for punishment and sometimes contemplation of suicide;
3. retarded depression in which there is chronic apathy, feelings of being demoralized and overwhelmed;
4. elation which is characterized by overactivity, lack of feelings of loss and adventurous, foolish behavior; and
5. phobic—anxious states characterized by panic attacks about dying that are extremely debilitating.

It is obvious that many of the manifestations of these types of pathological mourning are exaggerations of feelings and behaviors common to normal grief.

Shontz[30] has described maladaptive responses to physical loss by identifying where failures occur in the grief process. First, there can be failure to experience the emotional impact of a loss because of denial or a defense comparable to Pradhan's affect block and elation. It is important to realize that such failure can occur when impact or encounter is appropriate for the individual to experience. Second, there can be failure in retreat. The individual may retreat too soon or too late. If the retreat occurs too soon, there is a minimal drain-off of tension through grieving. On the other hand, delaying retreat prolongs intense grief and delays reconstruction and reorganization. Finally, there can be failure to begin acknowledgment, which implies failure to give up retreat. Health workers tend to worry about the patient who seems to continue to deny the realities of the situation despite much evidence. A paraplegic veteran of the Vietnam War spoke of a hospital social worker who insisted that he should get depressed, implying that he could not get over his loss until he did.

Failure to give up retreat is difficult to determine since the observer is dependent on what the griever is willing to share. One may be willing and able to acknowledge painful reality privately before being able or willing to make that acknowledgment public.

Pathological mourning generally requires intervention beyond what the nurse can plan and offer unless she or he has had special training. The nurse, however, is often in an excellent position to recognize grieving that seems to be ineffective in accomplishing separation from that which is lost. Early referral can result in more rapid and effective treatment.

Numerous methods of treatment have been established to facilitate grieving. Most of them have been developed to help persons who have lost a spouse. Some of the methods attempt to provide grievers with caring, understanding people in order to prevent pathological conditions. Widow to widow programs, for example, consist of periodic small-group meetings of people who have lost their husbands. The participants share feelings, problems and concerns as well as help each other with problem solving. Approaches have been many and varied, and thus it has been difficult to determine which are most effective. Investigators at Montefiore Hospital evaluated the relative effects of a specific type of unsolicited crisis intervention on the aged bereaved after the loss of spouse.[31] The treated group received support and assistance from a psychiatric social worker or a psychiatric nurse for six months or less. Assistance ranged from helping the bereaved express feelings and review the relationship to helping with chores, financial matters and other specific tasks.

V. D. Volkan[32] has described a method of re-grief therapy used with pathological grievers which included short-term therapy designed to help the patients bring memories of and experience with the lost person into consciousness. The purpose of this was to test the memories and experiences against reality, to accept what has happened with appropriate affect and to free oneself from excessive ties to the dead. The patient was generally seen four times a week to promote intensity. Volkan warned therapists to help patients avoid transference neuroses and to keep gratification of patient instinctual demands to a minimum.

Although definitive measures of the effectiveness of various types of therapeutic methods are not yet available, it is encouraging to note the apparent increase in attention paid to problems encountered in grief. Because grief is such a common experience, it is imperative that methods be found to prevent and treat pathological states of grief.

FACTORS INFLUENCING GRIEF

It has already been noted that there are many individual differences as well as similarities in grief reactions. Understanding factors that influence grief and the nature of the effects is important in determining normal and abnormal grief, help that is or is likely to be needed and types of interventions that most probably will be successful.

Many objective characteristics, person variables and external resources were described in the last chapter as being influential to the perception of loss. These are expected to affect the grief process also. First, they influence grief through loss perception. Second, they exert effects by facilitating or impeding establishment of new meaningful goals, giving up of unattainable goals and development of new pathways to goals that are at least temporarily unattainable. There are additional factors to consider in understanding grief: nature of loss situation, variables and sociocultural factors.

Nature of Loss Situation

Suddenness of loss, anticipation of it, preparation for it, and the relationship of the grieving person to the lost object are important aspects of the loss situation. Anticipation, suddenness and preparation are closely related because a sudden loss decreases opportunities to anticipate and prepare.

Suddenness, Anticipation and Preparation: It is commonly believed that anticipation of negative events and time for preparation decrease the intensity of grief. This is not completely supported by research evidence. G. Epstein et al.[33] report no relationship between outcome of grief and length of time the death of a significant other was anticipated. A study of widows in the Boston area revealed that anticipation of death did not lessen grief.[34] Even when the widow was relieved that death had come she was desolate. However, a positive correlation was found between length of advance warning and eventual satisfactory adjustment to widowhood. When the death of the spouse was sudden and without warning, there was a greater tendency for the bereaved to show more unresolved grief after a year and to suffer anxiety after two to four years. These widows tended to dwell on the loss that had occurred.

Logically one could expect anticipation of loss to allow for preparation or prior experience with loss to prepare one for later losses, but it seems that preparation for the loss does not tend to occur and past experience with loss has variable effects. In the former case, it has been argued that a person cannot really prepare for a loss for fear that preparation might cause the loss to occur. For example, a woman who makes plans for life after the death of her husband may fear that her preparation is causing his death. Acceptance of death and understanding of the grief process, however, do seem to help somewhat. Considerable anxiety can be relieved simply by realizing that the symptoms of grief are normal.

> The mother of a nurse was critically injured in an automobile accident. Her daughter cared for her 16 hours a day, every day for several weeks. The mother remained comatose and eventually died.
>
> Weeks later, the daughter continued to go over everything she had done while caring for her mother. She was searching for signs and symptoms that might have been there that she did not see. She wondered if she had done the wrong thing in caring for her mother.
>
> When she described this process several months later she said that she considered

herself extremely fortunate to have taken a course in graduate school in which she studied the processes of grief and mourning. This helped her to understand that what she experienced was normal. She realized that she would have experienced guilt if she had not cared for her mother.

In the case of the dying person, knowledge of impending death can open up opportunities to talk about it, prepare for it and enjoy what life remains. Two examples illustrate this.

A 60-year-old mother of four discovered quite suddenly that she had cancer of the colon that had already metastasized to the liver. She worked daily at sorting through clothes, papers, etc., throwing away things that had been saved for years. Her colostomy did not disrupt her social life as many thought it would. In fact she did more things than she had. She said she wanted to do as much as she could for as long as possible and indeed she did.

A 40-year-old man was diagnosed as having cancer of the pancreas after many months of pain. At first his wife didn't want him to know. Her visits to him in the hospital were terribly tense. She was burdened with keeping the secret while feeling personally devastated, and he was confused by the signs of tension. Finally, he was told and they were able to share the burden together and move on to experience great closeness and acceptance of the approaching death.

In both of these examples, anticipation of death allowed the individuals involved to prepare in ways that made their experiences more satisfying and apparently less frightening. Too often knowledge about impending loss is kept from the principal people. Such a practice robs the persons of time to prepare.

Anticipation and preparation can affect responses to other losses also. The writer interviewed a man in his thirties who was left paralyzed by a spinal cord injury. He had suffered a great deal from internal tissue damage and bleeding from dislocated hips and ectopic bone formation. After a few years, he had one leg amputated at the hip. His health improved greatly. At the time of the interview he was anticipating the amputation of the other leg. He had had time to prepare and consider the pros and cons. Also, his past experience with ill health and improvement subsequent to a similar operation probably contributed to his positive attitude toward the pending surgery. In terms of goal achievement, loss of limb improved his situation rather than making it worse.

This example shows how important it is for health workers to assess the impact of past events rather than make assumptions based on those events. Past experience with loss events is not one variable but involves many. Type of loss event, age at which the event occurred and number of such events experienced are but three critical aspects of past experience. It has been reported that early childhood separation from significant others can strongly influence relationships formed later in life.[35] The young child who has been separated tends to learn about the transiency of life and the finality of loss.

In summary, the relationships of suddenness of, anticipation of and preparation for loss to each other and to the nature of the grief response are unclear. A more clear-cut definition of variables and further research should facilitate greater understanding.

Relationship to Lost Object: The relationship of the grieving person to the object that is gone is another complex factor encompassing a number of variables. Parkes[36] described several: strength of attachment, security of attachment, reliance and involvement. Involvement is the extent to which an individual's roles, plans, methods of problem solving and the like depend on the lost person or object. In other words, to a great extent, involvement determines the amount of disruption in goal achievement or the extent of loss. Marris[37] points out that involvement with a person object is not to be equated with love. One can be very dependent on or involved with a person one does not love. A person's feelings toward one who has died, especially if they were ambivalent, can influence the progress of grief. Ambivalence may give rise to guilt for the negative aspects of the conflicting state.

Relationship to lost object can be viewed from the standpoint of its importance for goal achievement. The greater the importance of the object, the greater the subjective loss as well as the subsequent grief are likely to be. Consider, for example, the face as an object used to achieve goals (see Norris's description, p. 24). The face is important in most, if not all, face-to-face interactions with people. Any or all of these interactions may be altered or terminated by visible scars and deformities of the face; therefore, any goals involving other people may become less attainable. The importance of accurately comprehending the relationship of the grieving person to the lost objects (disruption in goal achievement) cannot be overemphasized.

Person Variables

The person variables that may influence the nature and course of grief are quite numerous, though few have been tested empirically. Any variable that facilitates finding, developing and accepting new methods to achieve goals or finding new goals that are meaningful should facilitate progress through the grief process. As mentioned earlier, variables described in the chapter on loss are also relevant here. In addition to these there are age, sex, beliefs and values, personality characteristics, prior experiences, socioeconomic status and many more.

Age: Age is important because of developmental tasks that tend to occur at particular ages or stages of life. There are many descriptions of stages. Any of these can be helpful to the nurse by providing information about what is common or usual—not what is "normal"—at a particular time in life. Erik Erikson[38] has developed a set of tasks, crises or struggles that are dominant at particular times, which he calls the "eight ages of man": basic trust versus basic mistrust, autonomy versus shame and doubt, initiative versus guilt, industry versus inferiority, identity versus role confusion, intimacy versus isolation, generativity versus stagnation, and ego integrity versus despair.

It is probable that the dominant task or stage influences which events are perceived as losses as well as the nature of the grief that follows a major loss event. The more tasks one has managed successfully, the more equipped he or she is likely to be to progress through grief without complication. A major loss may alter one's progress in resolving the major crisis of one of the eight ages. Loss of the mothering one during the trust versus mistrust age may increase the likelihood of a mistrust resolution or lack of confidence in self and others. Loss of sexual functioning due to spinal cord injury or disease probably has great implications for the person, male or female, who is in the age of intimacy versus isolation. The purpose here is not to describe all of the ways that age influences grief and grieving but to call attention to the importance of including age in nursing assessment, planning and the like. Failure to consider age when observing and analyzing behavior frequently leads to erroneous interpretations.

Sex: The sex of the one who has experienced a major loss is very influential to the grief that follows. A study of widows and widowers during the first year of bereavement found similarities and differences in the grieving of the two groups.[39] Women tended to define the loss as abandonment whereas men defined it as dismemberment. Men tended to be unable to display grief and wanted help in controlling feelings rather than in expressing them. Men were less likely than women to admit to feelings of depression. Emotional recovery did not occur more quickly for men; however, they did move toward reestablishing a stable life organization more quickly than the widows. Men tended to date sooner and could see no benefits to restricting behavior. Women tended to feel a certain loyalty to the deceased was necessary and this required "proper" behavior. These and other findings suggest that many of the differences are due to differences in male and female roles in Western society. It will be of interest to see if differences diminish as a consequence of the women's movement.

Little information is available about differences between the sexes in response to losses of other types. It seems reasonable to anticipate that differences would be comparable to those found in widows and widowers in many respects. Verification of this will require considerable investigation.

Prior Experience: Prior experience with loss has been covered somewhat in the discussion of characteristics of the loss situation. Little is certain about circumstances under which prior experience strengthens one's ability to cope or hampers such ability. Some experience with misfortune may be necessary to develop methods of coping with it; however, the kind, severity and number of events that lead to such development are yet to be determined.

Beliefs and Values: An individual's values, goals, beliefs about self, the world, life after death and faith in a Supreme Being are only a few person variables. Goals are critical to one's perception of loss and reflect a person's values and beliefs. If a person believes that the world is a hostile place over which one has little control, grief is probably more intense than if the individual views the world as more positive and modifiable. Belief in God and life after death provides great comfort for many in various loss situations. Expectation of eventually being reunited with the dead person may make a difference in grief following death. This does not mean, however, that the loss is not severe nor the grief acute. Consider Mr. R. who quite suddenly lost his wife of 40 years. He had great faith in God and believed that he would be reunited with her. One day about a month after his wife had died he said:

> I finally figured out a way to communicate with Mary. God is in communication with Mary. I talk to God. So, I tell God what I want Him to tell Mary and that way I'm talking to her.

Faith in God was also an important variable that influenced a 20-year-old missionary's reaction to becoming quadriplegic following a diving accident.

> Jim Scott was doing missionary work in a foreign country when he was hurt. He was flown to the States for surgery and rehabilitation. His injury left him with sensation over his entire body, severe spasms of the lower extremities, minimal movement of upper extremities and no voluntary finger movement. A nurse acknowledged the terrible frustration he must be experiencing due to his injury and rigorous, repetitive rehabilitation program. Jim said that he did not find the situation frustrating especially when he compared it to situations he had encountered on the mission field. Jim thought that his condition might be improved if God so willed and he knew his injury occurred for a purpose which he planned to learn and try to fulfill.

Some would say that Jim was denying the realities of his loss; however, that seems unlikely. He tended to face things squarely. His parents kept talking about him being cured, but Jim acknowledged that his condition very likely was permanent unless the Lord willed otherwise.

The effects of one's beliefs on grief depend a lot on the specific nature of the beliefs. Some believe losses or misfortunes are forms of punishment from God. Such losses might be experienced as relief from guilt or the source of much anxiety over future punishing events.

Regardless of the reader's beliefs, it is important to assess beliefs and values of individuals who are experiencing or about to experience a major loss. This information can facilitate understanding of behavior as well as point to resources that can be used to help overcome grief.

Personality Characteristics: Many personality characteristics have already been described. Personality includes such things as beliefs and values, coping style, motivation, assertiveness, conceptual style, attitudes, and communication style. Any of these characteristics that tend to facilitate reestablishment of meaningful goals or development of new methods to achieve goals that have become unachievable because of the loss event are expected to decrease the intensity and duration of grief. For example, the visibly disabled person who is assertive may be better able to manage tension in interpersonal situations (see Blackwell's discussion of the discredited, p. 44) and thereby open or maintain pathways to goal achievement.

Socioeconomic Status: Socioeconomic status was found to be a significant variable influencing the outcome of grieving after the death of a spouse.[40] Interviews conducted three to six weeks after the death of the husband showed that the grief of widows from high and low socioeconomic statuses was equal in intensity. A year later, higher socioeconomic status was associated with better outcome. Generally, many resources are more available to those of higher socioeconomic status. Money may not buy happiness, but it can open doors to education, purchase the best treatment of mental and physical illness or disabilities available and make possible many pathways to goal achievement not possible for those of lesser means. Regardless of the nature of the object that is lost, socioeconomic status is a potentially significant variable influencing the nature and duration of adjustment.

The reader can probably think of many other person variables that may influence the grief experienced following a major loss. An exhaustive listing and discussion of such variables is beyond the scope of this chapter.

Sociocultural Variables

Differences in needs from one phase of grief to another and the indicated nursing intervention in each phase were discussed previously. Grieving persons can be helped or hindered in their coping by the availability and behavior of persons in their environment. Sociocultural rituals and expectations also have the potential to exert powerful effects on the grieving individual.

Social Network: The social resources available to a person who has experienced a significant loss are likely to be critical to the nature of the recovery.

Following a major loss of a person, body part or something else, the individual often is stigmatized. Parkes[41] described a change in attitude toward the bereaved following a death. People who were once very friendly become embarrassed or strained. The writer interviewed several men who were paralyzed as a result of spinal cord injuries, and many of them described a similar change in their friends.

At first, following an injury or a death many people are often around to help or visit. The number of visitors or helpers generally diminishes quickly because the person just does not "fit in" anymore. The widow no longer fits in a couple's world and a paralyzed, former motorcycle racing star no longer fits with his former circle of friends. They no longer share common goals. Disruption of one's social network adds more loss, hence the intensity of grief may increase. Follow-up contact by caring other persons will be very welcome to the griever even though this may not be expressed.

Sociocultural Expectations: Sociocultural expectations include standards of behavior for the person experiencing a loss of someone or something significant as well as for persons with various relationships to them. Expectations may take the form of custom and ritual following a loss and determine what should be done, when, how, and for how long.

Nurses and other helping persons can be more helpful to the grieving individual if they understand the person's sociocultural background. Such understanding is not easily achieved by an "outsider." Although there are similarities in customs, there are numerous overt and subtle differences between and even within societies and cultures. The more astute nurse will look for the similarities as well as the differences in doing an assessment and planning intervention.

Custom and rituals seem to be most precise and clear when the loss event that has occurred is the death of a loved one. P. G. Rosenblatt[42] described the uses of ethnography in understanding grief and mourning in 78 societies. It is common for societies to have customs and ceremonies related to death. These free the bereaved from having to make decisions about how to behave. Emotionality tends to be most common in persons close to the deceased and, in most cases, women are more likely to cry than men. Overt anger and aggression were reported to be less common in societies with specialists such as undertakers who managed many things up to the time of disposing of the body. Such persons also, perhaps, relieve the bereaved from having to make numerous decisions. Self-control is prized in American culture as well as in Nordic societies. Italian and Jewish societies tend to be more emotional. Greek peasant women who lose their husbands are expected to remain widows and wear black for the rest of their lives. These women often are sedated for the first three months of their bereavement. In contrast, traditional Navajo customs allow for only four days of grieving.[43] Only during this time is discussion of the loss allowed and expression of feeling condoned. After the four days, the bereaved is expected to resume usual activities and refrain from any discussion of the loss. Discussion is curtailed because of fear of the power of the dead person. In addition to the above requirements, there is a prohibition against the conscious experience or overt expression of aggression. Occurrence of painful somatic symptoms is frequent in the bereaved and may be due to the repression of anger and displacement of anger to the self. Finally, Smith[44] has described a custom of many widows in Japan. The Shinto and Buddhist religions permit the bereaved to maintain contact with the deceased. Widows often have family altars made to the dead husband. Thoughts and feelings are discussed there. This is a source of comfort because the widow has not lost all interaction with the deceased.

These sample descriptions of noted variations are included to convince the reader of the importance of customs and rituals in the grief process and of the fact that those appropriate to one person may be totally inappropriate to the next. For example, if the bereaved person is from a society where expression of emotion is encouraged, interventions that facilitate emotional ventilation may be very helpful. On the other hand, the same interventions may be a hindrance to someone from a society in which self-control is valued.

Knowledge of effects of specific sociocultural variables on reactions to loss is dependent on further research in practically every area. At this point, all that can be said with assurance is that social and cultural factors are significant to grief and grieving.

NURSING PROCESS

The relevance of the concept of grief to nursing is obvious. Whenever significant losses occur in the lives of individuals, grief follows. Grieving persons are seen in every area where nursing is practiced. The griever may be a patient, parent, spouse, friend, child, nurse, aide, physician. All are vulnerable to the loss experience. Some will grieve openly and others will try to hide their distress. The professional nurse has many opportunities to influence the grief process and facilitate patient goal achievement through recognizing the influence of grief on one's physiological state, perceptual acuity, ability to process information, attention span and the like.

Assessment

The assessment of loss described in the last chapter is useful to the nurse in helping maintain alertness to signs of grief as well as providing information that gives potential meaning to behavior being observed. Caution is suggested, however, to avoid forcing grief on an individual or interpreting behavior as indicative of grief because of inadequate information or because of the nurse's subjective evaluation of the meaning of an event to a patient, parent, colleague, or anyone. Recognition of specific behaviors that are commonly exhibited at various stages of grief (crisis) can be an aid to nursing assessment as long as the nurse realizes that behaviors seldom match phases perfectly. Assessment is a continuous process. First, the nurse observes the client's behavior and tries to note themes or patterns. The next step is to try to infer meaning. For example, it might be inferred that the patient is angry, denying reality, anxious, or is feeling loss of self-esteem, helpless, or frustrated. Following this initial assessment the nurse proceeds to try to verify the inferences and determine factors contributing to the client's situation. Numerous contributing factors to loss and grief have been considered in the last two chapters and are listed below.

Objective characteristics of the loss situation
- Visibility
- Duration (temporary, permanent, uncertain)
- Abruptness (suddenness)
- Extent of change (functional deficit)
- Time required for treatment, reestablishing goal achievement, etc.
- Financial requirements

Person characteristics
- Preloss factors
  - Goal characteristics (basic and acquired needs)
    - Number of goals
    - Clarity
    - Centrality of particular goals
    - Number of pathways
    - Compatibility of goals
  - Personality characteristics
    - Beliefs
    - Openness
    - Flexibility
    - Coping style
    - Motivation
    - Communication style
    - Attitudes and values
    - Other
  - Cultural background
  - Past experience

- Age
- Sex
- Socioeconomic status
- Education or occupation
- Current status
  - Change in goal characteristics (temporary or permanent)
  - Personality factors
    - Changes in personality characteristics
    - Influence of personality characteristics on situation
    - Other

External Factors
- Sociocultural factors
  - Values and expectations
  - Attitudes toward disabled, bereaved, etc.
  - Rituals for loss and grief
- Physical surroundings
  - Accessibility
  - Safety
- Support network
  - Availability of family and friends
  - Amount and consistency of help provided
  - Agencies available
  - Other
- Changes in external situation (any of above)

Information about these factors enables the nurse to make a much more accurate nursing diagnosis. Knowledge about loss and grief may aid in giving observations meaning and reaching a nursing diagnosis. The greater the precision in the diagnostic statement, the more useful the diagnosis will be in planning appropriate patient goals and interventions ("Grief: patient is denying the consequences of disease" is more meaningful than just "Grief" as a diagnosis).

Planning and Intervention

Planning includes setting patient or client goals (with the client whenever possible). It is useful to state these goals using descriptions of patient or client behaviors that will be exhibited by a given time. For example, if the patient is in a panic state, crying, screaming, trembling, running, and so on, goals may be stated in terms of measurable reduction of these behaviors immediately or in whatever period of time seems reasonable. If a patient has experienced the impact of loss and a problem of withdrawal has been determined, behavioral goals that indicate a reduction of the withdrawals should be considered: patient will sit with others watching TV one hour a day by next Monday; patient will eat meals with other patients or staff within two weeks. Such precise statements are more useful than general goals when there will be relatively long contact with the client. The behavioral statements provide evaluation criteria for nursing intervention and the time dimension helps to arrange goals in steps.

Planning involves setting goals that will represent the client's progress in reestablishing equilibrium in whatever aspect of life has been disrupted. It also includes deciding on the strategies most likely to facilitate the progress. Some may be direct actions involving the client while others involve manipulating the physical and interpersonal environments (removing stressful stimuli or teaching family members how to be helpful to the patient). Information about the client and his or her situation (objective, person and external factors) described previously should be taken into account when establishing goals and determining the most effective methods of nursing intervention. Goals should reflect the values, abilities and resources of the client rather than those of the helping person. Goals also should be realistic according to stage of grief, as described earlier. Nursing activities that will help one person may hinder another; therefore, these same factors as well as the skills of the nurse should be taken into account in deciding on methods of nursing intervention.

Evaluation, the last part of the nursing process, is continuous as is assessment. Progress in meeting goals is a criterion measure of success. Failure leads the nurse to reassess goals and methods of intervention.

NURSING RESEARCH

There has been more intensive study of the grief process following death of spouse than the process following other types of loss. Many of the findings have been discussed in this chapter. The assumption has been made that the process following major losses is essentially the same. Longitudinal investigations of reactions to different loss situations will reveal the extent of similarity and perhaps some important differences.

Many loss situations affect more than one person. The loss of a family member through death, illness or other cause influences all members. What happens when the affected people are at different phases of the grief process? For example, what happens when the father of a boy with a spinal cord injury continues to deny the permanence of his son's paralysis while the son has moved on to acknowledge the reality and adjust to it?

Research that demonstrates which variables are most influential in the successful adjustment to loss may provide guidelines for the nurse clinician. For example, the writer in a study of paraplegic and quadriplegic men found that conceptual abstractness was positively associated with life satisfaction.[45] More research is needed and findings might suggest that clients should be encouraged to change conceptual style. Nurses may be unable to change many characteristics of the client's situation; therefore, it is important to know target variables or characteristics that can be manipulated to facilitate adjustment.

When the loss event involves loss of a body part or function, the client is faced with many physical goals as well as goals related to recovery from the emotional devastation. Physical goals are often achieved much faster than in years past and before the grief process has been completed. What are the effects of more rapid discharge from agencies on adjustment to such losses?

These are but a few areas that need to be researched to better understand and plan effective nursing care for clients experiencing grief. Much has been done, but far more is still to be accomplished.

CONCLUSION

The chapters on loss and grief can be used to establish a framework for understanding much of the behavior that follows significant events. Defining loss as interruption in goal achievement makes it a very personal situation, since there are many variations in goals and methods used to achieve them. The meaning of events for the individual is critical.

Knowledge about grief and common phases in reactions to loss provides a *general* guide for assessing others as well as ourselves. This guide can only be effective if it is viewed by the user as a set of generalizations that will apply to some but not all who grieve. Even if only one person is different, has needs that vary from those suggested in the guide, has unique customs, the goal for the nurse is to recognize the differences and plan nursing intervention accordingly.

REFERENCES

1. Switzer, D. K.: The Dynamics of Grief. New York, Abingdon, 1970, p. 12.
2. Marris, P.: Loss and Change. New York, Pantheon, 1974, p. 4.
3. Reed, A. W.: Anticipatory grief work. *In* Shoenberg, B., et al. (eds.): Anticipatory Grief. New York, Columbia University Press, 1974, p. 347.
4. Parkes, C. M.: Bereavement: Studies of Grief in Adult Life. New York, Basic Books, 1972, pp. 182-95.
5. Reed, Anticipatory grief work, p. 347; Moss, S. Z., and Moss, M. S.: Separation as a death experience. Child Psychiat. & Human Develop. 3, 3:187-94, 1973.
6. Freud, S.: Mourning and melancholia. *In* Collected Papers, Vol. 4. New York, Basic Books, 1959, pp. 152-70.
7. Bowlby, J.: Attachment and Loss. Vol. I, Attachment (1969). Vol. II, Separation, Anxiety and Anger (1973). New York, Basic Books.
8. Glick, I., Weiss, R. S., and Parkes, C. M.: The First Year of Bereavement. New York, John Wiley, 1974, Chap. 1.
9. Smith, C. R.: Bereavement: the contribution of phenomenological and existential analysis to a greater understanding of the problem. Br. J. Social Work. 5,1:75-92, 1975.
10. Kübler-Ross, E.: On Death and Dying. New York, Macmillan, 1969.
11. Engel, G. L.: Psychological Development in Health and Disease. Philadelphia, Saunders, 1962.
12. Fink, S. L.: Crisis and motivation: a theoretical model. Arch. Phys. Med. Rehabil. 48:592-97, 1967.
13. Bowlby, J.: Processes of mourning. Int. J. Psychoanal. 42:317-40, 1961.
14. Parkes, Bereavement, Chap. 3-7.
15. Shontz, F. C.: The Psychological Aspects of Physical Illness and Disability. New York, Macmillan, 1975.
16. Davis, F.: Passage Through Crisis: Polio Victims and Their Families. Indianapolis, Bobbs-Merrill, 1963.
17. Parkes, Bereavement, Chap. 4.
18. Kübler-Ross, E.: On the use of psychopharmacologic agents for the dying patient and bereaved. J. Thanatology. 2:563-66, 1972.
19. Parkes, Bereavement, Chap. 5.
20. Ibid., p. 59

21. Glick, Weiss, Parkes, The First Year of Bereavement, p. 56.
22. Parkes, Bereavement, p. 165.
23. Clayton, P. J., Herjanie, M., Murphy, G. E., and Woodruff, R., Jr.: Mourning and depression: their similarities and differences. Canad. Psychiatric Assoc. J. 19:309-12, 1974.
24. Glick, Weiss, Parkes, The First Year of Bereavement, p. 211.
25. Marris, Loss and Change, p. 27.
26. Shontz, Physical Illness and Disability, p. 174.
27. Ibid., pp. 174-75.
28. Ibid., p. 175.
29. Pradhan, S. N.: Basis for psychopharmacotherapy of the dying and the bereaved. J. Thanatology. 2:820-33, 1972.
30. Shontz, Physical Illness and Disability, pp. 168-72.
31. Gerber, I., Weiner, A., Battin, D., and Arkin, A.M.: Brief therapy to the aged bereaved. *In* Schoenberg, B., et al. (eds.): Bereavement: Its Psychosocial Aspects. New York, Columbia University Press, 1975.
32. Volkan, V. D.: Re-grief therapy. *In* ibid.
33. Epstein, G., Weitz, L., Roback, H., and McKee, E.: Research on bereavement: a selective and critical review. Comprehensive Psychiatry. 16, 6:537-46, 1975.
34. Glick, Weiss, Parkes, The First Year of Bereavement, p. 32.
35. Moss and Moss, Separation as a death experience.
36. Parkes, Bereavement, pp. 120-22.
37. Marris, Loss and Change, p. 33.
38. Erikson, E.: Childhood and Society. New York, Norton, 1963, pp. 247-69.
39. Glick, The First Year of Bereavement, Chap. 13.
40. Parkes, C. M.: Determinants of outcome following bereavement. Omega. 6, 4:303-23, 1975.
41. Parkes, Bereavement, p. 8.
42. Rosenblatt, P. G.: Uses of ethnography in understanding grief and mourning. *In* Schoenberg, et al. (eds.): Bereavement: Its Psychosocial Aspects.
43. Miller, S. I., and Schoenfeld, L.: Grief in the Navajo: psychodynamics and culture. Int. J. Social Psychiatry. 19, 3-4:187-91, 1973.
44. Smith, Bereavement, p. 87.
45. Carlson, C. E.: The relationship between conceptual style and life satisfaction following spinal cord injury. Submitted to Arch. Phys. Med. Rehabil., March, 1978.

Section II

Responses to Changes in Health Status: Concepts with Negative Connotations

INTRODUCTION

The four chapters in this section focus on phenomena generally described as unpleasant, uncomfortable or negative: alienation, hostility, boredom and restlessness. Many of these have been covered to some extent in the chapters of the first section. Grief, for example, includes a variety of subjective states and behaviors. Restlessness, hostility, alienation and even boredom are likely to be observed at various times following a loss. Catherine Norris noted the self-hate or hostility associated with obesity. Also, alienation is implicit in the stigmatizing process. Numerous ties can be made between concepts, and as these connections are described and tested, theories are built.

Each of the four concepts has a ring of familiarity. Most people would say they know what they are, what they mean and the feelings associated with them. But a closer look at each one reveals a great deal of complexity in these familiar phenomena. Norris's article on restlessness is an excellent example of how elusive the understanding of everyday events can be. She describes the tedious process of trying to give clear meaning to events. The process began with a clinician raising questions about insomnia. Pursuit of answers led down many pathways, including the study of bird migration patterns and biological rhythms. A major conclusion reached was that there is need for much descriptive data before restlessness can be understood. The same need exists for all of the concepts.

Alienation is defined by Dorothy Bloch as a multidimensional concept involving discord between perception of the real and the ideal or between aspirations and achievement. Alienation is subjective and dependent on the individual's value system. The five meanings or dimensions of alienation are powerlessness, meaninglessness, normlessness, isolation and self-estrangement. Evelyn Char defines boredom as an unpleasant experience of feeling captive in a dull situation. It is subjective and always unpleasant. Sister Martha Kiening defines hostility as a feeling of antagonism accompanied by the wish to hurt or humiliate others. Norris defines restlessness as a universal, discontinuous, animal behavior evidenced by nonspecific, repetitive, unorganized, diffuse, apparently nonpurposeful motor activity that is subject to limited control. Feelings include boredom, meaninglessness, emptiness, tension, uneasiness and impatience.

Each of the authors addresses the issue of cause of the respective phenomena. Bloch notes that numerous social and psychological factors, such as limited resources or failure to accomplish maturational tasks, may contribute to states of alienation, although further investigation is needed to identify specific causes. Restlessness is thought to be caused by such factors as role deprivation, boredom, fatigue, pain, anxiety, and certain disease states. Boredom, according to Char, may be caused by reduced or monotonous stimulation or a situation devoid of interest. It may be used to hide anger or to avoid close relationships. Hostility is thought to be a consequence of unfulfilled or frustrated needs or wishes. According to Kiening, normal hostility occurs in the face of justifiable fear or real danger; therefore, it has a defensive or protective purpose. Norris suggests that the purpose of restlessness may also be defense. It may be one of the early responses to change, strangeness or threat and lead to hypervigilance.

Each of the four concepts may operate in a variety of situations and examples are given for each of them. It is important that specific behaviors indicative of alienation states, boredom, hostility and restlessness be identified and described through careful observation. When this is accomplished, each phase of the nursing process and research related to the respective concepts will be facilitated. Norris reports progress in describing the nature and course of restlessness. Three phases of restlessness have been described: small muscle activity, gross muscle activity and aggressive behavior.

Nursing process is carried out despite gaps in knowledge and lack of definitive behavioral descriptions of phenomena. Patients feel alienated, express hostility, become bored and restless and need to be cared for now. They can not wait for the systematic descriptive and testing processes to be completed before they are relieved of unpleasant experiences. Thus nurses, as other professionals, use skills based on the knowledge currently available and incorporate new knowledge as it is developed in providing nursing care. Nurses also add to knowledge through sharing their observations of others and trying to understand them. Norris shows what a critically thinking nurse detective can do to add to knowledge.

Bloch describes several ways in which knowledge about alienation can be useful to the nurse. Estrangement of clients may lead to over- or underutilization of preventive health services. The nurse as a teacher can be more helpful to the client if she or he realizes that a powerless person tends to be less knowledgeable than others and that lack of knowledge leads to powerlessness. Increased knowledge, therefore, may decrease feelings of being powerless. Bloch describes how pervasive alienation is among patients wherever they are encountered. She provides examples of each dimension of alienation in clients as well as in the role of professional nurse. Such useful ways of decreasing alienation as development of client power are described.

Char points out that boredom occurs in patients and nurses. Recognition of anger and its relationship to boredom may make it possible for the nurse to deal more effectively with anger and boredom in nurse-patient situations.

Total care of the patient includes assessment of all his or her needs. If the patient is bored and this is recognized, the nurse can help by trying to find activities that will relieve the boredom.

Kiening reminds the reader that nurse assumptions about behavior need to be validated before they are acted on. Often the basic cause of hostility cannot be identified. If the nurse can help the patient identify the threat, perhaps assistance can be given to facilitate resolution. The dynamics of hostility are often very complex, but understanding is needed to determine the best nursing approach. Sometimes it is difficult to distinguish between assertiveness and behavior motivated by the desire to hurt. Kiening notes that acceptance of the person exhibiting hostility does not imply acceptance of the behavior. Free expression is not always helpful and it is the nurse's responsibility to set reasonable limits. Numerous examples are given to illustrate various aspects of hostility.

These four chapters provide the reader with a wealth of information about concepts and concept development. Many guidelines are provided for the clinician and many researchable questions are raised for the researcher.

6 ALIENATION

Dorothy W. Bloch

Mr. Morris is scheduled for exploratory surgery on the following day. When the nurse enters the room, he says, "Having bad health is just a matter of luck. If it's time for me to die, there just isn't much I or anyone else can do about it."

When Mrs. Jones and her infant daughter Jane are visited by the public health nurse, Mrs. Jones tells the nurse about her feelings of loneliness and rejection. She indicates that she perceives her family and friends as less interested in her.

These two examples introduce the concept of alienation. This popular concept is frequently used to explain many of our current social problems. Alienation, which has been called one of the five "essential unit-ideas in sociology"[1] and is often used to label persons who do not fit into society,[2] has enjoyed a rich, but often ambiguous use in the behavioral sciences. If alienation is such a pervasive concept, in what ways does nursing need to be concerned with the meanings, expressions and alleviation of alienation?

WHAT IS ALIENATION?

Alienation has been studied and described from the perspective of various behavioral scientists, including psychologists, sociologists, theologians and historians. Historically, the term alienation has been used to refer to both social structure and individuals.

One means of decreasing the confusion about the meaning of alienation is to distinguish between alienating conditions and states of alienation. As proposed by Eric and Mary Josephson, conditions leading to alienation are phenomena like work conditions, social interaction and the distribution of political power. Within this definition, Emile Durkheim's description of anomie is paramount. According to his analysis of suicide as a social phenomenon rather than an individual behavior, anomie is a "state of deregulation," which refers to the breakdown of regulatory mechanisms or norms which control behavior.[3]

States of alienation, by comparison, are viewed as the feelings of individual persons as they are dissociated from self, others or society. Conditions of normlessness, social isolation or social disorganization may lead to alienation, but not in every case.[4]

Accepting that alienation can include several dimensions leads to Melvin

Seeman's work as a useful starting point from which to seek out the subjective meanings of alienation or the states experienced by the individual. In his classic article he presented five states of alienation: powerlessness, meaninglessness, normlessness, social isolation and self-estrangement.[5]

Powerlessness

One of the most widely used meanings of alienation, powerlessness originated in the Marxian view of the conditions of the worker in a capitalist society. This conception of alienation refers to the feeling of being separated from or external to one's work and its products rather than a creator or contributor to one's work activities. Thus, the worker feels powerless or unable to control the outcomes of his or her own behavior.

This analysis of the individual's relation to the larger social order is closely related to the belief in internal versus external control, as developed by Julian Rotter.[6] Briefly, this variable is defined as an expectation that the outcomes of one's behaviors are determined either by what one does (internal control) or by the influence of outside forces, such as luck or chance (external control). The person with an external orientation would feel powerless to determine the consequences of his or her behavior, as illustrated in the example of Mr. Morris.

Meaninglessness

Under the rubric meaninglessness, Seeman summarized those conditions in which the individual experiences lack of clarity concerning what should be believed. The person experiencing meaninglessness cannot choose with confidence from among alternative explanations and is unable to predict the outcomes when acting on a given belief. With Mannheim's concept of meaninglessness occurring as society becomes increasingly concerned with efficient task specialization, there is a concomitant decrease in the opportunity to choose appropriately from alternatives and to act intelligently.

Normlessness

This aspect of alienation relates directly to the concept of anomie delineated by Durkheim. A state of anomie, referring to the problems of social control, is a situation in which the social norms have broken down or ceased to be effective; values are in conflict or absent. Thus, anomie denotes a social state of normlessness. The American phenomenon Robert Merton selected to illustrate anomie is the incongruity of culturally prescribed goals of success and means available to attain it.[7] Normlessness develops when socially unapproved behaviors are needed to achieve the goal—in this case, success.

Isolation

Feeling apart from society, the alienated person who is isolated does not place high value on beliefs that are usually highly valued by society. The individual does not expect to be included and accepted, and thus may have feelings of rejection or loneliness similar to those expressed by Mrs. Jones in the previous example. This concept of isolation closely resembles the form of adaptation to anomie Merton called rebellion. This attitude directs the person to seek the creation of a social structure which would be free from the present norms and goals.[8]

Self-estrangement

The last type of alienation, as formulated by Seeman, is self-estrangement. This refers primarily to the individual's inability to find his or her activities rewarding. In the words of Erich Fromm, the self-estranged experiences "himself as an alien."[9] A discrepancy exists between the self-estranged individual's ideal and actual self.[10]

Summary

Alienation can be viewed as a multidimensional concept with multiple variants of emphasis and sources. In this chapter, alienation will be viewed as:

1. discordance between an individual's perception of the real and ideal or between one's aspirations and one's achievements;
2. a subjectively perceived state of the individual, not an objective variable of the social structure;
3. dependent on an individual's particular value system; and
4. having at least five operational meanings—powerlessness, meaninglessness, normlessness, isolation and self-estrangement.

FACTORS CONTRIBUTING TO ALIENATION

As a variable of an individual's personality, the development of alienation can be traced to a number of antecedent events. One approach is to look toward developmental theories for explanatory notions.

According to Erikson, developing a sense of identity—that is, knowing who one is, having a feeling of well-being and being oneself—is the major developmental task of adolescence.[11] Donald Oken, in his attempt to understand adolescence from the viewpoint of alienation, points out that identity is the mirror image of alienation. Identity represents the opposite of the self-estrangement or alienation.

This developmental perspective suggests that alienation, or the lack of ego identity, can be avoided as an enduring personality trait through experiences and relationships which assist the developing person to accomplish the tasks of psychosocial maturation. In the struggle toward ego identity, adolescents will experience periods of alienation as a part of the identity crisis. Thus, adolescence can be a factor contributing to alienated behavior as the adolescent experiences the normal identity crisis.[12]

Viewing alienation as related to the discrepancy between one's goals and the opportunities to achieve them, Luther Otto and David Featherman suggest that persons with fewer resources and options may tend to experience more alienation. In this group of disadvantaged persons are included the poor, persons with little education and the psychologically impaired. A potential intervening variable between these people and alienation, of course, is socialization. Persons of sufficient wealth and education to achieve goals could still be alienated if inadequate socialization leads to inaccurate perceptions of their resources and aspirations.[13]

The relationship between alienation and the environments of adult social integration, specifically social participation and socializing, was also proposed in the Otto-Featherman model. Their assumption was that social integration produces a closer congruence between the perceived self and social environment.[14]

Considering any of the five variants of alienation may also suggest factors leading to alienation. For example, studies on powerlessness reveal the economic and social deprivation so often a part of the history of the powerless.

In sum, both social and psychological factors can be cited as contributing to states of alienation. Further exploration is needed to pinpoint causal factors which can then lead to intervention.

ALIENATION AND HEALTH CARE

Health science researchers, including nurses, have recognized that the concept of alienation has potential for explaining certain behaviors in the health care domain. To what extent and in what ways might an understanding of alienation be useful to a health professional, especially the nurse?

Preventive Health Care

Health professionals' awareness that some people are underutilizers or nonutilizers of preventive health services has stimulated a search for an explanation. An assumption that feeling estranged or separated from the mainstream of social institutions may lead to decreased use of these institutions has prompted some research on how feelings of alienation influence one's behavior in seeking preventive health services.

In a study reported by Philip Moody and Robert Gray, participation in a state-sponsored polio immunization program was investigated. One hypothesis was that the subjects who scored high on alienation would have a lower rate of participation in the immunization program. Alienation was measured on a scale including the concepts of powerlessness, normlessness and social isolation. This hypothesis was supported by data from 959 mothers. The existence of alienation in these women was an important antecedent of their unwillingness to participate in this prevention program.[15]

In her research on the utilization of preventive health services, Bonnie Bullough adopted a somewhat different definition of alienation as embracing the feelings of powerlessness, social isolation and hopelessness. In this survey of mothers' behaviors, preventive services included were pre- and postnatal care, dental care and family planning. Since both hopelessness and powerlessness have been found to be associated with a subculture of poverty, it is important to differentiate the influence of socioeconomic status on the utilization of preventive services from the effects of alienation. When this sample was divided into those above and those below the poverty level, alienation was found to be related to family planning behaviors for both groups.[16]

Other research aimed at linking alienation to low utilization of preventive care has revealed that mothers with high scores of powerlessness and social isolation obtained fewer immunizations for their babies.[17] Helen Nakagawa found similar results in predicting who secured immunizations for their children with the scores on the Srole anomie scale, which measures social malintegration. Anomic women were also slower in seeking prenatal care.[18]

Based on these studies, it might appear that a direct relationship exists between alienation and utilization of preventive health services. Lack of satisfaction with that simple explanation has encouraged further research. For example, Sue Hoppe and Peter Heller studied lower-class Mexican-Americans and their health care utilization with a more complex definition of alienation. They described alienation as a variable including both a subjective element, the feelings of powerlessness or social isolation, and an objective element, the discrepancy between one's aspirations and one's achievements frequently experienced by the poor and ethnic minorities. Based on previous research showing that lower-class persons tend to feel powerless over the outside world and are more involved in family relationships than in community activities, Hoppe and Heller hypothesized that familism may be a coping mechanism which reduces objective and subjective alienation among lower-class Mexican-Americans. Further, the intervening variable of familism would result in increased health care use. Although familism tended to encourage prenatal care, it was negatively related to seeking a physician when ill. This finding, as well as the negative relationship between powerlessness and the timing of prenatal care and the positive relationship between powerlessness and consultation when ill, suggests that the preventive and curative aspects of health care may need to be differentiated in studying the influence of alienation.[19]

Alienation, one means of describing a person's relationship with society, has been studied from several vantage points in an attempt to understand health care use. The studies cited indicate the potential usefulness of alienation as an explanatory variable. Because of the complexity of the meanings of alienation and its relationship to such factors as poverty, continued research is necessary to establish to what extent alienation does predict health care utilization.

Alienation and Learning

From an analysis of definitions of nursing practice, the teaching role of the professional nurse appears to be clearly established. Of importance to the nurse, therefore, is the identification of those factors which enhance or hinder the teaching-learning process of clients. Alienation has been considered as one of those factors.

A study of tuberculosis patients focused on the alienation of the learner. The hypothesis guiding Seeman and John Evans was that a high degree of alienation, as measured on a scale of powerlessness, was associated with less knowledge. Their rationale was that persons who believe that chance or luck controls events would be apt to consider acquisition of knowledge unimportant. As predicted, the patients who were low in the alienation scale had more information as well as greater satisfaction with the knowledge.[20]

This relationship between alienation and learning could also be approached from the other direction. For example, could the lack of knowledge the client had about his or her condition, medication and expected course of treatment lead to increased feelings of powerlessness or social isolation? If so, one way to ameliorate feelings of powerlessness could be to provide the alienated person with increased information and knowledge. Hence, the oft-quoted statement "Knowledge is power" may be a useful guideline regarding the importance of teaching.

At this time, empirical work providing adequate support for the association between alienation and learning is lacking. For nurses interested in how their teaching may influence the client, this relationship between alienation and learning remains open for further study.

Alienation and Patients/Clients

The alienated state, often exemplified by powerlessness, describes patients and clients in a variety of settings and circumstances. It is generally believed that persons who are deprived economically, socially and educationally are most likely to feel they lack power and control or feel separate or lonely. In our society, the poor, the ethnic minorities, the uneducated, females, the handicapped, the elderly and the ill are those most likely to be alienated. This generalization suggests that all nurses practicing in a clinical setting who provide care to the public can be expected to encounter alienated persons.

In addition to these groups of persons likely to be alienated, some specific subgroups have been singled out for closer scrutiny. Among these are the mentally ill. The association between alienation and paranoid behavior was developed by one psychiatric nursing specialist from her therapy with a paranoid patient.[21] Theoretical support for this association was provided by Herbert McClosky and John Schaar. Their research revealed a correlation between anomie or normlessness and inflexibility, anxiety, low ego strength and generalized aggression.[22] Based on the rationale that unchecked feelings of alienation can ultimately lead to paranoid behavior, therapy consisted of supporting the client leaving his or her job, the source of alienation. The relationship with the therapist provided the client with someone to relate to in discussing feelings of loneliness and apartness from others.[23]

To establish a relationship between alienation and the acting out behaviors, alcoholism and suicidal behaviors have likewise been studied from the perspective of alienation. In a study of alcoholics, alienation, particularly the social isolation component, was found to exist. Among alcoholics participating in an alcoholic rehabilitation program, the most alienated were less successful in being rehabilitated.[24] Similarly, a significant correlation was found between suicidal behavior and alienation when suicidal patients were asked to rate their alienative behavior. Self-estrangement, as well as separation from parents, characterized this group of suicidal persons.[25]

With the increased use of marijuana and other drugs, particularly among young adults, the relationship between alienation and drug use has become a frequently tested hypothesis. Although conflicting findings have been reported, more evidence exists for a relationship between marijuana use and societal alienation than personal alienation. Societal alienation is defined as alienation from the social institutions and mores or, in Seeman's terms, normlessness.[26]

These multiple, varied empirical studies relate one or more forms of alienation with some particular diagnosis or clinical phenomenon. A few broader clinical pictures might also be suggested.

The "multiple-problem" family is well-known to most nurses. Typically, this term refers to a family in which nearly all members of the household present a medical or social problem which has brought the family to the attention of some care-giving agency or agencies. The family members may have need for medical and nursing care, economic resources, legal services, and so on. The clients appear to be powerless as they move among the involved care givers to obtain help. An unending cycle of dependency can occur as the family is rerouted from one agency to another because not all the needs can be met by one service.

The disabled person is another example of the alienated client. The disability over which the person has little or no control contributes to a feeling of powerlessness. No matter what the person tries or wants to do, his or her efforts may have little effect on altering the condition of disability. The disabled may also face normlessness if societal norms concerning his or her deficiencies do not exist. Other people do not know how to respond to or what to expect from the disabled. Only recently have concerted efforts been made to provide for societal norms such as freedom to pursue an education and opportunities to seek a variety of occupations or social activities. Elevators, ramps, doors wide enough to accommodate wheelchairs, and public transportation for wheelchair users now enable some of the disabled to overcome the alienative effects of their handicaps. For many disabled, meaninglessness develops as others, particularly well-meaning professionals and family members, set goals and make decisions for them. Rather than being encouraged to make their own decisions from among the possible alternatives, they may be told by others "what is best." The isolation aspect may occur as the disabled feel rejected and alone or expect to be excluded.

Constantina Sofilios-Rothschild also described alienation in the form of self-estrangement, which occurs in some situations regarding monetary compensation for the disability. Contradictions may arise when the physician attests to the disability and subsequent inability to work while the employer may believe the injured person is able to return to the job. And the insurance company may also offer a differing opinion while the disabled tries to reconcile his or her ideal self and actual self.[27]

Through these examples of different kinds of illness and disability, the forms of alienation which can be experienced become more vivid. It appears likely that some degree of alienation is sustained by every ill person. Entering a health care system for help places the client in a situation of depending on the care giver. This relationship also implies that the care giver can have a certain degree of power over the client, rendering the client powerless to some degree. The powerlessness the ill person already feels because of the inability to control the symptoms of his or her illness can thus be reinforced by the need to succumb to the powerful authority of the health professionals. *Power and Illness* provides a careful analysis of the influence of the powerful on the powerless in America's health care system. A change in the present system is suggested as the only way to alter the balance of power and provide essential health services for all.[28]

The Alienated Health Professional—The Nurse

As a worker in the large bureaucratic structure of a hospital or health department, the nurse is frequently a target for alienation. Powerlessness is the most common mode of alienation, occurring when nurses experience a discrepancy between the power they think they have and what they believe they should have.[29] Adding to this source of alienation is the fact that nurses in many health care facilities also are faced with responding to the hospital administrator's power, as well as the physician's authority. The result may be alienation: a feeling that one cannot control one's own destiny.

The powerlessness of the nursing profession has been the focus of writers such as JoAnn Ashley[30] and Elliott Krause.[31] A dominant theme in these analyses is the power exerted by medicine over nursing, and thus the constant struggle by nursing to develop its latent power and use the power to make significant changes in practice.

Nurses have been described as subject to other types of alienation as well. For example, meaninglessness may come about as the nurse is forced to perform various tasks which comprise nursing care that are not holistic and patient-centered. The bits and pieces of care assigned to the nurse seem meaningless. Self-estrangement, or feeling separated from one's role, and normlessness due to a lack of clear-cut, accepted norms may also be observed.[32]

Thus, nurses within the health care system also may be among the alienated. Recognition of this possibility points to the need for the nursing profession to develop its power base and become an autonomous professional group in control of and responsible for its own practice.

NURSING INTERVENTIONS IN ALIENATION

The multifaceted definition of alienation can be useful in approaching the question, what can be done to eliminate, alleviate and prevent alienation?

Development of Client Power

Taking the approach that powerlessness is a key aspect of alienation leads one to consider the development of or increase in power as a means of decreasing alienation. Low income persons, minority groups and the disadvantaged are usually the recipients rather than the dispensers of the authority and power of others. In order to decrease their feelings of powerlessness, certain strategies may be employed by the nurse, as well as other health professionals.

For example, within the field of community mental health, nursing has joined with other professional groups in supporting the use of indigenous nonprofessionals. These persons are selected from among the groups being helped as a means of bridging the social distance between the professionals and the clients. These peers of the clients act as links between the middle-class professionals and the lower-class clients who are often suspicious, resentful and alienated from the health system. Services are improved as the nonprofessional brings the professionals and clients closer together, making the therapeutic interventions more beneficial and the clients feel more in control of their therapy.[33]

Another strategy for intervening in the powerless position of the patient is consumer advocacy. Stimulated in part by the desire to develop nursing's potential and uniqueness, nurses have become politically active supporters of such issues as national health insurance, health maintenance organizations, the Equal Rights Amendment, the patient's bill of rights and quality assurance programs.

The movement toward more active consumer involvement in directing health care was propelled largely by the legislation requiring consumers to become members of various policy-making groups, such as neighborhood health center boards. At about the same time, the power of the consumer was strengthened by legislation and professional codes of ethics which required informed consent before the patient/client could become a subject for research. In research nursing has also taken a strong position that the client cannot be kept in a powerless position, subject to the needs of the researcher. Rather, the client is protected by the right to control his or her own participation and responses in the research. Further, an increase in power has been afforded the research subject when the results of the research are shared, allowing the subject to benefit from the increased knowledge.

In 1976 the revised American Nurses' Association Code for Nurses spelled out in more detail the importance of client self-determination. No longer can the professionals wield the power to decide what the client should or should not do. Instead, nursing agreed to encouraging the clients' right to determine their own participation in care.[34]

Patient Teaching

Patient teaching remains as probably one of the most effective means of increasing the client's power. The diabetic patient provides an extreme example of how teaching can increase the patient's power.

Imagine the position of powerlessness and lack of control over one's symptoms of diabetes the patient would be in without any teaching. If, while hospitalized, the diabetic is told what to eat and what not to eat without any knowledge about food and metabolism, he or she is forced into a position of being unable to exert control over the outcomes of the illness.

As suggested by the discussion of the disabled, the person with symptoms that prevent full active participation needs to be informed of the full range of alternatives available. A patient teaching program can do that while providing for the person to make decisions about how to use the information.

Patient teaching programs which will make essential information available can be developed. When patients have the opportunity to increase their knowledge about health status, treatment program, medications and their effects, and prognosis, they will be in a position to make choices for themselves and thus have more control over their health. For the patient who is in the situation of being permanently disabled, the range of choices may be small. Yet, knowing what alternatives remain is still a means of exerting some control over one's destiny.

Nurses may not always know what information patients are most likely to need and desire. Questions to the patients may often elicit from them what knowledge they already possess and where gaps in information or further questions remain. In one study of medical and surgical patients and nurses, nurses and patients agreed on the importance of information about the illness and the patients' involvement in their own care, as well as information about symptoms. However, the patients were more concerned than the nurses about knowledge of chances of recovery, effects of medications and causes of their symptoms. Nurses, on the other hand, ranked information about the patients' care and what care and routines to expect higher than the patients did.[35] This study pointed out that nurses may make false assumptions about the information patients want. A successful teaching program will require some input from patients.

Clinical Examples

> The Smith family consists of a mother and several children. The father has recently moved out, and a divorce is pending. A nurse makes home visits following referrals to the mental health center from the schools and courts. The mother presents a myriad of problems—lack of financial resources, inability to cope with the teen-aged daughter's truancy, concern about the divorce and custody decision, difficulty in recognizing and understanding her son's increasing sexual awareness and interests, and a general inability to maintain a home for herself and her children.

The nurse, in recognizing the powerlessness and feelings of alienation of this mother, devised a plan for her and her children aimed at increasing their own resources and abilities to cope with their problems. The nurse assisted the mother in gaining more understanding of the normal growth and development tasks of adolescents and ways in which she might effectively meet these needs. To increase the mother's knowledge of general homemaking responsibilities, the nurse arranged for the mother to attend a day care center where opportunities for learning these skills, as well as planning a budget, existed. Through a long-term plan with consistent support provided by the nurse, the family began to show indications of less alienation and more coping skills. Consider, on the other hand, how alienation and powerlessness would have been maintained if the nurse had chosen instead to take over for the mother and provide the needed mothering activities herself.

> Mr. Barber had been in the coronary care unit for four days following a heart attack. During that time he had made considerable progress, and when an admission occurred during the evening shift, he was transferred rather suddenly out of the CCU to another unit. Later that evening, he complained to the nurse on the unit that he felt uninformed about his condition and wondered if he had been transferred because the doctors expected him to die. He remarked that he had felt stripped of all decision making since he had been hospitalized and had been told practically nothing about his condition.

The nurse's recognition of Mr. Barber's feelings of alienation and powerlessness prompted her to engage in an interaction with him in which she first helped him to express these feelings. She supported his feeling that not knowing what was occurring led to many concerns and questions. She followed this by attempting to teach him the temporary nature of the coronary care unit and what transfers out of that unit meant in terms of progress. She pointed out the indications that he was improving, and he agreed with her that those changes had taken place. She also encouraged him to ask questions about his heart attack and what symptoms, progress and outcomes he might expect.

By increasing his knowledge of the nature of the coronary care unit and the meaning of the abrupt transfer, the nurse provided Mr. Barber with information that could have been helpful to him as part of the coronary care unit teaching program. She also conveyed to Mr. Barber that he was an active participant in his own care and that knowledge about his progress could be shared with him.

CONCLUSION

If we are really in the age of alienation in which so many clients/patients feel alienated, the nurse must be cognizant of this. Alertness to the manifestation of alienation and ways in which it may be alleviated will result in a higher level of quality nursing care.

REFERENCES

1. Nisbet, A.: The Sociological Tradition. New York, Basic Books, 1966, p. 6.
2. Schimek, G., and Meyer, R. M.: Dimensions of alienation and pathology. Psychol. Reports 37:727-32, December 1975.
3. Durkheim, E.: Suicide. Trans. by J. A. Spaulding and G. Simpson. New York, The Free Press, 1951, p. 253.

4. Josephson E., and Josephson, M. R.: Alienation: contemporary sociological approaches. *In* Frank Johnson (ed.): Alienation: Concept, Term, and Meanings. New York, Seminar Press, 1973, p. 166.
5. Seeman, M.: On the meaning of alienation. Am. Soc. Rev. 24:783-91, December 1959.
6. Rotter, J. B.: Generalized expectancies for internal versus external control of reinforcement. Psychol. Monographs: General and Applied. 80, 1:1-28, 1966.
7. Merton, R. K.: Social Theory and Social Structure. Rev. and Enlg. Ed. New York, The Free Press, 1957, p. 139.
8. Ibid., p. 155.
9. Fromm, E.: The Sane Society. New York, Rinehart, 1955, p. 120.
10. Otto, L. B., and Featherman, D. L.: Social structural and psychological antecedents of self-estrangement and powerlessness. Am. Soc. Rev. 40:703, December 1975.
11. Erikson, E. H.: Identity and the life cycle. Psychol. Issues. Monograph 1, 1, 1:101-64, 1959.
12. Oken, D.: Alienation and identity: some comments on adolescence, the counterculture, and contemporary adaptations. *In* Frank Johnson (ed.): Alienation: Concept, Term, and Meanings. New York, Seminar Press, 1973, pp. 83-110.
13. Otto and Featherman, Social structural and psychological antecedents, p. 704.
14. Ibid., pp. 705-06.
15. Moody, P. M., and Gray, R. M.: Social class, social integration, and the use of preventive health services. *In* E. Gartley Jaco (ed.): Patients, Physicians and Illness: A Sourcebook in Behavioral Science and Health. 2nd Ed. New York, The Free Press, 1972, pp. 252-61.
16. Bullough, B.: Poverty, ethnic identity, and preventive health care. J. Health and Social Behavior. 13:347-59, December 1972.
17. Morris, N. M., Hatch, M. H., and Chipman, S. S.: Alienation as a deterrent to well-child supervision. Am. J. Public Health. 56:1874-82, November 1966.
18. Nakagawa, H.: Family health care patterns and anomie. *In* Bonnie and Vern Bullough (eds.): New Directions for Nurses. New York, Springer, 1971, pp. 199-208.
19. Hoppe, S. K., and Heller, P. L.: Alienation, familism and the utilization of health services by Mexican-Americans. J. Health and Social Behavior. 16:304-14, September 1975.
20. Seeman, M., and Evans, J. W.: Alienation and learning in a hospital setting. Am. Soc. Rev. 27:772-82, December 1962.
21. Aaronson, L. S.: Paranoia as a behavioral manifestation of alienation. Perspect. Psychiatr. Care. 15, 1:27-31, 1977.
22. McClosky, H., and Schaar, J. H.: Psychological dimensions of anomy. Am. Soc. Rev. 30:14-40, February 1965.
23. Aaronson, Paranoia as a behavioral manifestation of alienation, p. 31.
24. Calicchia, J. P., and Barresi, R. M.: Alcoholism and alienation. J. Clin. Psychol. 31:770-75, October 1975.
25. Leonard, C. V.: Self ratings of alienation in suicidal patients. J. Clin. Psychol. 29:423-28, October 1973.
26. Knight, R. C., Sheposh, J. P., and Bryson, J. B.: College student marijuana use and societal alienation. J. Health and Social Behavior. 15:28-35, March 1974.
27. Sofilios-Rothschild, C.: The Sociology and Social Psychology of Disability and Rehabilitation. New York, Random House, 1970.
28. Krause, E. A.: Power and Illness. New York, Elsevier, 1977.
29. Clark, J. P.: Measuring alienation in a social system. Am. Soc. Rev. 24:849-52, December 1959.
30. Ashley, J.: This I believe . . . about power in nursing. Nurs. Outlook. 21:637-41, October 1973.
31. Krause, Power and Illness.
32. Zungolo, E. H.: A study in alienation: the nurse practitioner. Nurs. Forum. 7, 1:38-49, 1968.
33. Reiff, R., and Riessman, F.: The Indigenous Non-professional. Monograph 1. Community Ment. Health J., 1965.
34. Hadley, R. D.: ANA code for nurses revised, greater focus on nurse, client. Am. Nurse. 8:5, October 15, 1976.
35. Dodge, J. S.: What patients should be told: patients' and nurses' beliefs. Am. J. Nurs. 72:1852-54, October 1972.

7 HOSTILITY

Sister M. Martha Kiening

Hostility is a concept which seems to be receiving increasing attention in contemporary medical and nursing literature. This is particularly true since the phenomena of aggression and violence, two of its outward expressions, have escalated to the point of major areas of world concern. Hostility is, perhaps, one of the most difficult barriers for nurses to overcome when they encounter it in their work with others. It is a common human trait, which can operate not only between nurse and patient, but between the nurse and members of the patient's family, among members of the professional team and, not uncommonly, between family members and the patient. In the larger society, it operates within groups to impede their work and among groups to hamper and impair progress toward desirable social goals. Most important, it operates within individuals, often unconsciously, making them unaware of the hostile wishes and impulses that form the motives for many of their actions. The perceptions that individuals have of others can thus be distorted by their own hostile outlook on their life situations.

In its broadest sense, hostility may be seen as a continuum, the manifestations of which range from overly polite behavior to extreme forms externalized in murderous rage or homicide or internalized as depression or suicide. During the past decade, there have been efforts by some authorities to make more careful distinctions among hostility, anger and other related affective states such as aggression, violence and rage.[1] Albert Rothenberg states that there are many inconsistencies in the definition of hostility and reliable test measures for hostility, anger, aggression, rage and violence are not available.[2] It is to be noted, however, that violence as a cause of increasing concern in our society is also becoming the object of more concentrated study by mental health professionals.[3] Others are beginning to take issue with the classical psychoanalytic theory that inwardly directed hostility leads to depression. They see hostility as a defense against the depression rather than as a cause of it.[4]

Most problems which the nurse encounters in day-to-day contacts with patients, families and coworkers stem from covert hostility or the milder types of aggressive behavior that signal its presence. This chapter attempts to focus on hostility as a symptom or sign of unmet nursing needs which then forms the basis of an emergent nursing problem.

The degree to which nurses are aware of their own hostile impulses and wishes, and of the behavior patterns they have adopted to cope with them, are crucial factors in determining how effective nursing intervention will be in dealing with a patient's hostile behavior. Because hostility is so often an automatic response, this awareness is not easily achieved, and when the hostility springs from the very early developmental period its sources are probably not recognizable at all.

Webster defines hostility as unfriendliness or animosity. Martin Symonds distinguishes hostility from aggression, seeing hostility not as an act but as an attitude.[5] It must also be borne in mind that aggression may be constructive as well as destructive. Rothenberg makes careful and meticulous distinctions between anger and hostility. He states:

> . . . hostility always has a destructive component whereas anger does not. Feeling hostile always involves the wish or intent to inflict harm, pain or actual destruction on another person or object. Being hostile always involves inflicting or trying to inflict some type of destruction, psychological or physical upon another.[6]

Anger is usually short-lived and is compatible with love. For the purposes of this chapter, it may be useful to define hostility as a feeling of antagonism accompanied by a wish to hurt or humiliate others which may produce feelings of inadequacy and self-rejection from loss of self-esteem. This feeling may be repressed or dissociated or expressed in various kinds of covert and overt behavior.

Hostility is thought by many authorities to be the result of frustrated or unfulfilled needs or wishes; according to Karen Horney, repressed hostility is one of the major sources of anxiety.[7] Originally part of a basic, biological mechanism through which the individual adapted to threats, irritations and frustrations, hostility is not a disorder or a disease of itself, but rather one of our necessary human endowments. For primitive humans, withdrawing from or destroying a threat to one's basic biological integrity may have spelled the difference between extinction or survival. Normal hostility derives from justifiable fear of real danger; irrational hostility originates in anxiety. Hostility becomes a disordered response when it is kept alive to generate anxiety, the energy of which is then expended futilely rather than constructively. Such is the case when hostility is used to strive toward immature goals or substituted for understanding and cooperation in dealing with problems. The person who becomes the "patient" in a medical system is a person under stress, who attempts to alleviate anxiety or deal with hostile feelings in ways that have previously proved at least partially effective. The regression engendered by illness makes it all the more necessary for the person to revert to earlier childhood patterns of response and defense.

Whether or not a rudimentary form of hostility can be traced back as far as the fourth month of gestation in the fetus, it is certain that the early roots of hostility can be discerned soon after birth. Babies will turn their faces away from a threatening stimulus or even "attack" it by crude attempts to push it away. Later, infants may use the power of locomotion to physically remove themselves from the threat. As children grow older, threats begin to come from the environment as a reaction to something that they have done which brings disapproval from significant others. They may then externalize hostile feelings in the form of angry behavior, such as defiant looks at the reproving or punishing adults. Or, they may project this hostility onto the other persons and behave as though the "badness" were in the others, thus justifying their own anger. In later development this overtly hostile behavior may be replaced by shyness, retreat and withdrawal. Three-year-olds have already developed the ability to anticipate blame or punishment from an adult and to protect themselves by retiring to a safe area. They feel weak and inadequate in the face of a powerful person against whom they cannot openly vent hostile feelings. These frustrated or unmet needs for status, prestige or power form one of the bases for hostility in adult life. This type of hostility operating in the hospitalized patient, with paratactic distortions of earlier childhood experience, may reactivate childish, hostile impulses against the nurse who is seen as an authority figure.

In very young children, the need to repress hostility comes chiefly from two sources:

1. Fear of jeopardizing parental relationships:
   a. They depend on these powerful adults for their very existence.
   b. They fear them in the face of their own weakness and inadequacy.
   c. They desperately need and crave parents' love and approval.
2. Reflected self-appraisal:
   a. They reject the "bad-me," the components of personality that have previously brought disapproval from significant adults.
   b. This rejection leads to further anxiety and an attempt to disown or dissociate the hostile feelings by projecting them onto others or pushing them out of awareness.

This is, of course, an oversimplification of a complex dynamism, but it should help to develop an understanding of why certain childhood situations evoke hostility in adult life. Persons who find it intolerable to acknowledge their hostility or anger tend to perceive the world as hostile, unfriendly and dangerous.

Although social and cultural standards demand that controls and limits be set on aggressive tendencies, healthy self-assertion is a mark of maturity. If the child is constantly required to repress all expression of these tendencies, the impotent anger thus engendered eventually becomes dissociated, but the hostile inpulses and wishes remain in the unconscious generating anxiety and guilt. This process then becomes a cycle in which anxiety based on a felt threat provokes reactive hostility which, if repressed, may again create anxiety.

The disapproval with which our society views the outright expression of anger, particularly in polite social settings, makes it difficult to maintain one's right to healthy self-assertion. What is sometimes labeled as "demanding," "uncooperative" or "unreasonable" behavior of a patient may be a normal and even commendable attempt to maintain dignity as a human being, in a highly institutionalized, impersonal setting. A person whose needs for growth and self-realization are really threatened is acting in a mature way when taking a stand. The nurse needs to be perceptive in order to assess what is healthy and necessary for this person. The nurse also needs to feel reasonably free from bureaucratic and institutional pressures in order to individualize the patient's care. Much has been done in recent years to recognize the fact that the hospitalized child has a need to protest openly and even angrily, but social pressures within the system still operate all too effectively in silencing the adult who feels aggrieved and angry at an unwelcome—and often unforeseen—situation.

Viewed operationally, then, the development of hostility may be described as follows:

1. A person has experienced frustration, loss of self-esteem or unmet needs for status, prestige or love in the past.
2. A situation occurs in which the person holds certain expectations of self or others.
3. Expectations are not met.
4. The person feels inadequate, hurt or humiliated.
5. He or she experiences anxiety in the form of hostility.
6. The person may then act in one of three ways:
   a. repress the hostility and withdraw.
   b. disown the feeling and overreact by being extremely polite and compliant.
   c. engage in some type of overtly hostile behavior, either verbal or nonverbal.

The influence of hostility on the cause and progress of disease has long been recognized. In ancient time, imbalance of the bile or choleric humor was believed to produce certain bodily diseases. Washington Irving's classic character, Rip Van Winkle, came home to learn that his shrewish wife had finally "burst a blood vessel in a fit of anger." Early investigators in the field of psychosomatic medicine, notably F. Dunbar and F. Alexander, focused on the role that hostility plays not only in the so-called "psychosomatic" illnesses, but to some extent in most or all disturbances of physiology as well.[8] Although earlier theories concerning hostility as the cause of certain specific diseases have not always been borne out by the available data, hostility can in no way be discounted as an important factor in both the etiology and the progress of illness. It would seem to be particularly important in such conditions as hypertension, rheumatoid arthritis, asthma and neurodermatitis, to name but a few. G. Engel maintains that even pain can sometimes be traced to guilt feelings about expressing aggressive impulses or wishes.[9]

More pertinent for the nurse, perhaps, is the literature dealing with situations that seem to have a fairly high potential for hostility. As previously noted, there is now a greater awareness of the need for the hospitalized child to express grief and frustration by angry outbursts and tears. What is not so universally recognized, however, is the fact that most adults experience some degree of hostility during a period of enforced illness and hospitalization. The initial reaction to any illness is anxiety, which may be expressed as hostility. The dependency feelings that accompany acceptance of the illness may lead to feelings of hostility if this is the pattern the patient usually follows in attempting to cope with stress. The period of convalescence may be prolonged if the patient has repressed resentful, hostile feelings toward medical personnel during the period of accepted illness.

Patients with certain types of illness or physical disabilities seem to exhibit more hostility than others. The preoperative cancer patient may displace hostility toward the surgeon onto nurses, social workers or family members. Postoperatively, particularly when the illness is terminal, the nursing staff may experience even more hostile reactions from the patient's family than from the patient. The now classic work of Elisabeth Kübler-Ross on death and dying has demonstrated very clearly the role hostility plays as the person goes through the final phases immediately preceding death itself.[10] The amputee and the hemodialysis patient are particularly prone to feelings of hostility as one way of coping with dependency and feelings of helplessness. The tendency to focus frustration on others may lead to serious problems in the care of the chronically ill. This can prove particularly damaging to relationships between patients and family. As patients begin to realize that some of their basic emotional needs cannot be satisfied, they may become quite disturbed. Persons close to them, such as devoted family members, may then become the objects of jealousy and displaced hostility. Early recognition of this danger and frank discussion of the realities of the situation with patients lead them to greater self-understanding. Attempts to assist patients in reaching a balanced satisfaction through appropriate and satisfying activities within their capacities and limitations will help prevent unhealthy focusing of hostility onto others.

Regardless of the type of illness for which the person seeks medical help, the circumstances surrounding the event are usually sufficient in themselves to call forth a great deal of anxiety and, in most instances, varying degrees of hostility. The person is placed in much the same situation as when early childhood experiences first evoked a hostile response. He or she is again weak and inadequate in a world of powerful authority figures who must be depended on to ward off danger or threat, painfully aware of being dependent, with needs for love and approval intensified by stress, and his or her very self-identity threatened by the alien, impersonal world of the hospital. The highly organized routines through which the person's medical care is delivered only augment the ego-alien stimuli. Individuality is denied and personhood is negated by this assembly line approach. Resentment at being casually classified and thus deprived of his or her uniqueness and difference from all others causes anger which serves to protect this identity.

Not all people are alike in their ability to feel or express anger. Likewise, it is seldom possible to assess the degree of hostility present by the directness or intensity of its expression. Behavior indicative of hostility varies considerably with the individual. Even the ways in which people express or act out hostility may differ according to the circumstances in which they find themselves and the degree of stress they are undergoing. Nor is it always possible to detect who is really the focus of the patient's hostility, for the tendency to displace this feeling on those less threatening and less able to retaliate is a common one.

Unless in a psychiatric setting, a nurse rarely encounters the violently aggressive behavior signaling that the person has temporarily lost control. Should such a situation occur, it must be dealt with as a psychiatric emergency. The nurse must be able to recognize when patient behavior begins to signal a crisis and should summon help as quickly as possible. In many hospitals, psychiatric services and consultation are available. These services and an ongoing relationship with the psychiatric department and its nursing staff are valuable resources which should not be neglected or overlooked.

Covert expressions of hostility may be frequent, but are not always easily identified. Patients may be silent because they are resentful, withdrawing from a perceived threat, or seething with anger to such a degree that they dare not trust themselves to speak. They may be depressed, a sign of hostility turned inward upon the self. A perceptive nurse picks up many nonverbal cues indicating that the patient may feel hostile; facial expression and bodily posture often betray inner turmoil. The nurse may wonder why the patient is so placating and obsequious or finds it necessary to adopt so ingratiating an attitude toward those who care for him or her. The nurse can only surmise what the patient is trying to communicate, unless he or she can express these feelings. The nurse cannot act directly on assumptions or hunches without having validated them with the patient. What the nurse perceives as dangerous, threatening or discomforting may not be felt in this way by the patient at all. Often, the basic cause of a person's hostility cannot be identified, nor is such "depth psychotherapy" either appropriate or necessary in order to deal with a presenting problem. If the nurse can help the patient identify what it is in the here-and-now situation that seems threatening, she or he can help the patient deal with the problem at hand and resolve the hostility, or at least prevent it from interfering with needed care. In cases in which a real personality problem exists, psychiatric consultation should be sought so that professional psychotherapy can be instituted if it should be indicated.

Overt expressions of hostility may take the form of sarcastic, abusive or rude remarks. Freud tells us that a hostile joke is one way to satisfy an instinct by circumventing an obstacle that stands in the way of this satisfaction.[11] The person may be argumentative, demanding, verbally attacking or threatening. Rejection and fault-finding are other indications of a hostile attitude. Such behavior is usually motivated by fear and a distorted perception of a threat to the self or the self-image. The hostility thus generated is then displaced onto another object which in some way symbolized the danger.

Resentful silence or deliberate avoidance needs to be dealt with gently but directly before any meaningful communication or therapeutic nursing intervention can take place. The nurse may tell the patient that she or he observed the patient's silence or avoidance and inquire if something has happened. Recognition of the fact that the patient appears troubled will convey the nurse's concern and willingness to help. Regardless of whether this brings only further silence or an angry outburst, the nurse must be prepared to accept the patient as he or she is and to continue to meet the nursing needs in every way possible.

Accepting the patient does not in any way imply that the nurse should abdicate responsibility to set reasonable limits or controls, should this become necessary. Occasionally, the free expression of hostile feelings may excite the patient instead of relieving the tension. The subsequent feeling of guilt then tends to be projected in the form of hostility, onto the nurse, whom the patient sees as responsible for his or her behavior to some degree. Some patients, especially those with strong authoritarian traits, respond to limit-setting much more readily than they do to discussion and ventilation. Their anxiety is lessened when they feel that the "danger-control persons" show no signs of weakness, but seem to be really in control and can be depended upon to help them preserve their self-respect. Only a sound understanding of the dynamics of human behavior, derived both from theory and clinical experience, will enable the nurse to make the discriminating judgments necessary in deciding upon the most helpful approach for any given individual. The following clinical examples illustrate a variety of approaches, most of which seemed to be of some help in reducing the patients' anxiety and enabling them to begin to cope with their situation in a more constructive manner.

One of the most difficult of all situations for nurses to face and to deal with occurs when overt hostility, which they had in no way anticipated, is focused directly on them. When the hostility is anticipated, some thought and planning can be given to dealing with the problem. However, when such open hostility and verbal abuse are unexpectedly encountered, nurses are placed in a very difficult position as they try to deal with their own anxiety and the patients' evident antagonism and rejection. The following incident exemplifies such a situation:

> The A family had been scheduled for a routine clinic appointment, but failed to keep it. A nursing student who had been working with the family visited the home to ascertain the reason for the missed appointment. Greatly to her surprise, she was received with unmistakable signs of hostility. At first, they refused to open the door and, when they did, they blocked the entrance to her. When she gained reluctant permission to enter, both family members placed their legs up on the available chairs in such a way that she was prevented from being seated. The mother accused the nurse in loud, angry tones, stating that she had not contacted the clinic to clarify the patient's appointment as she had said she would. The father spoke to the mother in loud tones saying (about the nurse) "She is

no help . . . you see you can't depend on her." Both expressed a wish to have the nurse discontinue her services to the family. The nurse attempted to calm both parties and to encourage description in sequential order of the wife's missed appointment and her understanding of the arrangements. Both patients resisted these attempts and continued to express their hostile feelings. At this point, the nurse realized the futility of attempting to discuss the matter and permitted them to verbalize their hostile feelings. Upon leaving, she stated she would contact them at a later date.

After conferring with the mental health consultant, the nurse wrote a letter to the family, explaining the misunderstanding and saying she would call them the following week. It was decided that a letter would be the best approach at this time, because it would give them something concrete to refer to and would also give them time to prepare for the visit. When the nurse telephoned the home to confirm the appointment, the mother was still taciturn and monosyllabic. However, when she did make the visit, both clients were very friendly and open, even to the point of prolonging the visit beyond the scheduled hour.

In retrospect, it can be said that the nurse used the only approach open to her at the time of the initial visit: she accepted the persons as individuals by permitting them to talk without retaliation and counterhostility. Possibly the most important factor in reestablishing working relationships was the nurse's concern for the welfare of her clients. She demonstrated by her actions that she considered them important and would proceed with any nursing intervention they needed if they would permit it. Her letter not only presented whatever factual information was necessary to clear up the misconception, but again acknowledged their importance as people who had a right to an explanation.

Hostile relationships among patients can pose a ward problem that, once it is identified, calls for a creative and consistent approach on the part of the nursing team. An attempt must be made to reduce hostility-provoking stimuli and to provide a measure of acceptance and security for these patients. The following is an example of overt hostility which was, nevertheless, indirectly expressed:

Two elderly ladies occupied beds next to each other in a four-bed ward in a general hospital. One carefully kept her curtains drawn all day, thus creating for herself an area of isolation which could not be disturbed without vociferous protest. Because each took a considerable amount of nursing time, they were usually assigned for care to two different nurses who worked simultaneously. During the time each was receiving morning care, one of the patients kept up a running line of comments about the "old lady in the next bed. She's really not all there, you know." . . . "She doesn't like anyone." . . . "She's pretty sick, do you think she'll make it?" Meanwhile, the other patient was remarking to her nurse about that "mean old woman in that bed over there." The problem was discussed at a team conference. It was noted that each of the participants in the "feud" could communicate with the other only indirectly. By using the nurses as deflectors of a sort they were able to establish at least a negative relationship with each other. Because direct confrontation might have proved too traumatic and resulted in a need to save face by still further strengthening of defenses, it was decided to try an indirect approach, which would provide opportunity for the two patients to speak with each other directly while both nurses were present, to facilitate the process and to provide a feeling of security.

The following morning, both patients were taken in wheelchairs to the lounge area by their respective nurses. They were formally introduced to each other and both nurses sat down to engage them in friendly conversation. This became a daily event and, as they began to know each other better, nursing personnel were able to gradually withdraw. The two ladies found a number of common interests and began to enjoy each other's company, even within the ward situation.

One might conjecture at length on the basic motives for the original hostility. As it was, for some reason, each of these patients had felt in some way threatened by the other. When the misperceptions began to be cleared and they had additional firsthand information about each other, the hostility between them seemed to be resolved. Accepting their need to communicate through a third person and working from this knowledge was the approach chosen by this particular nursing staff. Other alternatives might have been tried, but the basic principle from which nursing intervention was derived is that of recognizing the hostile behavior, accepting the patient's need to deal with a perceived threat, and trying in some way to reduce the threat by clarifying the misperceptions from which it seems to emanate. When the unknown became the known, the fear had no further foundation in reality.

Most patients find it difficult to express anger or hostility toward authority figures, particularly if they themselves are authoritarian personalities. If the patients have invested the nurses with an authority role, nurses may need to be even more perceptive in recognizing distress signals that appear in the guise of hostility. They may find, too, that the patients need considerable encouragement before being able to trust their nurses enough to voice what is distressing them. One such incident is recounted below:

> A highly successful professional man had been hospitalized and placed on bed rest. A new nursing supervisor was struck by the apparently hostile feeling of the nursing staff toward this patient. He was described as "impossible," "with a chip on his shoulder" and "sarcastic." When the supervisor entered his room, she found a very unhappy, taciturn man in the bed; his wife sat quietly by with a worried expression. The nurse introduced herself and the patient remarked sarcastically:
>
> Patient: Oh, so they sent the supervisor.
>
> Nurse: I've been trying to get acquainted with the patients. How is everything with you, Mr. B.?
>
> P.: (sarcastically) Oh, everything is just fine.
>
> N.: That's not the impression I get, Mr. B. Something seems to be troubling you.
>
> P.: Oh, no, nothing at all. There's no use going into all that! Just forget about me. I guess I'll be OK.
>
> N.: You don't sound very convincing to me, Mr. B. Is there something I can do to help?
>
> Here, the patient began to pour out, in an angry and aggrieved tone, all the frustrations he had been brooding over for the past few days. At this point, his wife placed her hand on his arm, admonishing him not to complain. The nurse continued to encourage him to describe and clarify. Some of his protests were legitimate struggles against complete helplessness and dependency. Added to this was the stress of apparently trying to live up to his wife's expectations of what a good patient should be and do. After a nursing conference, adjustments were made in the plan of care, thus individualizing it more. Time was also set aside during which he could talk about the things that were disturbing him, and an effort was made to respect his needs and preferences as much as possible. By the time he was discharged the following week, his anxious, hostile behavior had abated, and a better understanding was beginning to develop between him and the nursing staff.

The initial reluctance to speak displayed by this patient in the presence of an authority figure was overcome by the encouragement and acceptance that the nurse conveyed. Empathy and sensitivity are especially important in a situation of this kind. Pushing a patient into revealing what he or she is not yet ready to discuss can be harmful and it may result in intensification of the anxiety that caused the problem in the first place. The patient needs time to learn how far he or she can trust and may need more than one visit to feel free enough to speak about the trouble. The nurse can inquire directly what the problem seems to be, but the patient must be ready before a productive working through can take place. In the example just cited, mutual withdrawal of the patient and the nursing staff from each other had become progressively more pronounced and would have continued, had the intervention not been direct and prompt. This patient was behaving in a way that was alienating and rejecting the very people on whom he most depended for help at this time.

The following incident illustrates what can occur when nurses are unaware that their actions are not only one cause of the patients' hostility, but actually reinforce the hostile, resentful behavior patients adopt in an almost last-ditch fight to defend their self-image and punish those who seem to deprive them of the esteem and approval they so sorely need.

> Mrs. L. occupied the first bed next to the door in a five-bed ward. Mrs. K., the patient next to her, was a very sweet, compliant person, with many friends and visitors, and was well liked by everyone except her next-bed neighbor, Mrs. L. This neighbor's rude remarks frequently reduced Mrs. K. to tears, yet she never fought back. Students assigned to Mrs. K. were indignant with Mrs. L. for her seemingly unjust attacks on Mrs. K., but were at a loss to know how to deal with Mrs. L.'s hostile behavior. In an effort to comfort Mrs. K., they redoubled their efforts to give her tender, loving care and withdrew still more from Mrs. L. The problem was discussed with the psychiatric consultant, and the students were helped to see what a vicious cycle had unwittingly been set in motion. As Mrs. L. saw herself more rejected, her anxiety rose, and, with it, the need to defend herself in the only way she knew: hostility and verbal attack. As a first approach, it was suggested that each nurse who passed her bed would acknowledge Mrs. L. by a friendly, "Good-morning, Mrs. L.," being careful to use her name, or by a smile or nod of recognition. An attempt was made by Mrs. L.'s nurse to spend time with her daily, talking with her in a friendly, relaxed way. The staff were also helped to recognize the psychological harm being done Mrs. K. by the reinforcement of her neurotic, compliant behavior and her attempt to control the situation by playing the martyr. Through their strong positive response, they were providing effective feedback, which encouraged this behavior still more. As the plan went into effect, Mrs. L.'s sarcastic, biting remarks became less frequent, and nursing personnel were agreeably surprised to find her a friendly, humorous person, who now dealt with them on a much more mature level.

Covert hostility, of which the hostile person is not aware, may be unwittingly translated into behavior that is perceived by the other person as hostile. The following is an interesting example of how the nurse's own unconscious may betray her or him into an automatic, hostile response:

> Mrs. X. had undergone extensive surgery for a radical mastectomy. While the nurse was assisting the physician for the first postoperative dressing, the patient started to look down at the unsightly incision. Quickly but gently, the nurse placed her hand on the patient's cheek, turning her head to prevent her from seeing the wound. The patient accepted this submissively, without comment. Several weeks after she had been discharged from the hospital, the patient met the nurse during one of her return visits for a check-up. She remarked to the nurse: "Do you remember the day you slapped me? I'd never have believed you would slap me, but you did." Surprised at this misinterpretation of what had been meant as a kindly gesture, the nurse protested that she had not slapped her. No amount of explanation, however, would convince this lady that it had not been a slap. Not a very hard one, of course, but still a slap.

One might, as a first reaction, say that the patient's own hostility caused her to project these feelings onto the nurse and thus see the nurse as hostile. However, as the nurse began to look at herself more honestly, she asked herself a number of questions: Why did she react so automatically to the patient's gesture? What would have happened had she permitted the patient to look at the wound? Was she being overprotective? If so, perhaps this reactivated the patient's childhood feelings about an overprotective parent. Or, to be still more honest, perhaps the nurse saw her own self-image as the good nurse or the "good mother" threatened by some imaginary harm to the patient for which she might be responsible. If this were really the case, the hand that she placed on the patient's cheek might not have been as gentle as she liked to think. The answers probably lie somewhere in between, for the complex dynamism of human behavior usually does not admit any simple explanation. It does point up, however, the fact that hostility can be unconscious, and that it may be a reciprocal process of which neither of the persons involved is fully aware.

Each person who exhibits hostile behavior has a unique background and reasons for behaving that way. If the hostility results from the illness or from some existing situation, it usually subsides as the person becomes better or the situation improves. If the hostility is deep-seated and part of the person's life-long pattern of defense, it will require professional psychotherapy. In either case, nurses must be able to recognize the cues that signal hostility. Their first action should always be to look at themselves and their own feelings. Just as a patient may misperceive or distort a situation, the nurse, who belongs to the same human race, may have childhood experiences and images reactivated by something in a situation.

It is not always easy to distinguish between hostility (which is motivated by the wish to hurt or humiliate) and healthy self-assertion, which is part of the normal human process of the exercise of individual rights. One of the marks of emotional maturity is a healthy striving toward self-actualization. This implies the ability to perceive reality correctly in relation to one's own life situation and to assume personal responsibility for one's own actions. This self-assertion, which is part of the growth process, may be difficult to exercise within the structure of our highly efficient automated health systems. Persons who do assert themselves for justifiable reason, refusing to surrender their independence, may fail to conform to what is expected of patients. The staff may criticize them accordingly.

Nurses who have learned to recognize their own feelings and to bring them under conscious control are usually able to respond in a professional and disciplined manner to the patients' hostile expression of underlying fears. The nurses' response reflects acceptance and understanding; usually the attack is not so much against them personally as it is a reaction to the whole frustrating situation as the patients see it. Nurses need to keep in mind, however, that there may be times when they find themselves under a real emotional strain in trying to cope with particularly trying patients whose hostility seems to be chronic and who are beginning to wear down their own emotional reserves. This is an occupational hazard for which nurses need counsel and support from those professionally qualified to help. The nursing supervisor, mental health consultant or other qualified person should be available in order to lend whatever assistance and support is needed at this time to carry out therapeutic nursing intervention. If nurses are able to demonstrate sincere concern for patients and their welfare, they help patients meet and resolve the crisis; once the anxiety is allayed, patients can begin to stabilize and use the proferred assistance in constructive ways. Nurses can only do this if they feel relatively comfortable in this anxiety-laden situation.

An understanding of the dynamic bases of hostility—and the behavioral processes which hostility activates—is essential for the competent nursing practitioner. When nurses perceive behavior that seems to indicate hostility, they need to check out their observations with someone else in the situation whenever possible. The first necessary step in effective nursing intervention is for nurses to validate their assumptions with the patients, assist them in the description and clarification of what they are experiencing and the possible reasons behind these feelings. To be aware of their own reactions, to accept the patients without giving either approval or disapproval, and to avoid value judgments will sometimes be difficult for nurses, but these are the essential ingredients of therapeutic nursing. Skill in detecting the patients' unspoken wish for limit setting and the ability to control without being punitive or retaliating demand maturity and professional acumen. Most important of all is the effort nurses exert to ameliorate the circumstances causing the hostility and to enable the patients to maintain pride and self-respect. Working in this way, nurses truly assist patients to grow in self-understanding and achieve optimal health and self-actualization.

REFERENCES

1. Schless, A. P., Mendels, I., Kipperman, A., and Cochrane, C.: Depression and hostility. J. Nervous and Mental Disease. 159, 2:91-100, August 1974; Rothenberg, A.: On anger. Am. J. Psychiatry. 128, 4:454-60, October 1971; Novaco, R. W.: Stress innoculation: a cognitive therapy for anger and its application to a case of depression. J. Consulting and Clinical Psychol. 45, 4:600-08, 1977.
2. Rothenberg, On anger.
3. Bach-Y-Rita, G., Veno, A.: Habitual violence: a profile of 62 men. Am. J. Psychiatry. 131, 9:1015-17, 1974; Penningroth, P. E.: Control of violence in a mental health setting. Am. J. Nurs. 75, 4:606-09, 1975; Lion, J. R., Madden, D., Christopher, R.: A violence clinic: three years experience. *In*: Scientific Proceedings in Summary Form: 128th Annual Meeting, American Psychiatric Assn., 1975, pp. 109-10; Isle, W. P.: Malpractice liability of the mental health professional. Professional Psychol. 6, 4:399-412, 1975.
4. Schless, Mendels, Kipperman, and Cochrane, Depression and hostility.
5. Symonds, M.: Psychodynamics of aggression in women. Am. J. Psychoanal. 6, 3:195-203, Fall 1976.
6. Rothenberg, On anger.
7. Horney, K.: The neurotic personality of our time. *In* Collected Works of Karen Horney. Vol. I. New York, Norton, 1937, p. 63.
8. Dunbar, F.: Emotions and Bodily Changes. 4th Ed. New York, Columbia University Press, 1954; Alexander, F.: Psychosomatic Medicine. New York, Norton, 1950.

9. Engel, G.: Psychogenic pain and the pain-prone patient. Am. J. Med. 26:899, 1959.
10. Kübler-Ross, E.: On Death and Dying. New York, Macmillan, 1969.
11. Freud, S.: Jokes and Their Relation to the Unconscious. Trans. by J. Strachey. New York, Norton, 1961, p. 101.

ADDITIONAL READINGS

Adler, G., Shapiro, L.: Some difficulties in the treatment of the aggressive acting-out patient. Am. J. Psychotherapy. 27, 4:548-56, 1973.

Berkowitz, L.: The case for bottling up rage. Psychol. Today. July 1973, pp. 24-31.

Bird, B.: The patient with hidden anger. *In* Bird, B.: Talking with Patients. 2nd Ed. Philadelphia, Lippincott, 1973.

De Rossi, H. A.: Supervision of the first year psychiatric resident. Part VII: Hostility toward the family. Psychiat. Q. 45, 4:559-73, 1971.

Gerber, L.: Countertransference with a hostile, dependent patient—what the books don't tell you. Voices. 10, 4:56-60, 1975.

Gil. D.: Violence against Children. Cambridge, Mass., Harvard University Press, 1971.

Henderson, I. W. D.: Hermes and beyond. J. Thanatology. 1, 6:468-83, 1971.

Jeglijewski, J. M.: Nursing the amputee. Am. J. Nurs. 73, 6:1024-27, 1973.

Lion, J. R., Pasternak, S. A.: Countertransference reactions to violent patients. Am. J. Psychiatry. 130, 2:207-10, 1973.

Milberg, I. L.: Pinpointing emotional factors in skin diseases. Pract. Psychol. for Physicians. 3, 1:49, 53-56, 1976.

Novaco, R. W.: The functions and regulation of the arousal of anger. Am. J. Psychiatry. 133, 10:1124-28, 1976.

Pasternak, S. A.: Violence and Victims. New York, Halstead, 1975.

Reichsman, F., Reichsman, L., and Norman, B.: Problems in adaptation to maintenance hemodialysis. Arch. Intern. Med. 130, 6:859-65, December 1972.

Weismann, M. M., Klerman, G., and Paykell, E.: Clinical evaluation of hostility in depression. Am. J. Psychiatry. 128, 3:261-66, 1971.

Wunderlich, R. A., et al.: Psychological considerations in physical therapy for obese patients. Phys. Ther. 53, 7:757-61, 1973.

8 RESTLESSNESS

Catherine M. Norris

Once upon a time a curious nurse became fascinated with the subject of insomnia—that indescribable misery suffered by so many persons under stress. Patients and nurses, she had noted, reported many reasons for not sleeping, such as restlessness, inability to relax, weakness, chill, nausea, overtiredness, and listlessness. But, when put to it, the nurse found she could not define these terms and, to her amazement and chagrin, she could not even describe the behavior they represented. This is when she really became curious.

Starting with the word, restlessness, she found nursing notes liberally sprinkled with reports of this phenomenon. "Patient restless; unable to sleep." "Restless night." "Restless after 3 A.M.—tossing and turning." Clarifying the meaning of restlessness seemed only as far away as the dictionary. But, to the nurse's surprise, two commonly used medical dictionaries neither listed nor defined the word.[1] She then turned to indices of health literature, only to discover that restlessness was not even indexed.[2] Nursing and medical literature seemed to be written with the assumption that everyone already *knew* what restlessness meant.

So the curious nurse found herself thinking, "If thousands of nurses (and doctors) have been using the word during a century of enlightened practice, I should know restlessness when I see it." On the other hand, she thought, "If a word is not defined and little can be found in the literature about the behavior the word represents, how can one recognize it? What kind of communication values does it have? How can nurses do research and teach nursing when there are no adequate definitions or descriptions of the phenomena of nursing?"

The curious nurse decided that neither she, the clinicians nor the researchers knew what they were talking about. With this conclusion she felt a sense of urgency for nurses who are at the bedside to *observe* and *describe* nursing events, until nurses, wherever or however they work, have the data they need to recognize and assign meaning to the phenomena of nursing.

Our curious nurse clinician tried talking with colleagues about where one

Copyright February 1975, The American Journal of Nursing Company. Reproduced, with some additional material, with permission from Nursing Outlook, Vol. 23, No. 2.

goes and what one does to identify an undefined, undescribed behavioral phenomenon. After much discussing, going to the dictionary, searching the literature, and asking nursing experts, she abandoned this mode of investigation as having little payoff. In fact, she began to entertain the idea that restlessness occurs so frequently and is characteristic of so many conditions that its presence has little or no usefulness in communicating about people.

A BEGINNING

Then, as she sat gazing out the window one October day, she noticed a tree full of birds fluttering and hopping as they flocked for their flight south. Suddenly a neon light flickered, then flashed: Restlessness. Our nurse detective searched the literature on migration and found many articles on migration of both land and sea animals.[3] Migratory creatures, she discovered, characteristically become restless before they organize and take off for other homes. Hibernating animals also become restless as they organize themselves for the long sleep.

While the internal organs of the body produce the vast amounts of energy required for restless behavior, it is thought that the environment provides the triggering mechanism. Changes in food supply, temperature and length of the photoperiod, deprivation of shelter, increasing population density, storm activity and other environmental conditions involving barometric changes have been identified as triggering mechanisms and studied by animal physiologists. All the published reports of restlessness that the nurse reviewed indicated that change—often change that threatens habitual practices, rhythms, personal space or physiological homeostasis—was in some way the triggering mechanism for restless behavior.

CLINICAL MANIFESTATIONS

Our curious nurse now began to get a feeling for the subject and, because she is a clinician, went back to the clinical area, where she reviewed her nursing practice, talked with other nurses and observed restless patients. She discovered that there seems to be several kinds of restlessness. Many of the nurses, for instance, believed they could differentiate between the kinds of restless behavior associated with such widely varying conditions as impending death, incipient insulin shock, diabetic coma and mania. Some said they could even distinguish between the restlessness stemming from boredom, associated with anxiety, signifying possible internal hemorrhage and shock or indicating intracranial pressure.

Some nurses said they used restlessness as a diagnostic sign or early predictor of complications or danger. When asked for the data used to make these determinations, however, they were unable to specify the critical behavioral variables. While this may have been due to poor observation, a more likely explanation is the intuitive nature of much of nursing practice or the possibility that much of the data of restlessness is auditory—the sounds, for instance, of a person tossing in the bed, creaking beds, tapping fingers, sighs—and nurses are not as carefully prepared to hear as to see.

Restlessness seems to be expressed in many ways: by tossing, turning or twisting in bed, by pacing, tapping with fingers or feet, picking with the fingers, scratching, or other motor activity of a repetitive, seemingly urgent and not purposefully controlled or directed nature. Facial expression may be tense, watchful or fearful. The rate or amount of speech may increase. Dilated pupils may accompany restlessness as may skin temperature and color changes, but whether they should be considered part of the phenomenon is not certain since nervous and vasomotor changes in restlessness are unknown. Time may be distorted, with the restless person finding time slow or "losing track of it."

SOME INITIAL GENERALIZATIONS

Even with this description our nurse could not identify the phenomenon so everyone would know exactly what it is. The indicators were not constant enough in a sufficient number of cases to permit naming. So our nurse detective tried to narrow it down by asking: *Who is restless?* Restlessness seems to be a universal phenomenon in animal life. The most fruitful descriptions were found in the literature on migration of birds and animals, hibernation, and animal sexual behavior.

Next she asked: If everyone is subject to restlessness, *when does it occur?* Restlessness seems to occur only under certain conditions. In lower animals it appears to be fairly specific to the species. Changes in light, food supply, air turbulence, environmental temperature and barometric pressure, singly or in combination, trigger restlessness. Intimate association with pets can verify this observation.

In humans restless behavior seems to occur in response to internal as well as external stimuli related to change, the unexpected, the unknown or other circumstances that might present a threat. Seasonal rhythms affect humans as well as animals; one nurse mentioned "spring fever." It probably originates in complex relationships among geophysical and electromagnetic fields with physiological processes.

As our nurse delved still further, she asked: *How does one experience restlessness?* Restlessness does have feeling or perceived aspects, but one may or may not be aware of being restless. And one may be unable to specify how it feels. Some people express it as feelings of tension, uneasiness, excitement, anticipation, impending doom, danger or the sense that all is not well. It may be accompanied by impatience and an urge to be "doing something." Feelings of boredom, meaninglessness and emptiness may also occur.

Some people are aware of the motor aspects and recognize that constant activity makes the uneasiness tolerable. It may be that much of the experience of restlessness is at the "gut" rather than the perceptual level. The phenomenon appears much more complex as one talks with nurses and patients than when one studies migratory behavior.

Human restlessness seems to be related to a person's perception of others, events or his or her situation, but it may originate entirely from within the body. It may be related to the inability to receive or understand external messages put into the system as well as messages originating within the system. This would then be cause-effect related to perception.

RESTLESSNESS VERSUS REST

Our nurse now had some beginning information about population, occurrence, appearance and experience of restlessness. But she had nothing which indicated its function and little information about cause and effect. She reached a stalemate with colleagues and patients at this point and started grasping at straws, one of which was the concept of rest. If restlessness is a state of nonrest, she reasoned, then contrasting it with the state of rest might be productive.

Four general ideas—all positive values—are associated with rest. One idea expresses a state of peace, tranquility, mental and spiritual calm, refreshing quiet, or emotional ease. A second idea is that of an absence of motion, inactivity, quiescence or being quiet. A third idea contrasts rest with some other state, such as inactivity after labor, freedom from troubles or disturbances and cessation of motion or action. Last, rest is seen as the result of a specific action, as "to rest my eyes on" or "rest against something."

Restlessness as a condition of nonrest, then, could be characterized by a negative mental state which is *not* tranquil, peaceful, or refreshing; by a state of motion and activity; by an inability to relax after work, to cease motion and activity, plus a continuing burden of troubles or problems; and, finally, by the absence of specific rest-creating objects or experiences. Thus analyzed, restlessness is characterized by inability to remain at rest; uneasiness, unquiet, unceasing activity; and the absence of, or the inability to perceive or respond to, quiet and inaction.

WORDS AND VALUES

Thinking about some of those words, our nurse clinician was struck by what the English language did to the words "rest" and "restless." If language influences and guides ideas and the way people think about these ideas, she reflected, one could look at the kinds of values and impressions that are commonly associated with restlessness.

A restless person in our society is apt to be a nonconformist, a questioner, a complainer, and maybe an activist or an "actor-outer." This is bad for the orderly conduct of a group-oriented, bureaucratic society! People who are restless in their jobs may not be dependable or steady—which is bad! Adolescents who are restless may take drugs, become sexually involved, drop out of school or bum around the country—which is bad! People who are restless under stress may be unpredictable, not in control, and this is bad! People who are restless in their professional careers may be searching for the unattainable and chronically unhappy, and this is bad!

Restlessness, our nurse realized, has many negative connotations. In contrast, symbols conjured up by the words restful and resting suggest coolness, serenity, calmness, comfort and ease. These are good! When nurses call a patient "restless," therefore, the negative values associated with the word may prevent them from seeing restlessness as possibly beneficial, helpful, protective or useful.

(These value attributes may be true only in our own culture, however. In countries where childbearing practices include swaddling, bundling and strapping onto cradleboards that restrict free, random physical activity for long periods of time, one might expect restlessness to have different values and meanings than where physical activity is allowed and encouraged in infancy and childhood.)

CAUSE, EFFECT AND PURPOSE

But if restlessness is to have meaning for clinical nursing, our nurse detective reasoned, then she would have to identify or speculate about cause, effect and purpose. Remembering her exploration into restlessness in animals, she began by observing that some human restlessness is triggered by the same environmental changes that cause premigratory animal restlessness. She also noted that some human restlessness is triggered by changes beginning and occurring in internal surfaces of the body—for example, hemorrhage or toxicity. (This may be true for animals, too.)

In addition, because of humans' highly developed intellectual apparatus, our *perception* of changes and conditions as strange, incomprehensible, threatening, exciting or challenging would need to be considered restlessness-producing. In both animals and humans, disturbances or disruption in biological rhythmicity, especially circadian rhythm, could cause restlessness.

Some people make some fairly specific correlations of certain conditions or events with restlessness. Fatigue and boredom are commonly said to predispose to restlessness. Role deprivation might be another cause. Certain disease conditions are accompanied by or characterized by restless behavior: for instance, thyrotoxicosis, the manic and sometimes the depressed phases of manic-depressive psychoses and epilepsy just before seizures. Some physiological conditions are also correlated with restlessness: internal hemorrhage, drug idiosyncracy, hyperinsulinism, impending diabetic coma, elevated body temperature. Pain and anxiety also correlate with restlessness.

But how to find meaning in all this? How to bring the large number of instances of restlessness and the wide variety of behavioral variables into some cause-and-effect, purposeful relationship? Taking a wild conceptual leap, our nurse clinician theorizes that restlessness may be one's first, or one of the first, responses to change, strangeness or threat.

It is already known that the first response to disease or emotional disturbance is often some modification in the sleeping-waking diurnal cycle—loss of sleep, restless sleep or increased duration of sleep. Neurophysiologically, sleeplessness is accompanied by increased cortical vigilance. Restlessness, whether in sleep or awake, is also accompanied by increased vigilance, but whether there is some relationship between inability to sleep and restlessness is not known. The same cortical-hypothalamic mechanism might be operating in both types of experience.

Restlessness may belong to a group of disturbances in rhythmicity (insomnia, loss of appetite, irritability) which herald dis-ease or a newer, higher level of functioning. It may have a warning function. Restless behavior, then, may have defense as its purpose—beginning defense at least, or initiation of a coping process. While the activity itself may seem random and without observable purpose, it may be a tooling-up phase in relation to human coping activities.

In fact, restless behavior might be viewed as a transitional state between change and problem-solving, or between one homeostatic state and the development of a new dynamic equilibrium. In view of the role of activity in energy demand and production, this idea makes sense. It also makes sense in view of the idea that intuitive knowledge can be very perceptive and accurate. Thus restlessness may be a primitive defensive response to a primitive perception of danger, as diagrammed in Figure 8-1. In terms of health, it may represent the generation of the energy needed to cope.

THE COURSE OF RESTLESSNESS

It has been observed that restlessness may begin with small muscle activity. A variety of finger gestures involving one or both hands includes rubbing, folding, tapping, playing and pill-rolling activities. Fingers may also be used to scratch, pick or run through the hair. The clicking of ball point pens at conferences and meetings is becoming a classic sign of restlessness among nurses. When the toes are visible they may be observed wiggling.

If restlessness is not relieved in this phase, gross muscle activity develops. People may be observed to shift weight from one part of the body to another—moving from side to side, resting face on hand supported by elbow, pacing, wiggling, startling easily (becoming jumpy), changing posture, kicking the air, crossing and uncrossing legs, sliding down in chair or bed, picking up and dropping or spilling something. Also, reapplying one's makeup, changing or continually smoothing clothes or thrashing around in bed are typical signs of restless behavior.

Some nurses think that if restless behavior is not resolved in this phase there is a third phase, characterized by aggressive behavior. This may include getting up and leaving, making a noise, putting on one's light, saying the

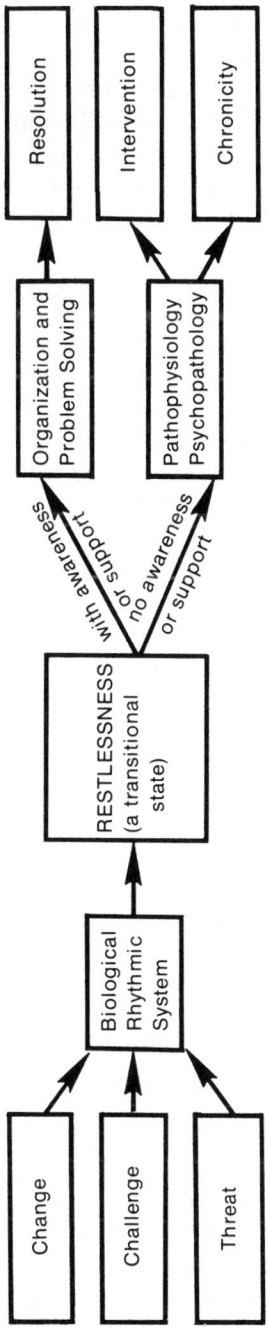

Figure 8-1. *Process of Model of Restlessness*

session is over, making some kind of mess or demanding something. It has been suggested that disorientation may be one pathological resolution of this stage. The activities representing restlessness are repetitive and may be rhythmic.

There are nurses who conceptualize small muscle activity as sending a small or weak message, large muscle activity as sending a strong message and aggressive behavior as sending a demanding message. When messages arise from inside the body, the later phases might be characterized by action but also by hypotension, shock or some form of physiological crisis.

A TENTATIVE CONCEPT

Our nurse clinician theorist now had quite a lot of information, but restlessness was still standing alone, unrelated to nursing or any other body of knowledge. She thought of tying it to anxiety but that was too narrow, to adaptation but that seemed too broad; so she tried to relate it to human rhythmicity. She abstracted the major ideas and attempted to organize them logically to provide another view of the concept of restlessness.

1. One characteristic that all life has in common is rhythmicity.
2. All physiologic activity, as an aspect of life, is characterized by some kind of rhythm.
3. Biological rhythms are a function of the internal environment (physiological), external environment (geophysical, electromagnetic, social) or both.
4. Biological rhythms for each species or each type of living organism are essentially specific to that particular species or group of organisms.
5. Some rhythms are genetically determined while others are learned.
6. Whether learned or genetically determined, biological rhythms may have behavioral as well as critically related physiological variables.
7. Maintenance of the organism's existing rhythms—again, whether learned or genetically determined—is essential to the well-being of the organism.
8. Interference with or change in the organism's normal biological rhythms signals the need for adaptation of some kind at some level.
9. This need for adaptation is manifested by an increase in energy production and energy expenditure.
10. The first visible evidence of energy production and expenditure due to change in a biological rhythmic process is restlessness.
11. The first experiential evidence of threat to a biological rhythm may be felt as restlessness.
12. Restlessness is an apparently nonspecific, nonpurposeful, nondirectional, randomly diffuse human activity, but with the real purpose of preparing the organism to cope (see Figure 8-2).

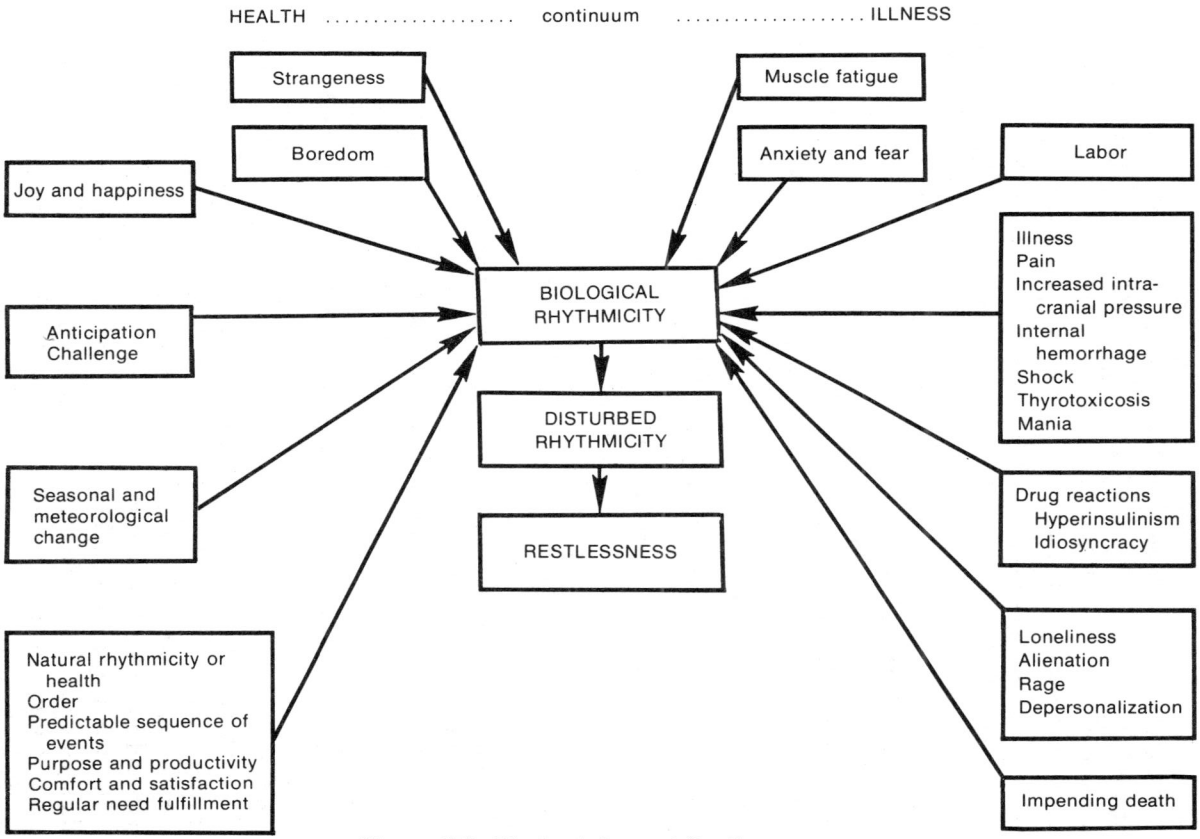

Figure 8-2. *Rhythmicity and Restlessness*

This explanation would not be complete without a definition, for there probably would have been no exploration if the dictionary had defined restlessness. Our nurse clinician says:

> Restlessness is a universal, discontinuous, animal behavior evidenced by nonspecific, repetitive, unorganized, diffuse, apparently nonpurposeful motor activity that is subject to limited control.

Nurses using this definition still would not be able to say, "This patient is restless!" The question remains: "How will I know it when I see it?"

When all the behaviors our nurse observed were summarized, there seemed to be only five indicators of restlessness that are always present. Even these may not hold up in the face of rigorous research. But for the moment, if (1) *increased,* (2) *repetitive,* (3) *apparently purposeless skeletomuscular activity* is present, accompanied by (4) *urgency in repeating the activity,* and (5) *increase in muscle tonus of the body, face or both,* our nurse clinician theorist says the patient is restless.

NEED FOR DESCRIPTIVE DATA

There are many more chapters to this story but they are not yet written. Our nurse clinician would be happy forever after if hundreds of observational and phenomenological descriptions of restlessness were done by clinicians in any place where they work. Different types of restlessness need to be described.

How does the restlessness of the dying patient differ from that of the patient who has hyperinsulinism or the patient who is bored? Can we come up with descriptions of the urgency to pick the bedclothes, the darting, faraway eye movements, the getting out of bed attempts, the listening gestures, and the urgency for speech represented by the words without sound or with muffled sound that are often discernible in the mouth and lip movements of the dying patient?

Can we describe better the eyes darting around fearfully looking for help, the handwringing, arm and leg rubbing, uneasiness of the patient having an insulin reaction? Can we delineate more effectively the gross tossing, thrashing, turning, heaving, big muscle activity of the bored person, with the half groan, half moan, the impatient thrust of the pillows or yank at the sheets, and the indignant flashes of the eyes? We need so many of these descriptions if we are to give reliability to the word "restlessness."

Interestingly, experiences involving great joy, enthusiasm or anticipation that require changes in behavior are often characterized by extremes in restlessness. But in terms of rhythmicity, one might expect restlessness as a component of any required change in whatever direction. According to some reports by patients and nurses, it takes as much energy to experience happiness as it does to deal with a negatively perceived threat.

SPECIFIC RESTLESSNESS SITUATIONS

There is some agreement among nurses who work in intensive care units that there is a characteristic restlessness that precedes myocardial infarction and cerebrovascular accident. They describe the patient's eyes as darting back and forth to the clock. The patient talks a lot, jumping from one subject to another, asks for things, asks to be checked—for example, intravenous site, catheter, dressing—licks his or her lips, asks about the welfare of other patients, and very often ultimately asks to sit on the edge of the bed or to get out of bed. Nurses indicate that these restless behaviors may start as long as 24 hours before the infarct or stroke.

Substantial information about restless behavior could be generated by data from patients in coronary and intensive care units under constant electronic monitoring. These circumstances allow nurses to examine the events preceding the restlessness, those coincident with it, and the coping behavior which follows it. Restless movements more often than not produce artifacts in the monitor readout. Many coronary care units and intensive care units routinely monitor patients on videotape in addition to the monitor readout. One step might be to start correlating restlessness with other variables from banked videotapes.

In infants restlessness is seen as expressing an unmet need, such as hunger, interpersonal comfort, or coldness. Infants squirm, wiggle, rock their bodies from side to side, rock their heads from side to side as well as flex and unflex arms and legs. Yawning or whimpering may accompany the restless motor activity before the infant moves to a more aggressive form of behavior—crying.

DEFENSES AGAINST RESTLESSNESS

Some nurses believe they observe people who eat when they are not hungry, smoke more than usual or do repetitive sublimation-type activities such as knitting, sewing, crocheting or playing solitaire to defend against their restlessness. This observation again raises the question of the relationship between restlessness and anxiety.

NURSING CARE IN RESTLESSNESS

Some nurses take the position that restlessness is uncomfortable. They believe it becomes increasingly uncomfortable if it is unrelieved and procedes to gross motor or aggressive activity. These nurses believe that nurses should intervene in restless behavior in the earliest possible phase. In the intensive care unit assessment of vital signs, including blood pressure, and reporting both the signs and the restless behaviors may permit medical decisions that will prevent serious pathological outcomes. Nurses try to reassure by communicating, "I am watching the monitor; I am taking care of you. You are never alone. I am here."

Nurses identify offering food, a snack or warm drink as one kind of intervention if the person feels this would be helpful. Food or snack also provides a change of focus or diversion when people are bored as well as symbolizes one of the most primitive sources of comfort. It provides a change of pace from routine activity. Warm bathing and baths may be useful with both adults and children in hospitals or at home. Nurses identify verbal reassurance and support as useful for people who feel fearful, alone and lonely, and this includes many older people. Companionship, which has its roots in the sharing of bread, may be enough by itself to intervene in much restless behavior. Touch, massage and cuddling where appropriate have all been used by nurses to intervene in restless behavior.

If the assessment of restless behavior indicates high probability of drug idiosyncracy or side effects, nurses are in a position to seek medical collaboration in intervening, that is discontinuing the drug. Providing a night light may relieve restlessness during the hours of darkness. Orders for small dosages of tranquilizers are sought by some nurses to relieve restless behavior.

One nurse made an interesting observation about restlessness in groups of people who are not acquainted with each other. She noted that people move toward the center of the restlessness as when a crowd is waiting for the theater or a department store to open. It makes one wonder about the function of restlessness in mob development and action.

There are still questions about where restlessness fits into the scheme of things. Is it related to anxiety and fear or part of them? If it is related to anxiety and fear, what is the nature of the relationship? How important is restlessness as a human behavior and how important is it to eliminate? Where should it be placed in the priorities of nursing care? To what extent is restlessness learned? Is it just the external behaviors, or is the whole process, including feelings, learned from significant others? Which accompaniments of restlessness are causal and which have other relationships? What is the nature of cause in restlessness? More nurses are needed to observe it!

Those nurses who work with patients and ask the meaning of what they see; those who allow themselves the luxury of following where their questions lead them; those willing to consider the apparently incongruous and ridiculous; those who can tolerate the messiness and imperfections of the whole process of concept development—only those nurses can describe, define, categorize and identify nursing phenomena and their meaning and develop effective nursing interventions for them. These are the nurses who will form the base on which the science of nursing will build.[4]

REFERENCES

1. Dorland's Illustrated Medical Dictionary, 25th Ed. Philadelphia, Saunders, 1974; Taber, C. W.: Cyclopedic Medical Dictionary, 11th Ed. Philadelphia, F. A. Davis, 1969.
2. Cumulative Index Medicus. Bethesda, Md., Department of Health, Education and Welfare, 1972, 1973; International Nursing Index. New York, American Journal of Nursing, 1971, 1972, 1973; Psychological Abstracts. Lancaster, Pa., American Psychological Association, 1972, 1973.

3. Natural History. New York, Journal of the American Museum of Natural History, 1971, 1972, 1973; The Living Wilderness. Washington, D.C., Wilderness Society, 1970, 1971.
4. I want to identify and express appreciation to nurses in my classes whose observations and reporting extended my understanding of the concept of restlessness:

Sister M. Alphonse
Judy A. Bartle
Evangeline D. Broaddus
Edith A. Bush
Wilma Delores Campell
Maxine Chambers
Ruth R. Curtis
Connie R. Fleming
Charlotte Hamilton
Barbara F. Keller
Sandra S. Laird
Carol J. Lattimore
Connie Myers
Wanda Irene Newman
Christine M. Orwat
Paula M. Patrick
Sandra S. Shelton
Martha C. Skelton
Ruth A. Strong
Janis L. Heart
Carol A. West
Elizabeth Wood

9 BOREDOM

Evelyn Char

A glance around the room reveals fixed expressions on the women's faces. Most are turned in the speaker's direction, but one has the impression that they are not actively listening. Their eyes seem to be focused on the same person but there is a dullness in them. Others are squirming ever so slightly and silently shifting in their chairs. Two seem engrossed in handwork, their heads bent over their crocheting or needlepoint. The observer may conclude from the lack of excitement and activity and the flatness of the facial expressions that the ladies are bored.

The nurse stands at the foot of the patient's bed, poised to leave, equipment in hand, a look of impatience and flight about her. The patient continues speaking, the nurse nods her head, but her body language expresses impatience. In the utility room she remarks to a coworker that she is bored by the patient she has just left.

The young man holds the newspaper before him, utters "uh-hum" at frequent intervals, while his mother sitting next to him is talking. His responses seem mechanical and uninterested. His mother leans toward him as she speaks and he continues to turn the pages of the newspaper, seemingly skimming the articles and not paying attention to her. One may speculate that the young man is bored.

The observed behaviors just described can be examined in light of the mental health concept that all behavior is purposeful, has meaning and can be understood. Situations in which people report feeling bored include meetings where the discussion leader did a poor job of conducting, the topic being discussed was uninteresting and the individual present felt time was being wasted. Students complain about attending uninteresting or poorly taught classes because they are dull and not meaningful. The older child required to attend church services whispers to parents "this is boring." Production line workers doing repetitive tasks daily have a high incidence of boredom.

WHAT IS BOREDOM?

Webster defines a bore as a dull, tiresome, annoying person or something that is monotonous, wearisome and tediously devoid of interest. Boredom is the state of being bored.[1]

Erich Fromm says that boredom is a paralysis of our productive powers and the sense of being unalive. All humans need to have stimulation and excitation, and lack of stimulation results in boredom.[2] In today's society many people are chronically bored and seek relief by participating in a great many activities which prevent them from consciously feeling bored. These attempts to escape boredom include alcohol consumption, watching television, taking a ride, going to parties, engaging in sexual activities, taking drugs and being attracted to reports of crime or accidents.[3]

Boredom is the unpleasant experience of feeling captive in a dull situation or with an uninteresting person. It is the individual's subjective perception of the situation or other person as lacking or providing little interest, stimulation or excitation, or being monotonous or tedious. The experience is always unpleasant and undesirable. The bored person has the introspective feeling of being oppressed and captivated, and the resulting anger at being captive is felt as boredom. The feeling of being captive may involve perceived role requirements, such as the student required to attend class, the person with a repetitive job, a committee member attending meetings, the dutiful child, the hospitalized patient, the nurse responsible for that person's care, or the patient on a specific medication or treatment regimen.

Outward signs of boredom that may be readily observed are yawning, fidgeting, inattention, disinterest, restlessness or dullness in facial expression. Subjective symptoms are more difficult to observe and are usually exhibited through body language or verbal communication. Body language may give a truer indication of what is being said or communicated because it is more difficult to exert conscious control over this aspect of behavior than the spoken word. Posture can be a means of punctuating a conversation. A shift in position so that the listener is no longer facing the speaker may mean the listener is finished or turning attention elsewhere. The teenager who has had enough of a parental lecture accompanies the verbal "yeah, I know!" with a physical turning away that signals, "Enough, let me go!" He or she may remain immobile with a bland, bored facial expression, but closer scrutiny reveals eyes that hide smoldering anger.

RESPONSES TO BOREDOM

In a situation that has low stimulation or interest, the individual can attempt to obtain stimulation or excitation by increasing or changing the activity, such as switching from reading to playing tennis. However, in an uninteresting situation in which the individual is captive, the sense of a forced physical presence gives rise to anger or hostility. One may attempt to control the anger, suppress it, hide it, or express it consciously or unconsciously. The anger may be with the perceived captor as, for example, asking hostile questions of the teacher or displaying passive resistance to the group leader; or it may be with oneself for becoming involved in the situation and not knowing how to extricate oneself. Anger liberates energy which can be useful. Full expression of affect gives one a sense of completion and readiness to move forward, while limited or covert expression leaves one feeling incomplete or unfinished. An example is resentment as unexpressed anger. Breaking the awareness barrier between parts of the person frees energy, allowing the person more self-expression in a coordinated way.[4] Energy which is expended to control the anger may sometimes be observed in the form of fidgeting, restlessness or daydreaming, and may result in weariness and dullness, even dozing.

The term stressful boredom has been applied to extended periods of immobilization, such as that endured by astronauts, nuclear submarine crews and patients hospitalized for long periods of time.[5] The intensity of reactions which may be caused by unrelieved boredom gives us an indication of the power of the impulses engendered by it. Acts of aggression have occurred during prolonged periods of boredom, as when crews mutiny on long ocean voyages or striking laborers become violent.

In less stressful situations the individual may be able to escape from the boredom by changing jobs, leaving the class or meeting, or leaving the hospital without the physician's consent. When physical presence is mandatory, the person may attempt to escape by daydreaming, being inattentive or sleeping. In a captive situation one may seek tangential stimulation, such as doing a handicraft project of embroidering during a meeting, doodling while listening or watching television when confined to a hospital bed.

Another response to boredom could be seeking something of interest central to the situation or person. If the speaker's manner is dull, the topic may be interesting; if the surroundings are monotonous, the people present are each unique. Taking responsibility for doing something about a boring situation or discovering why a certain person is boring are positive measures to dispel boredom.

Ennui is a sense of weariness or dissatisfaction but without the feeling of being captive. A vacation day with no plans and everyone sitting around wondering what to do is an example of ennui. This condition is readily improved by finding something to do which is appealing. Ennui is differentiated from boredom in that the individual does not feel restricted or forced to be physically present.

WHEN THE NURSE IS BORED WITH A PATIENT

Mr. G., an elderly patient on the orthopedic floor, related the story of his injury several times over to every nurse who attended him. The details were elaborated and the tale became longer with each telling. His loneliness was relieved when furnished with an audience, but his attempts to maintain social contact became tedious and boring. The unpleasant feeling of boredom causes one to find ways of avoiding and escaping it and the nurses soon began to find excuses to leave before Mr. G. could recount his story again.

When a patient, or anyone, behaves in ways which are perceived by others as boring, that behavior has meaning. It is a result of highly personalized perceptions and deep meaning that exists within the context of what is happening inside and outside of the individual at the moment. Behavior has meaning and significance to the behaver and receiver.[6] Nurses who recognize boredom in themselves or others have the opportunity to seek the meaning of that behavior.

A nurse once remarked, "Patients don't bore me, I try to find out what they are saying." If the nurse practitioner utilizes that viewpoint, her or his effectiveness will greatly increase.

William Schutz related using his awareness of being bored as a cue that the other person is using boredom as a defense. He suggests taking responsibility for discovering the causes for the negative feelings and initiating action to improve the situation.[7]

A chronic bore is a very angry person, veiling the anger by exhibiting boring behavior.[8] Mrs. S. always complained about minor items and especially about the elevator noises at night preventing her from sleeping. She spoke in a whiney tone, repeating her grievance about matters which seemed insignificant and dull to the nursing staff. A nurse new to the unit was assigned to give Mrs. S. care. Other team members commented with relief that they would not have that "boring lady," which served as a challenge to the new nurse to discover reasons for Mrs. S. seeming so insipid to the nurses.

> MRS. S.: Could you change the sheet before you leave? I spilled some tea on it this morning when I was leaning over to get it. They put the tray so far away from me that I could barely reach it. After not sleeping at all last night I was very shaky and my hand was unsteady. Those elevators are so loud at night that it's just impossible to get a decent sleep.
>
> NURSE: You're having difficulty sleeping at night?
>
> MRS. S.: Yes, it's bad enough to be sick and in the hospital without noisy elevators keeping you up all night.
>
> NURSE: Could you tell me about your need to be in the hospital?
>
> MRS. S.: Well, I didn't think I needed to be in the hospital but my doctor said I should, so here I am. My son says the doctor knows what's best and he brought me here last Tuesday. He phones every day, but he's got so many things to do he can't come to visit. He's been here only once since last week. I tell him it's OK and that the nurses take good care of me. Could you move that over here, please? It's so heavy for me. Thank you.
>
> NURSE: What reasons did the doctor give you for your hospitalization?
>
> MRS. S.: Well, I'm really not too certain, he said something about tests and then deciding what to do. I'm afraid to ask. I don't want to be a bad patient. My son talks to the doctor, but he hasn't visited me for a week. I know the people here are trying to take care of me even though they disturb my sleep at night.

We can speculate that Mrs. S.'s complaints and boring behavior represented anger at her son, doctor and being hospitalized. If an individual does not feel safe in expressing anger because of fear of retaliation, it may be displaced. The anger may not be directed toward any particular person; instead the individual may experience feelings of irritability, tension, restlessness, sadness, apathy, hopelessness or depression.[9]

The anger is much closer to consciousness in boredom than in depression. However, we rarely introspect to the point of consciously feeling the anger, so what we experience is boredom.[10]

Avoiding relationships because they are too frightening or dangerous may be another cause of seemingly boring behavior. Conversations with a patient who is evading close personal contact can be monotonous and insipid. The vagueness and dullness tire the listener and discourage forming a significant relationship. A woman diagnosed as schizophrenic for many years repeatedly conveyed the picture of a very dull, routine, daily existence. She bored her nurse therapist by describing her inactivity until the therapist realized that she and the patient were mutually palled. The nurse therapist's sense of boredom was an attempt to mask her anger at being forced to listen to the patient's prosaic descriptions, while the vapid atmosphere was less hazardous for the patient because she did not have to explore painful feelings or risk entering into a new relationship. Awareness of the situation enabled the nurse therapist to redirect the interviews, resulting in much more productive sessions and the patient becoming more actively involved in her daily living.

A nurse describing her early attempts to obtain information by using open-ended questions found herself "listening to the patient's trials and tribulations beginning with his first day of life" because she did not know how to redirect the conversation. To avoid manifesting her impatience at having to remain there listening to the patient, she allowed her mind to wander and felt bored.[11]

Hidden anger in nurses is that which is not expressed. By denying its presence nurses purposely create a semblance of all being well without being fully aware of doing so. It is a mental function which does not mean they do not know they are feeling angry. It means they do not choose to know—or choose not to know.[12] An attempt to bring it clearly into expression may be of great value.

If nurses understand the concept of anger, understand their own patterns of reacting to and dealing with anger-provoking situations, and learn to recognize anger in others, then they will be able to deal more effectively with anger in relationships with patients.[13]

A nurse may become bored hearing a patient reiterate an episode over and over. Mr. K. described his grandchild's visit in great detail, even repeating what he said to her and how she replied.

> MR. K.: Susan came running up to me with the can of cookies. She said she helped her mother bake them. She's so tiny I was afraid I would squash her when she hugged me.

When the nurse recognized that she was bored by hearing the story repeated daily, she explored the meaning more fully to grasp its significance. She discovered that Mr. K. lived in a nursing home miles away from relatives and friends and he savored the semi-annual visits from his grandchildren. When Susan brought him the home-baked cookies and hugged him, the outward manifestation of truly caring was deeply touching to Mr. K. The high symbolic value of the experience was not initially evident to the listener.

WHEN THE PATIENT IS BORED

Holistic care of patients includes consideration of their activity and emotional responses to being ill. Many hospitalized patients are bored. Confined to bed or a miniscule room, shifted from their usual environment to one that is strange and frightening, restricted in variety of food, activities and social interactions, they are captive in a situation intended to be beneficial.

A person accustomed to a great deal of physical activity may feel severely constrained when hospitalized. An avid reader who has a medical problem which interferes with vision may be distressed at his or her plight. The decrease in interest, stimulation and meaningful activity in addition to the sense of imprisonment can easily result in boredom. The nurse's recognition and awareness of the patient's subjective perception of the situation can lead to attempts to learn what would be of interest and helpful in relieving boredom. Some patients escape the boredom by leaving the hospital despite their physician's advice.

A woman isolated for tuberculosis was extremely lonely because of limited contact with others and long periods of solitude.[14] In curtailing exposure to the patient, social interaction is also severely decreased. Affording some activity or interest to the patient, such as books, television, radio and magazines, can be of great value in helping him or her pass the sequestered hours. Quality nursing time spent in direct contact with the patient can include meaningful social interaction to fulfill some of the emotional needs of the patient. In hurrying to complete nursing tasks, the nurse sometimes forgets the patient's need to talk.

Some hospital visitors bring items to relieve the patient's boredom, such as knitting, needlepoint, magazines, puzzles, books and candy or other snacks. For the less fortunate patient who does not have visitors, the nurse can attempt to provide similar relief by asking patients to share their magazines or puzzles when they have finished with them.

Occupational therapy facilities are a bonus, and the nurse can request such services for patients or suggest they be ordered by the physician. Their immense benefit is sometimes more appreciated by the patient than the medication or unfamiliar treatment.

Nursing can learn from the airlines, which have done much more to provide relief from monotony and tedium, though their passengers are captive for a much briefer time than patients. The passenger in flight is wined, dined and kept occupied almost from the moment the wheels leave the ground until they set down at their destination.

SUMMARY

Boredom occurs when a person is in a situation that is monotonous, tedious, low in or devoid of interest or with another individual who is dull or tiresome. It is the person's subjective perception of being captive in the situation and the resulting anger that is felt as boredom. The person may attempt to leave or escape from the situation, either physically or by finding something of interest within the situation. He or she may endeavor to control, suppress or express the anger.

Total care of the patient includes consideration of all the patient's needs. If decreased activity or interest is causing the patient to feel bored, the nurse can attempt to help the patient by providing or finding activities which can relieve the boredom. The nurse who is feeling bored can examine the situation and the behaviors of him or herself, the patient or both to gain an understanding of what is occurring and to make possible changes.

REFERENCES

1. Webster's Third New International Dictionary, unabridged. Springfield, Mass., Merriam, 1966, p. 256.
2. Fromm, E.: The Anatomy of Human Destructiveness. Greenwich, Conn., Fawcett, 1973, p. 272.
3. Ibid., pp. 274-76.
4. Hays, D.: Anger: a clinical problem. *In* Burd, S., and Marshall, M. (eds.): Some Clinical Approaches to Psychiatric Nursing. New York, Macmillan, 1963, p. 114.
5. Selye, H.: Stress without Distress. Philadelphia, Lippincott, 1974, p. 86.
6. Chapman, J., and Chapman, H.: Behavior and Health Care. St. Louis, Mosby, 1975, p. 15.
7. Schutz, W.: Here Comes Everybody. New York, Harper, 1971, p. 155.
8. Rubin, T.: The Angry Book. New York, Macmillan, 1969, pp. 139-40.
9. Travelbee, J.: Interpersonal Aspects of Nursing. Philadelphia, F. A. Davis, 1971, p. 36.
10. Glasser, W.: Mental Health or Mental Illness? New York, Harper, 1960, p. 31.
11. Balch, C.: Breaking the lines of resistance. *In* Riehl, J., and Roy, Sr. C.: Conceptual Models for Nursing Practice. New York, Appleton-Century-Crofts, 1974, p. 132.
12. Bird, B.: Talking with Patients, 2nd ed. Philadelphia, Lippincott, 1973, p. 89.
13. Hays, Anger, p. 113.
14. Bullough, B.: Where should isolation stop? Am. J. Nurs. 62:86, October 1962.

Section III

Responses to Changes in Health Status: Concepts with Positive Connotations

INTRODUCTION

The six concepts included in this section embrace feelings, thoughts, processes and situations that tend to be considered positive or to generate feelings of well-being. These were developed independently; however, there are various characteristics that some of them seem to share. Trust and hope are similar in that they refer to attitudes or beliefs about positive things. Denial and humor are mechanisms or processes that can be, and often are, used to ward off unpleasant feelings. Privacy and relaxation are experienced as positive or tend to contribute to positive outcomes for the individual.

Mary Thomas defines trust as a general attitude of contentment and confidence resulting from an assumption that life is pleasant and will remain manageable. Good is expected by one who trusts. When trust is impaired, negative things are expected. Hope, as defined by Silvia Lange, consists of a collection of feelings and thoughts centering on the belief that there are solutions to needs and problems. Hope is different from a wish or an expectation, and in early childhood it is closely related to the formation of trust.

Trust and hope are contrasted with their opposites by these authors. Thomas contrasts the effects of trust with mistrust. Those who trust tend to be comfortable with self-awareness, share awareness with selected others, accept new experiences and persons who differ from themselves, demonstrate consistency between words and actions and be able to delay gratification. On the other hand, those who mistrust are uncomfortable with self-awareness and sharing awareness with others, try to get others to behave in familiar ways, avoid new experiences, demonstrate inconsistency in words and actions and are unable to delay gratification. Lange contrasts opposite poles of a hope continuum. The positive side of the continuum is characterized by hope, confidence, faith, inspiration and determination. Associated behaviors are activation, comfort, moving toward people and competence. The negative pole of the hope continuum includes feelings of despair, helplessness, hopelessness, doubt, depression, apathy and grief. Imcompetence, moving away from people, hypoactivity and discomfort are behavioral correlates of this end of the continuum.

Thomas points out that the nurse's trustworthiness needs to be established before the patient can be assisted to trust, and she provides examples of where trustworthiness might be threatened. The remainder of the chapter is focused on the process of development of trust and examples of helping the patient to trust.

Lange describes helplessness as the overwhelming sense of losing control over the external world and hopelessness as the sense of overwhelming defeat or loss of control over oneself. Behavior indicative of the two look similar to behavior observed in early phases of grief. One can feel helpless and hope. If it is concluded that a person is feeling hopeless it may be useful to assess the individual's hope structure. Lange describes the hope structure as the process by which hopes are maintained. It is made up of an affective component and cognitive functions.

Lange also describes tasks of hoping (reality surveillance, encouragement, worrying and mourning), operational definitions of hoping and despairing and provides the reader with many ways to apply the concept of hope to nursing in any setting. She suggests the importance of nurses being aware of their own feelings about the meaning of life, illness and death and of knowing the fluctuations of these feelings. Finally, she describes seven major coping skills that are used in adjusting to illness and suggests that hope facilitates the use of all of them.

The authors of the next two chapters on humor and denial of illness describe what might be called mechanisms to maintain comfort or to prevent emotional discomfort. Vera Robinson describes humor as a form of communication that is used as a coping mechanism. Sister Martha Kiening describes denial as a defense mechanism. More completely, Robinson defines humor as communication perceived by interactants as humorous and leading to laughing, smiling or the feeling of amusement. It is thought to have many purposes, such as to decrease social distance, satisfy repressed impulses or relieve hostility. Kiening defines denial as the kind of behavior that indicates failure to accept obvious facts or their significance. The fact that perceived reality and actual reality are inconsistent when denial is used makes it a rather brittle defense. Both humor and denial seem to help people cope at least under some circumstances. Both free people from everyday realities.

Robinson focuses a great deal on the use of humor in nursing. She explores the use of humor to establish relationships, decrease anxiety, release anger in an acceptable form, avoid painful feelings and facilitate learning, and she points out that the evaluation of humor should be based on the needs it serves rather than the technique used. As is true with use of other concepts in nursing intervention, the use of humor should be individualized. Robinson suggests that the nurse carefully evaluate the lifestyle of the individual and his or her response to humor.

Privacy and relaxation are the final concepts developed in this section. Both of these concepts involve comfort. Dorothy Bloch describes comfort as the end goal of privacy. According to Sandra Sweeney, relaxation is a state that is free from "tension, toil, or strain" which is manifested in many ways. Relaxation is often equated with comfort or pleasure.

According to Bloch there are several aspects of measuring privacy. Privacy includes the right to exclude others from knowledge and information and the awareness that this applies to others. Amount of information, place, time and manner of excluding others may be important. Exclusion of oneself from others and the goal of comfort are other aspects of privacy. Privacy may refer to an event, lifestyle, personality or anonymity. There are also many dimensions of relaxation. Sweeney says that it may have a physiological or psychological origin and is psychologically controlled. It can be affected by both internal and external stimuli, is an active, conscious process and has both psychological and physiological behavioral manifestations. A review of the literature on relaxation is presented along with a summary of current trends in relaxation techniques and training.

Sweeney suggests that relaxation is necessary for mental and physical health. Like denial and humor, relaxation is perhaps an adaptive coping process. Bloch contends that privacy is universal and is necessary for life. There are rules in each society that tend to guarantee privacy for individuals and groups. Privacy is described as having many functions including: (1) personal autonomy; (2) emotional release; (3) self-evaluation; and (4) limited and protected communication. Privacy is a way of achieving goals and adapting and should be balanced with companionship and sharing to be effective. It is not viewed as an end in itself.

Authors of both of these chapters devote considerable attention to the application of the respective concepts to nursing. Bloch begins with a discussion of the Patient's Bill of Rights. She goes on to discuss privacy for patients and gives specific examples for each of the functions of privacy. Finally, she reminds nurses that they need to know functions of privacy, variables influencing privacy and individual modes of expressing the need for privacy and to remember that they too need privacy. Sweeney points out the need to identify the phenomena of relaxation and to determine various aspects of its use. She describes several situations in which relaxation techniques have been found helpful. For example, relaxation has been effective in treating anxiety. Relaxation techniques and strategies are described and the nurse is cautioned about their use. The nurse should be knowledgeable about relaxation techniques and realize the hazards that exist if they are used improperly.

These six concepts have been described as sharing positive connotations and comfort. Each concept encompasses negative phenomena too. Too much or inappropriate trust, for example, can have devastating effects. Likewise, denial can result in failure to take proper precaution for health and safety. Privacy in its extreme form may lead to isolation. There may even be negative outcomes from too much or inappropriate use of humor and relaxation.

10 TRUST

Mary Durand Thomas

Trust, which can bridge the gap between patient and nurse, is fundamental to full attainment of the purpose of nursing. The nurse, in assisting a person to move toward health, observes, diagnoses, intervenes and evaluates the results. But the nurse's observations, upon which the remainder of the nursing process is based, are inaccurate and incomplete unless they are made in relationship of mutual trust. For it is improbable that the patient who believes the nurse to be untrustworthy will share his or her true thoughts and feelings. Their interactions would then be a mere façade rather than a productive encounter between two trusting persons.

But helping the patient to trust is warranted on the basis of a broader consideration: the nursing goal of health promotion. For trust has been called "the cornerstone of a healthy personality"[1] because it allows the person to be open to and accepting of him or herself, thus furthering constructive growth.

DEFINITIONS OF TRUST AND MISTRUST

What is this "trust" that is so crucial? It has been described as "a global undifferentiated attitude, a contentment and confidence which stems from a deep assumption that life is pleasant and will not become unmanageable." The trusting person "operates on the tacit assumption that situations . . . will be of a piece with the stable known world." Such a person expects that people and situations will be good and that their hostility, danger or undependability have to be demonstrated.[2] On the other hand, the person whose trust is impaired is one "who expects bad from every new situation and to whom the kindness and dependability of people must be demonstrated."[3] This impairment has been variously termed mistrust[4] and suspicion.[5]

Crucial to the development of an operational definition are the effects of trust and mistrust on behavior. Thus the person who trusts:

1. is comfortable with an increasing awareness of self and his or her goals and motivations.
2. is able to share this awareness with appropriate people.
3. accepts others who deviate from his or her own ways of thinking, feeling and acting without intense needs to change them.

4. accepts new experiences.
5. demonstrates a consistency between words and actions that lasts over time.
6. is able to delay gratification.

Conversely, the person who mistrusts:

1. is uncomfortable with any awareness of self, goals and motivations.
2. is unable to share this awareness with appropriate people and, as a result, demonstrates various manifestations of loneliness.
3. does not accept others who deviate from his or her own ways of thinking, feeling, and acting, but instead often attempts to manipulate others to behave in familiar ways.
4. avoids new experiences.
5. demonstrates inconsistency in words and actions over time.
6. is unable to delay gratification.

The nurse, in interactions with patients, can use these behaviors as a measure of the extent to which both she or he and the patient tend toward trust or mistrust. One caveat should be offered, however. Neither, the nurse nor the patient is ever completely trusting or completely mistrusting. Rather, each person may be considered to be somewhere on a continuum between the extremes.

As can be noted from the effects of trust on behavior, two reciprocal aspects are implied: "reasonable trustfulness as far as others are concerned and a simple sense of trustworthiness as far as oneself is concerned."[6] Thus, as one is more self-accepting, one is more accepting of others who have different ways of behaving. And the degree to which persons are open to their own feelings and motivations influences the degree of their behavioral consistency as seen by others. Similarly, persons who mistrust will usually be seen as untrustworthy by others. Unable to delay gratification because they are not sure their needs will be met and unable to accept awareness of themselves, they avoid new experiences, are less accepting of others and demonstrate inconsistent behavior.

Trust and mistrust may be seen to be related respectively to those behaviors frequently termed interdependence and dependency. For trusting persons—who can accept themselves, others, and new experiences, who are capable of consistency and delayed gratification—can participate in relationships that are genuinely interdependent. Conversely, mistrusting persons—concerned that their needs will not be met, unable to communicate awareness of self, and not trusting others to meet their needs—demonstrate dependency behavior.

Before looking at trust and mistrust in nurse-patient interactions, it may be well to define the relationship between trust and gullibility. Is the gullible person one who tends to be too trusting? As a matter of fact, gullibility is more closely related to mistrust than to trust. Gullible persons, not open to what they really believe and feel, accept others' interpretations of events as their own. As they move from situation to situation and from person to person, accepting interpretations of others, their behavior can be seen as inconsistent and forsaking of their own trustworthiness.

TRUSTWORTHINESS IN THE NURSE

Before nurses can assist patients to trust, they must be trustworthy. They may assess the extent of this attribute in themselves by comparing their behavior in the nurse-patient encounter with the operational definitions of trust and mistrust. How comfortable are they with increasing self-awareness? Are they able to share this awareness with others? How accepting are they of others who think, feel and act differently from them? Are they open to new experiences? Is there a consistency in their words and actions within a situation and from one situation to another? Are they able to delay gratification while working toward a goal? The extent to which these questions can be affirmatively answered is an indication of a nurse's ability to trust.[7]

In nurse-patient interactions, there are two common situations in which nurses may feel their trustworthiness is at stake. When asked a question by the patient, the nurse, fearful of losing his or her trust, may hesitate to admit to a lack of knowledge. But trust is not measured by the vastness of knowledge. Instead, a reply of "I don't know, but I'll try to find out" could indicate that the nurse is a person who does not attempt to bluff but answers honestly—someone who can be trusted.

Another test of trust occurs when the patient says "I want to talk to you about something, but I don't want you to tell anyone." Because the nurse is pleased at being singled out and hopes to gain the patient's trust, the nurse may agree not to convey the information. But if something is learned that should be shared with other health team members, the nurse can be caught in a dilemma: either belie the patient's trust or prove untrustworthy in the nursing role. On the other hand, the nurse could respond: "If you tell me about something that is important for your care, I would want to share it with other nurses or with your physician." There is an obvious risk that the patient may be reticent about sharing the information or may withhold it. But what is of greater importance in this encounter is that the patient has had the opportunity to learn that the nurse is honest and will act consistently with what she or he says.

This is not to imply that nurses always would, or should, trust coworkers. They may enter a work situation expecting to trust only to find that they have to reconsider another person's behavior. For example, a nurse, having seen a coworker mishandle information shared about patients in the past, may then learn of a patient's minor infringement of a policy that was instituted for the protection of all patients. Would the nurse want to share this information with the coworker, knowing that the possible consequence would be some punitive response, such as stereotyping the patient as a "rule-breaker"?

Unfortunately, there are no established answers; rather, a judgment appropriate to each situation must be rendered. However, being gullible or naive about another's behavior should not be confused with being trusting, and being singled out by a patient should not be equated with being trustworthy.

PREVIOUS DEVELOPMENT OF TRUST

The nurse's trustworthiness establishes the degree of trust possible in the nurse-patient relationship. But even nurses who believe they are reliable may find—to their disappointment and irritation—that they have not gained the patients' trust. It is useful to remember that the most accepting and consistent nurse may be seen as untrustworthy by a patient whose prior experiences have led him or her to be mistrusting.

What are these previous experiences that have taught the patient to trust or to mistrust? During the first year or year and a half of life, infants are learning to trust both themselves and others in the world around them. As their internal world becomes differentiated from the external world, they are "constantly testing the coherence, continuity, and dependability of both."[8] This testing occurs through felt experiences within their environment. For example, as infants learn to control and adapt their movements they are gradually able to trust their own bodies. Similarly, their repeated experience of being hungry, communicating discomfort, and feeling comfort pursuant to nursing, assures babies that the world is a dependable place.

The experience of mutuality implicit in such incidents is a critical element in learning to trust. For it is in

> ...*getting what is given,* and in learning to *get somebody to do* for him what he wishes to have done, [that] the baby ... develops the necessary groundwork to *get to be* the giver.... Where this mutual regulation fails, the situation falls apart into a variety of attempts to control by duress rather than by reciprocity.[9]

Through all of their experiences babies are thus learning to what degree they can trust themselves and their environment. If they receive consistent understanding and love from parents, they are helped to develop a basic trust. If, on the other hand, they frequently experience parents' indifference, lack of understanding or annoyance, their trust will be impaired and they will tend toward mistrust and loneliness.

Although the individual's most poignant encounter with trust and mistrust occurs at the beginning of existence in the world, other situations later in life present the encounter in new forms. A child who calls out when alone in a dark room at night may wonder if someone will come; a child or an adult who gives a gift or extends him or herself to another person in some way may find that the other person reacts in an unexpected way; the ability to trust oneself and one's expectations of others may be called into question. Thus all persons, through continuing tests of their mastery of trust, find opportunities for the further development of this trust.

HELPING THE PATIENT TO TRUST

It has been noted that one of these opportunities for developing a mutually trusting relationship occurs in the nurse-patient relationship. However, as nurses provide patients with opportunities for learning to trust them, even the best-intentioned nurse may find the task difficult when confronted by the patient who cannot trust self, others, or the future. Some examples of patient situations will be discussed in order to view possible nursing intervention.

The Patient Who Attempts to Prove His or Her Expectations

Mistrusting patients, without being aware of it, may create situations that prove their expectations.

> Mrs. Adams was such a patient. After having been paraplegic for four years, she was admitted to the hospital for treatment of infected decubiti. She repeatedly said to members of the nursing staff: "You don't really want to take care of me . . . Nobody in the past wanted to and you'd rather not." Even though a nurse had cared for her several times, Mrs. Adams would still give specific instructions for turning the Stryker frame and caring for her decubiti. Her behavior indicated a lack of acceptance of others as well as the expectations that others would neither accept nor care for her. Rather than anticipating good from this experience of hospitalization, she expected that it would be like other situations in which she had perceived others as not caring.
>
> A nurse in this situation could easily have become angry and not wanted to care for Mrs. Adams, thus actualizing the expectations and increasing the patient's loneliness. Instead one nurse responded: "Have you noticed something that seems to mean I don't want to care for you?" Mrs. Adams was able only to say that she *knew* nobody would want to care for her even before she came to the hospital. Over an interval of several days similar conversations occurred, and each time the patient repeated the instructions for her care, the nurse asked such questions as "Are you wondering if I'll do this correctly?" Eventually the patient said: "You know, before I came in, I was sure nobody would want to wash out these sores, but I guess that really hasn't been true."

The nurse did not say to the patient "You can trust me"; for when the patient expects people to be untrustworthy, such statements are meaningless. Instead she manifested her trustworthiness by her consistent acceptance.

The Patient Who Says That Everything Is Fine

> Entering Mr. Davis's room, the nurse found him sitting in the chair, glumly looking out the window. In response to her question, he said that everything was "fine." The following conversation ensued:
>
> NURSE: You don't look like you're feeling fine. You seem sad to me.
>
> MR. DAVIS: No. (pause) Well, yes . . . I am blue.
>
> NURSE: Can you tell me what's wrong?
>
> MR. DAVIS: (talked at length of the restrictiveness of his diabetic diet and of having to attend classes with other diabetics) I know the doctor wants me to stay, but I'm thinking about leaving.
>
> NURSE: Has it been that difficult for you?
>
> MR. DAVIS: (again talked of the restrictive diet) The doctor wants me to lose about 30 pounds and get my insulin regulated so that I won't have complications.
>
> NURSE: But you don't know if it's worth it?
>
> MR. DAVIS: That's it. I enjoy eating and I've always just taken extra insulin.
>
> NURSE: And so the change is hard to make.
>
> MR. DAVIS: It sure is.

NURSE: What have you heard about possible complications in the classes that you've been attending?

MR. DAVIS: (discussed some complications) They do sound bad to me but it means giving up so much. (pause) Maybe it's worth it. I guess I'll stick it out for a while.

The nurse in this interaction noted the inconsistency between what Mr. Davis said and what he indicated nonverbally. He was unable to share his thoughts and feelings until she demonstrated by her responses that she would accept them. She also observed his difficulty in delaying present gratification for a future goal. While she helped him to become aware of, and to discuss, his feelings about the present restrictions, she was also encouraging him to trust that "sufficient satisfaction . . . [would be] sufficiently predictable to make waiting and 'working' worthwhile."[10]

The Patient Who Compares Notes

A patient who suspects that others are not trustworthy may attempt to verify this suspicion by "comparing notes." He or she may raise an identical question with a number of nurses and watch for any apparent or real inconsistencies. Or information received from personnel may be compared either with what other patients have been told or with what has actually occurred. For example:

Mr. Carnes, a patient in a tuberculosis ward, kept a list of patients who had been allowed passes from the ward, which privilege he correlated with their length of hospitalization. Inasmuch as he had been admitted prior to many of the patients on the list and yet had been unable to leave the ward, he was quite vexed and perplexed. A nurse, noting his frequent inquiries, said: "How come you've been wondering about how long people have been here?"

MR. CARNES: A lot of them haven't been here as long as I have—and they're getting passes.

NURSE: And you're feeling left out?

MR. CARNES: Well, sure. A guy has the right to get out if other people do. But the doc says I can't go yet.

NURSE: Do you understand why not?

MR. CARNES: Well, he said my kids would get my TB germs if I didn't wait for a while. But some of these guys have kids and they've gone out.

The nurse continued discussing with the patient his feelings and the reasons why his progress could not be compared with the progress of other patients on the basis of length of stay.

When the nurse shares observations of patients' behavior with them in such situations, they can be helped to discuss their expectations. Apparent contradictions may become clarified in the conversation, and real inconsistencies can be discussed with other personnel.

The Patient with Whom the Nurse Has Brief Contact

Because learning to trust is a slow process, it may seem an irrelevant consideration for nurses who have only brief contact with patients. It is true that these nurses may rarely have the satisfaction of seeing growth in the mistrusting patients' ability to trust them. But they *can* provide the opportunity for patients to trust and can know that at least they have not reinforced their mistrust.

CONCLUSION

Helping a patient learn to trust is a difficult, time-consuming process, which demands trustworthiness and effort on the part of the nurse. But such a relationship is essential to the entire nursing process. By experiencing the openness of trust, a patient is more able to share true feelings with the nurse, which in turn allows for greater accuracy in nursing observations and diagnoses and increased effectiveness in interventions. And it is by developing trust as a bridge in such a relationship that the nurse can assist the patient in moving toward health.

REFERENCES

1. The eight stages in the life cycle of man. *In:* Youth and the life cycle: an interview with Erik H. Erikson. Children. 7:45, March-April 1960.
2. Baldwin, A. L.: Behavior and Development in Childhood. New York, Dryden Press, 1955, p. 547.
3. Ibid.
4. Erikson, E. H.: Growth and crises of the "healthy personality." *In* Kluckhohn, C., and Murray, H. A., with the collaboration of Schneider, D. M. (eds.): Personality in Nature, Society and Culture. 2nd ed. New York, Knopf, 1953, p. 190.
5. Deutsch, M.: Trust and suspicion. J. Conflict Resolution. 2:267, December 1958.
6. Erikson, Growth and crises of the "healthy personality," p. 190.
7. Since the appearance of the first edition of this book, a scale has been developed to measure nurses' trust of patients: Wallston, K. A., Wallston, B. S., and Gore, S.: Development of a scale to measure nurses' trust of patients: a preliminary report. Nurs. Res. 22:232-35, May-June 1973.
8. Lynd, H. M.: On Shame and the Search for Identity. New York, Harcourt, 1958, p. 45.
9. Erikson, Growth and crises of the "healthy personality," p. 192.
10. Erikson, E. H.: The problem of ego identity. J. Am. Psychoanal. Assoc. 4:97, January 1956.

11 HOPE

Silvia Prodan Lange

> Man is, properly speaking, based upon hope; he has no other possession but hope; this world of his is emphatically the place of hope. — Thomas Carlyle

> Hope is a good breakfast, but it is a bad supper. — Francis Bacon

> When hope leaves man, despondency begins to subdue him. — Plato

Hope is a complex human experience. It is a mixture of feelings and thoughts which center on the fundamental belief that there are solutions to significant human needs and problems. Hope makes life under stress tolerable; it is "the light at the end of the tunnel." Hope is a way of being in the world which draws on previous life experiences of the self and with others. It is a way of dealing with the uncertainties of the present in anticipation of a future which will be more gratifying and closer to one's deeply felt needs, goals, aspirations, dreams and wishes.

The purpose of hope is to ward off despair. Despair is mental anguish, disorganization, helplessness and hopelessness. Hope is an essential concomitant to life and growth. Ija Korner emphasized the coping value of hope, stating:

> Man who knows that tomorrow he will meet the consequences of today's action cannot but be uncertain. The more uncertain, the more he needs a cushion, a defense against his fears and anxieties. If the outcome may involve disappointment, threat, destruction, and despair, man's need for protection becomes overwhelming. Hope induces a feeling of "assumed certainty" that the dreaded will not happen, that despair will not occur.[1]

Hope is regarded by many as a mixed blessing. Defending against despair, it enables an individual to tolerate difficult situations and maintain motivation. But hope has the potential for decreasing contact with reality so that a person does not deal with the here and now.

Greek mythology tells of Pandora, the first woman, who according to one version, was created as punishment for man. When she opened the forbidden box, she let out all the evils of the world including hate, greed, despair, shame, envy, guilt, sloth and disgust. The only thing remaining was hope. This raises the existential question—is hope the antidote to the world's evils or the greatest evil of all? The suspicion of evil lies in the danger of hope distorting reality, prolonging agony and relying on faith rather than taking specific measures to remedy a situation.

Ezra Stotland emphasized the positive aspects of hope, stating:

> The importance of hope for man has long been known to layman and professional. It is widely accepted that with hope, man acts, moves, achieves. Without hope, he is often dull, listless, moribund. Faced with a situation that threatens a loss of hope, he may desperately try to cling to it, to restore it, to protect it. Yet despite a common awareness of the role hopefulness plays in determining behavior, rarely has it been introduced into the mainstream of psychology and psychiatry.[2]

Recently, there has been an increase in the exploration and understanding of the complex behaviors of hope. This has been drawn from animal research, concentration camp and prisoner of war observations, institutionalized patients, suicidal behavior, sudden death, and behavior of critically ill patients and their families.[3] Erich Fromm discussed hope as an essential part of the world if technology is to become humanized.[4] Elisabeth Kübler-Ross, in her studies of death and dying, maintained that throughout the stages of the dying process hope remains as an essential element.[5]

A basic assumption of this chapter is that there is a relationship between hope and health. Loss of hope has a deleterious effect on the human being resulting in giving-up behavior which may lead to physical and emotional disequilibrium. Death, through the loss of the will to live, may result from resigned withdrawal or suicide. In many clinical situations the nurse plays a crucial role in recognizing, maintaining and restoring hope.

The purpose of this chapter is to examine the experience of hope in the context of health and illness. Hope, hopelessness and helplessness are defined and described. The psychosocial origins of these emotional states are discussed. An operational definition of hope is derived from the hope structure and the tasks of hoping. Application to nursing situations emphasizes how nurses can help the patient, the family, and themselves to sustain hope and combat feelings of despair.

DEFINITIONS OF HOPE

> Hope! Of all ills that men endure, the only cheap and universal cure; the captive's freedom, and sick man's health, the lover's victory and the beggar's wealth.
>
> Abraham Cowley

> Hope is the thing with feathers that perches on the soul. Emily Dickinson

> I suppose it can be truthfully said that Hope is the only universal liar who never loses his reputation for veracity. Robert C. Ingersoll

The definitions of hope are elusive. Although the word hope is one of the most frequently used in referring to emotional states, it is one of the least precisely understood.[6] Though often used synonymously, hope is not simply a wish, expectation, desire or the attitude of optimism or stoicism.[7]

Hope differs from wishes in the following ways. A wish reflects on unmet need, but one that is not vital to the person's existence. It has a low level of probability of coming true. If it does, the person is amazed and pleased. A hope is much more central to important needs and reflects wishes that might come true. When a hope is realized, the person experiences relief and satisfaction but rarely amazement. When hope is lost, deep despair results. In differentiating between a wish and a hope, Korner stated:

> A wish is something which *might* happen, but the person does not organize his behavior with the "expectation" that it *must* happen in order to avoid undesirable and disagreeable dreaded outcomes. In hope, however, it is exactly this quality of personal dependence on outcome which is its central characteristic. . . . The individual feels that hoped-for events *must* occur for the sake of his well-being; he may or may not be committed to his wishes, but he invariably is committed to his hopes.[8]

An expectation differs from a hope in that there is generally a high level of anticipated probability of the event, either positive or negative, coming true. There is much more of an emotional component to hope than to mere expectations.

The use of the word "hope" in relation to "desire" is similar to the misuse of love and like. People say, "I love ice cream" when they mean they like it very much. Similarly, they say, "I hope I'll get a new car" when they mean they desire a possession which is attractive but not essential.

Optimism is often a relatively superficial, Pollyanna attitude. The stoic, with rigid pride, denies reliance on others. Hope is much deeper than these attitudes and generally involves another person or a belief in a higher being or purpose. A person gives hope to another through inspiration. This is done by raising expectations, encouraging, patting on the back, heartening, reassuring, buoying up and making promises for future events.

Common expressions which convey the complexities of hope include hope for the best, hope against hope, don't count your chickens before they are hatched, high hopes, false hopes, catch at a straw, holding on to hope, and faint or lost hopes. Hopelessness is reflected in these words: shattered hope, futility, pessimism, despair, and despondency. The future is seen as dark and gloomy. Hopelessness is the state of acute or prolonged desperation which represents the feeling of being beyond hope—irredeemable, irreversible, incurable and incorrigible. Elements of helplessness are reflected in these words.

Fromm underscored the difficulty of describing hope with words:

> Too often, in the process of talking about love or hate or hope, one loses contact with what one was supposed to be talking about. Poetry, music, and other forms of art are by far the best-suited media for describing human experience because they are precise and avoid the abstraction and vagueness of worn-out coins which are taken for adequate representations of human experience.[9]

Yet Fromm continued to do the difficult with the comment that hope is a shared human experience in which one can use one's own experiences to understand another person. He stated that hope is paradoxical and that "it is neither passive waiting nor is it unrealistic forcing of circumstances that cannot occur. It is like the crouched tiger, which will jump only when the moment for jumping has come."[10]

THE HOPE CONTINUUM

The man who lives only by hope will die with despair. — Italian proverb

The idea of the hope continuum helps to explain shifts of feelings, thoughts and actions. On one end of the continuum is the hope syndrome, which includes hope, confidence, faith, inspiration and determination. At the other end is the despair syndrome, with despair, helplessness, hopelessness, doubt, depression, apathy, sadness and grief. A person may change position along this scale depending on his or her basic personality, external factors, perception of the situation and influence of other people.

Major differences between hope behavior and despair behavior include level of activity, comfort, relatedness to people and competence.[11] Table 3 describes these differences.

ORIGINS OF HOPE, HELPLESSNESS AND HOPELESSNESS

Hope

Hope is a much greater stimulant of life than any happiness. — Friedrich Nietzche

Peace of mind comes only when you have lost hope. — Arabic proverb

The origins of hope are in early childhood experiences, especially those related to the formation of basic trust. Erikson described this period as one in which the infant needs consistent, responsive care in order to learn to count on others to meet his or her basic needs in a loving way. He stated:

> Mothers create a sense of trust in their children by that kind of administration which in its quality combines sensitive care of the baby's individual needs and a firm sense of personal trustworthiness within the trusted framework of their culture's life style. This forms the basis in the child for a sense of identity which will later combine a sense of being "all right," of being oneself, and of becoming what other people trust one will become.[12]

The infant gradually begins to anticipate relief of suffering and gratification of needs and looks forward to his or her mother with eagerness and fascination. The infant experiences pleasure, joy and bliss when she comes, and anger, fear and helplessness if she does not come.

Fromm wrote about hope, faith and fortitude as essential elements of human life. The possible loss of these attributes is characteristic of human existence as "the vicissitudes of environment and accident begin to further or to block the potential of hope."

> Most of us had hoped to be loved—not just to be coddled and to be fed, but to be understood, to be cared for, to be respected. Most of us hoped to be able to trust. When we were little, we did not yet know the human invention of the lie—not only that of lying with words but that of lying with one's voice, one's gestures, one's eyes, one's facial expression. How should the child be prepared for this specifically human ingenuity: the lie? Most of us

are awakened, some more and some less brutally, to the fact that people often do not mean what they say or say the opposite of what they mean. And not only "people" but the very people we trusted most—our parents, teachers, leaders.[13]

Table 3
Comparison of Hope and Despair Behaviors

Hope	Despair
Activation	*Hypoactivation*
Feeling vitality, vibrancy	Feeling all excitement, vitality gone
Having energy and drive	Feeling empty, drained, heavy
Feeling inner buoyancy	Being understimulated
Seeming to be more alert and wide awake	Feelings seeming to be dulled
Experiencing everything fully	Feeling tired, sleepy
Feeling interest and involvement	Feeling dead inside
Feeling like singing	Feeling mentally dull
Comfort	*Discomfort*
Having a sense of well-being	Having a lump in one's throat
Feeling harmony and peace within	Sensing loss, deprivation
Feeling free of conflict	Heart seeming to ache
Feeling loose, relaxed	Not being able to smile or laugh
Feeling general release, lessening of tension	Having whole body tense, wound up inside
Feeling safe and secure	Having feeling of being trapped, boxed in
Feeling life is worth living	Being easily irritated, hypersensitive
Feeling optimistic about the future	Feeling under a heavy burden
Moving toward People	*Moving away from People*
Having an intense positive relationship with another	Having a sense of unrelatedness
Reaching out	Wanting to withdraw, be alone
Having a sense of being wanted and needed	Lacking involvement
Feeling much respect and interdependence	Not caring about anyone
Wanting to touch, hold, be close	Feeling a certain distance
Sensing empathetic harmony with another	Wanting to crawl into oneself
Competence	*Incompetence*
Feeling strong inside	Feeling that nothing one does is right
Having a sense of sureness	Sensing regret
Feeling taller, stronger, bigger	Feeling vulnerable and totally helpless
Being more confident in oneself	Feeling caught up and overwhelmed
Having a sense of accomplishment, fulfillment	Having no sense of control over situation
Really functioning as a unit	Longing to have things as they were
Being motivated	Feeling unmotivated and afraid to try

Fromm related hope and hopelessness to the broader society in saying that social classes and nations live through hope, faith and fortitude. If they lose these qualities, they disappear through lack of vitality or irrational destructiveness. He further stated that the development of hope or hopelessness in an individual is largely determined by the prevailing attitude of the culture. Hope can be rekindled or extinguished depending on what is going on in the larger society. Organized religious beliefs represent aspects of faith, trust and hope.

Helplessness

Helplessness refers to a complex syndrome of emotions, thoughts and behavior. It frequently occurs in situations where the events are uncontrollable. Everything that *can* be done *has* been done, and nothing that *is* done has a significant impact on altering the situation. Helplessness is the sense of being overwhelmed by the loss of control over the outside world.

Helplessness is experienced in early childhood as well as toward the end of life in critical illness and death. It is demonstrated in situations such as difficulty with motivation in school, responses to enforced institutionalization and anaclitic depression and infant death.

Arthur Schmale stated that helplessness reflects a loss of ego autonomy because of the feeling of deprivation from the loss of gratification desired from someone else.[14] The origins are in the early mother-child relationship. Undifferentiated anxiety is the basic emotional state in the infant experiencing physiological and psychological disequilibrium. The infant is truly helpless and must be cared for. He or she develops by repeated reaching out with eyes, hands, mouth and cries.

Development of anxiety into feelings of helplessness takes place during the end of the first year of infancy when the baby becomes increasingly aware of a separateness from the mother. Martin Seligman stated that mastery develops when the infant has a rich supply of synchronies between actions and outcomes.[15] This is developed through responsive mothering in which the mother pays close attention to the signals her child gives and matches her actions with the needs.

Inconsistent or inadequate mothering does not prepare children to develop enough trust to differentiate themselves from others. They may remain hypersensitive to all shifts in the external world and not achieve a sense of mastery, autonomy and self-reliance. In the future they will be particularly vulnerable to loss.

The syndrome of helplessness may occur at any time during life that a person experiences a real or threatened loss of someone or something which is a source of direct gratification, and there is no way to control or avoid the loss. This includes the loss of health. The terror of the crying, frightened baby, unattended and with no relief, is powerful. The helpless person feels like crying or calling for help, symbolically as well as behaviorally, but may not be able to do so.

The helpless person feels left out, let down and deserted, and does not feel capable of or responsible for doing anything. He or she feels that help must come from others. For many people the experience of illness and treatment stimulates massive feelings of helplessness.

Seligman did extensive research with animal and human subjects in experiments where the subject was prevented from exerting any effective control over the environment. He postulated a theory of learned helplessness resulting from situations in which the outcome is independent of the responses of the subject. This results in (1) a reduction of motivation to try to control the outcome; (2) interference with new learning of alternate responses which might control the outcome; and (3) feelings of anxiety as long as the controllability is uncertain and feelings of depression when the events are predictable but still not controllable.

Hopelessness

It is possible to feel helpless and still feel hope. Hopelessness reflects the sense of overwhelming defeat or loss of control over the self. The hopeless person feels a sense of devastating despair and futility. He or she feels unworthy of help and may reject it when offered.

William Lynch described hopelessness as the sense of the impossibility of life, stating, "what a man must do he cannot; no matter what he does it leads to a sense of checkmate; he is in a trap. . . . life is too much . . . what is the use? There is no goal, no sense, no reason; and so I do not hope or wish or will."[16]

Hopelessness involves the lack of a future orientation. The only wish of the person who feels hopeless is to give up. Such a person may sink into apathy which is marked by a negative attitude, noninvolvement, withdrawal, boredom and absence of feeling and concern. Hopelessness may lead to death or a life devoid of satisfaction and meaning.

Schmale regarded hopelessness as a loss of ego autonomy with the feeling of despair which comes from an individual's awareness of being unable to provide the self with gratification. He theorized that hope and hopelessness are developed primarily between the ages of four to six when the child is increasingly aware of sexual differences. Being able to make a positive identification with the parent of the same sex gives rise to feelings of hope—someday the child will grow up and be recognized because of individuality. The person will be capable of sexual and social gratification.

However, the child often has a grandiose feeling of omnipotence. Feelings of hopelessness aid in developing a more realistic self-concept and are therefore necessary to ongoing development. They are activated whenever one judges one's self as too inadequate or too bad to deserve satisfaction.

People who experience marked feelings of hopelessness often have rigid and narrow standards for the conditions under which they can receive gratification. They may have few satisfying interpersonal relationships and are markedly ambivalent, with a pseudoindependent, pseudoself-reliant attitude. Intense feelings of guilt and shame may prevent them from turning to others for help. Instead, they withdraw and insulate themselves from the environment.

Hopelessness and helplessness may occur together, indicating an actual, threatened, fantasized or reawakened unresolved loss for the psychic self about which nothing can be done for the present time. There is a self-judgment that the person cannot function without the lost love object.

The behavior of a person experiencing this syndrome includes reduced activity, passivity, a saddened expression, vegetative signs of depression (weight loss, appetite loss, sleep disorder, social and sexual deficits), lack of motivation, interference with learning, and diminished interest in and activity with external objects. Extreme behavior is muteness, motionlessness and general unresponsiveness. There are many similarities between the hopelessness-helplessness syndrome and some forms of clinical reactive depression.

A certain degree of feelings of helplessness and hopelessness is inevitable in the human experience of living. There are approaches to avoid the devastating and overwhelming impact of these syndromes.

The first approach is in the early child development stages through adequate, responsive mothering. The child can be encouraged to learn mastery and self-confidence which will later give support in the difficult experiences of loss and life changes.

Confidence is faith in one's own strength, capacity and potential to achieve goals, satisfy needs and avert or overcome danger. Confidence includes being able to rely on others—to love and be loved. The confident person looks to a future based on past satisfactions and successes. One feels sure of maintaining old relationships and developing new ones. With confidence, a person does not need to rely on hope.

The child can be gradually immunized against later feelings of overwhelming helplessness by repeated experiences of actions having a definite impact on the desired outcome. Having small, safe experiences with frustration and failure will help to build a structure in which the child exerts control over the environment, others and him or herself. Extreme feelings of hopelessness are warded off by successful child-rearing practices which help the child develop individuality, pride and the ability to relate to others.

When hopelessness is activated in the adult person, it is useful to examine the hope structure to determine how it is failing and how it can be restored. Many situations seen as hopeless are not. Many people who feel helpless are not. In these instances, the reality situation, past life experiences and present and future goals must be evaluated.

THE HOPE STRUCTURE

> Hope warps judgement in council, but quickens energy in action.
>
> Edward Bulwer-Lytton

> Hope is generally a wrong guide, though it is very good company by the way.
>
> Lord Halifax

The term hope structure refers to the process by which hopes are maintained. Hope is made up of affective components and cognitive functions. These occur in varying patterns to maintain psychological equilibrium.

Affective Components

The affective components of hope are on the faith-doubt continuum. Faith is a positive belief that unknown forces can be relied on. Fromm stated, "Faith is not a weak form of belief or knowledge; it is not faith in this or that; faith is the conviction about the not yet proven, the knowledge of the real possibility. . . ."[17]

He stated further that faith is based on the experience of living and of self-transformation. Because one experiences change, one has faith that others can change.

> In the sphere of human relations, "having faith" in another person means to be certain of his core—that is, of the reliability and unchangeability of his fundamental attitudes. In the same sense we can have faith in ourselves—not in the constancy of our opinions but in our basic orientation to life, the matrix of our character structure.[18]

The emotional elements of hope include faith, trust, confidence in self and others, and fortitude. These are shown in attitudes and behavior recognized as determination, motivation, inspiration and encouragement.

When faith weakens, the person may experience doubtful feelings which lead to despair. Despair is a complex of feelings and attitudes which include hopelessness, helplessness, sadness, depression and grief. There are nuances of similarities and differences in these feelings.

Cognitive Functions

The cognitive component of hope is the way in which a person perceives and processes reality. Korner called this "the rationalizing chain" which protects the affective components of hope from threatening reality facts. He stated:

> Hope is, therefore, the construction of a chain formed from bits of reality accompanied by and held together by logic and reasoning. The logic and reasoning, good or bad as they may be, reinforce and protect the belief elements from uncertainty, the cognitive support against internal doubts, the antidote for the anxiety generated by the possibility of a negative outcome. The rationalizing chain differentiates hope from just wishing and/or contemplating one's chances. Wishing permits the relative absence of reality principles; calculating chances enforces taking reality into account. Hope alone permits the best of both worlds—the freedom of the wish and some of the consolations of reality.[19]

The rationalizing chain is made up of selected information which will support the desired hope. If the contradictory facts become overwhelming, the person may utilize the defense mechanism of denial or simply fall back on increased faith. He or she may retreat from reviewing reality in terms of the future and concentrate only on the present.

THE TASKS OF HOPING

> Where there is no hope, there can be no endeavor. — Samuel Johnson

> Hope springs eternal in the human breast. Man never is, but always to be blest.
> — Alexander Pope

Hoping includes four tasks: reality surveillance, encouragement, worrying and mourning.[20] The first task is cognitive; the other three are affective.

Reality Surveillance

To sustain hope, individuals make certain sense out of their reality. They scan the environment for clues. As long as they *believe* they have grounds for hope, they feel reassured, whether or not the facts are realistic.

Methods of reality grounding include the following:

1. Environmental conditions—those that support the hope are emphasized. They may be present or future conditions. "Because they have moved me out of the intensive care unit, it means I'm going to recover."
2. Assets, abilities, and potentialities—the healthy, coping part of the person or situation. "Even if he is quite spastic, there is nothing the matter with his mind."
3. Comparison with others in a similar group or condition. "Here are photos of a patient with burns like yours, before and after treatment."
4. Consensual validation—turning to other people for agreement with the perception of the situation. "Your husband is saying that maybe something can be done about your marriage, after all. How do you see it?"
5. Responsible action—taking steps so that favorable conditions are maintained. "I've agreed to take Antabuse so that, even if I want to drink, I won't."
6. Denial of negative possibilities. "There's no *way* the transplant won't take—the match is perfect."
7. "If . . . then" conditional events—hope is dependent on certain events which may or may not occur. "If I don't have a reoccurrence of symptoms in a year, then I'll try to get pregnant."
8. Maybe, someday, something—possible future discoveries or happenings, "wishful thinking." "Maybe someday some drug will be discovered to cure autistic children."
9. Truism—an uncontestable generality which supports the hope because it refers to everyone. "He is capable of living as normal a life as possible with his disability."
10. Hope commendation—the hope is supported by affirming its value. "It would really be better for Mother to die than be in such misery."
11. Testimonial—supports hope by telling of someone in a similar situation who overcame the difficulty. "I know someone who is paraplegic. He got married and has a happy sex life."

These cognitive hoping styles are often used in combination and vary with the individual. An analysis of the particular style of a person may help to determine where and how to shift the hoping focus if this seems necessary. For instance, the nurse may ask patients about their assets and abilities if they are focusing only on limitations. The nurse might arrange for them to talk to former patients who have learned to cope.

Affective Tasks

Along with the cognitive reality grounding, a person uses three affective tasks in hoping. These are encouragement, worrying and mourning.

Encouragement results when the person finds some base on which to rest his or her hopes. This may be from others or from the self. It motivates, sustains and comforts the person to be able to keep going.

The task of worrying reflects doubt and uncertainty. The person is forced to think about the hoped-for and consider other possibilities and outcomes. It can be beneficial for finding supports for hope, considering alternatives and preparing for anticipated stress and substitute hopes.

Mourning is the task faced by the person who has to give up or drastically alter hopes. There may be a period of intense emotional suffering and involvement which will dissipate over time as the person reorganizes his or her life.

When important hopes are lost, the person goes through a tumultuous reaction of confusion, sadness and uncertainty. From this crisis, some individuals come out stronger and in better relationship to their world. Other people establish new hope systems. Loss of hope may result in devastating reactions of despair, apathy, "hardening of the heart," violence, revenge and death.

OPERATIONAL DEFINITIONS OF HOPING AND DESPAIRING

In all things it is better to hope than to despair. Johann von Goethe

The person has experiences in the past which are related to being able to trust, separate self from others, exert meaningful control of the physical and interpersonal environment, and establish a sense of identity. Out of these experiences the person develops various hopes, conscious and unconscious, for self and significant others in the ongoing present and the future. A stressor event or loss challenges or threatens these hopes. The person is uncertain about the outcome of the situation but anticipates an improved state, relief of distress and achievement of goals. The person attempts to strengthen hope by increasing faith or altering cognitive view of reality factors, which may result in:

Hoping	Despairing
1. The person reaches out to others for support, relief, encouragement and strength.	1. The person is not able to turn to others or alter his or her view of reality.
2. The person finds reassuring evidence from others that he or she can continue to struggle and master the current situation.	2. The person makes unfavorable comparisons of present distress/failure and anticipation of future relief/success.
3. The person feels neither helpless nor hopeless about the possibility of achieving goals.	3. The person sees no adequate or possible solution and loses faith in self and others.

4. Hope is maintained with the possibility of future goals and aspirations.	4. Hope is lost and the person experiences despair with hopelessness and helplessness.
5. Energy and motivation are mobilized.	5. Motivation is lost and energy is inhibited or depleted.

APPLICATION OF THE CONCEPT OF HOPE TO NURSING

For to him that is joined to all the living there is hope. Ecclesiastes 9:4

Confidence and hope do me more good than physic. Galen

The concept of hope has many implications for nursing. Because hope is such a complex and universal experience, it cuts across the human condition, especially during periods of acute distress and adaptation to major life changes. Because hope is a motivational force which maintains energy, it is essential to mobilizing forces toward health. Loss of hope leads to despair, which lowers the ability of the individual to deal with the ongoing physical and emotional crisis.

Hope in Maternal-Child Nursing

The concept of hope is important in understanding the significance of early childhood experiences. Most parents have conscious and unconscious hopes for themselves and their children. Mothers need help in learning how to give adequate psychological and physical care to their growing infants. Responsive mothering fosters the child's sense of mastery and self-reliance.

Maternal deprivation or separation may result in catastrophic reactions. The effect on the developing personality will be seen later in increased susceptability to loss, helplessness and activation of depression. The death of a parent has a long-standing impact on the young child.

Acute illness in a child may precipitate feelings of hope, helplessness and hopelessness. The specific long-term influence varies in relationship to the interference with age-related developmental tasks.

For children who are born with significant birth defects or develop chronic disabling illnesses, there is need for understanding the process and tasks of hope. The families of these children are faced with an enormous burden of adaptation and coping. Over time the tasks will shift or be reactivated. The families may experience a sense of chronic grief which becomes acute when reminded that their children are limited to living less fully than other children.

Proper balance of the tasks of hoping is maintained when family members are included actively in caring for a child who is acutely or chronically ill. The participation itself implies that goals are worth striving for and can be achieved with mutual cooperation. This also helps to resolve feelings of helplessness and guilt that the parents may have.

Parents and children can shift cognitive balance by seeking information, talking with the staff, sharing with other parents with similar problems, and seeing other children in various stages of illness and recovery.

Hope in Medical-Surgical Nursing

Severe physical illness or injury is a life crisis to a patient, the family and sometimes the treatment staff. Critically ill patients require dramatic and intensive care which may be life-saving. Or heroic efforts may still result in death, which activates feelings of hopelessness and helplessness.

People with chronic, disabling conditions go through stages of adaptation similar to those of any significant loss. Feelings of hope and despair fluctuate as the person works through the necessary changes.

There is speculation that the giving-up syndrome of helplessness and hopelessness may precipitate or exacerbate an illness. A person who is dying usually experiences many aspects of hoping and despair as do the dying person's significant others in dealing with the impending loss.

Rudolf Moos described seven adaptive tasks of the patient and family to severe illness or injury:

> 1. *Dealing with the discomfort, incapacitation and other symptoms* of the illness or injury.
> 2. *Managing the stresses of special treatment procedures and the environment,* especially in intensive care units with life-saving but frightening machines and activities. The patient may feel overwhelmed by helplessness and dependency on staff and equipment.
> 3. *Developing and maintaining adequate relationships* with medical, nursing and other care-taking staff. The patient vigilantly scans the staff for signs of hope and is sensitive to attitudes of helplessness or hopelessness in other people.
> 4. *Preserving a satisfactory self-image and maintaining a sense of competence and mastery.* Defining the limits of independence and resetting life goals are an important part of this task, and hope is vital to this process.
> 5. *Preserving a reasonable emotional balance* of the many disturbing feelings aroused by the illness and treatment. These include the sense of failure, anxiety, apprehension at not knowing outcomes, sense of isolation, and feelings of inadequacy and resentment. Maintenance of hope is essential for dealing with these reactions.
> 6. *Preserving relationships with family and friends* in spite of a changed role-identity of being a "patient" or a "dying person."
> 7. *Preparing for an uncertain future* in which significant losses are threatened.[21]

In describing this last task for patients and families, Moos stated:

> Ironically, new medical procedures which raise hope for patients with previously incurable illnesses may make this task more difficult. Patients must prepare for permanent loss of function while maintaining hope that restoration of function may be possible. When death seems likely, patients and family members must engage in anticipatory mourning and initiate the grieving process while maintaining hope that new treatment procedures may prove beneficial.[22]

The seven tasks of adaptation are dealt with by individuals in a variety of ways. These vary as to the illness or injury, the personality of those involved and the unique set of environmental circumstances.

Jerome Motto commented that current trends in health care are not conducive to creating an atmosphere of hope. They tend to deter the development of the trusting relationship so important to conveying and maintaining hope in a critical situation. "That suicide occurs more often in curable than in incurable diseases compounds the irony."[23]

The assessment of hopelessness may be the first step in influencing a patient's outlook for the future. Motto stated:

> It is not holding out false hope to maintain an attitude of quiet confidence, to discuss the details of a health problem with an understanding patient, to review the outcome and significance of diagnostic and therapeutic procedures, to acknowledge the limitations of determining prognosis, and to encourage the conserving of hope as well as preparation for any eventuality.[24]

The impact of the influence of hope has been studied in clinical situations of patients with severe burns, in acute care units, on hemodialysis and receiving treatment for cancer. Hope for the dying patient and his or her family is a significant area for nursing intervention.

Hope in Psychiatric-Mental Health Nursing

The relationship of hope to conditions which are primarily emotional in origin is especially pertinent. Much of the information about hope, hopelessness and helplessness has come from psychological studies of patients in various psychiatric situations.

For many years there was an aura of hopelessness about the treatment and prognosis of these people. It is now understood that much of the "hopeless" conditions and behavior was related to the phenomena of institutionalization and dehumanization. The concept of learned helplessness is directly applicable.

Hope has a relationship to the clinical entity of depression. The person who later develops significant reactive depression may have had disturbed childhood relationships. According to Ronald Drake and Joseph Price these include parents who are struggling with their own depression and dependency.[25] They overprotected their children, teaching them to "overtrust" others and "undertrust" themselves in dealing with developmental tasks. Later, the parents withdrew love and support as they expected higher levels of performance. The children felt bewildered, lost and helpless until they mobilized themselves to meet parental demands. They became pseudoindependent and pseudomature without the opportunity of having dependency needs recognized and met. Later in life, these persons may be especially vulnerable to approval from others and to loss. The latter often precipitates depression with feelings of helplessness and hopelessness.

The relation of suicidal ideation and behavior to depression has long been recognized. Aaron Beck et al. have isolated feelings of hopelessness as a stronger indicator of suicide potential than depression itself.[26] They define hopelessness operationally as having negative expectations. Hopelessness leads to an attenuated desire to live, which increases suicidal ideation and action. The suicidal person has a highly constricted view of the future or rates it negatively.

Hopelessness is often the catalyst in suicide. The hopeless person misconstrues experiences in a negative way, anticipating a negative outcome for any attempt to achieve major goals. The implication for treatment is the recommendation that attention be paid to the cognitive and attitudinal aspects of hopelessness and hoping.

Sidney Jourard wrote that suicidal behavior was the response to a real or imagined invitation to die.

> But a person lives only so long as he experiences his life as having meaning and value, as long as he has something to live for: meaningful projects that will animate him and invite him into the future, or entice him to pull himself into the future. He will continue to live so long as he has hope of fulfilling meanings and value. As soon as meaning, value, and hope vanish from a person's experience, he begins to stop living; he begins to die.[27]

Suicide under these circumstances may occur through an active step or a passive resignation resulting in sickness or accidents.

Stotland, a pioneer in the study of hope, focused on the therapy of hope to treat patients with psychoses.[28] The importance of a hoping environment among staff and other patients was emphasized as essential to recovery. Many therapeutic units are now developed with a concept of hope which emphasizes coping abilities and minimizes helplessness.

NURSING ACTION IN THE MAINTENANCE AND RESTORATION OF HOPE

> Hope is the most beneficial of all the affections, and doth much to the prolongation of life, if it be not too often frustrated; but entertaineth fancy with an expectation of good.
> Francis Bacon

> He is the best physician who is the best inspiror of hope. Samuel Taylor Coleridge

People strive to cope with the impact of serious illness in a variety of ways. These coping skills are used in combination and reflect the characteristic styles and current stresses. If the nurse is knowledgeable about the patient, family and illness situation, she or he is better prepared to maintain and restore hope.

To do this the nurse must be able to provide an atmosphere of hope which comes from self, other staff, patients and the physical environment. This is possible through exploration of one's view of the meanings of life, illness and death. Feelings of hope, helplessness and hopelessness are found in all nursing situations under certain circumstances. In addition to helping others with these feelings, the nurse may experience shifts along her or his own hope continuum.

If nurses feel hopeless or helpless in relation to a patient or family, they talk these feelings over with others to get encouragement and a clearer picture of the reality of the situation. If their hopes for the recovery of a patient are disappointed, they often feel bewildered, angry, confused and grief-stricken. They use the hoping tasks of worrying and mourning.

In some situations nursing staff members protect themselves from the hurt and despair of desperately or terminally ill patients by lack of involvement and emotional distancing. In these circumstances the staff needs ongoing encouragement and understanding to maintain a hopeful attitude to communicate to patients and family members. Even in situations where death is imminent, help can still be given.

Moos identified the following seven major coping skills that patients, families and staff use in reaction to the stresses and adaptations required in cases of significant illness or injury.[29] Hope helps to sustain the person in using these skills. And the use of coping skills has an impact on the degree of hope experienced. Nursing action is based on the coping skills and the hoping tasks.

The coping skills are the following:

Denying or Minimizing the Seriousness of the Crisis; Isolating or Dissociating Feelings Connected with the Condition

The mother of a premature infant maintains that the baby is "just a little early."
A man with a prior myocardial infarction regards new symptoms as "indigestion."
A nurse concludes that the suicide of a patient was "probably for the best."

This coping style maintains hope by not facing and becoming overwhelmed by the worst. It provides time for other coping resources to be developed. Reality factors are temporarily distorted to increase encouragement and decrease worrying. The first stage of mourning is shock and disbelief (see Chapter 5).

The nurse recognizes the need for this kind of reaction and does not directly confront it. She or he remains alert to cues that the person has shifted from the need for denial or insulation and prevents the patient and family from taking injurious action based on the denial.

Seeking Relevant Information which Can Relieve Anxiety Caused by Misconception and Uncertainty

A married couple asked for genetic counseling after their first baby was born with multiple physical handicaps.
A woman recently diagnosed as having diabetes asked if she had brought it on herself by eating too many sweets.
A depressed man asked if he would become addicted to his prescribed medication.

This coping skill can maintain or restore hope by providing information (reality factors) about the condition and successful treatment of other people (encouragement). It decreases the need for or answers the questions raised by worrying. It decreases helplessness by giving a time dimension in which specific events and emotions can be anticipated. With accurate information, goals can be better set. The act of seeking information can reduce feelings of uselessness and helplessness.

The nurse is knowledgeable about the given illness, treatment and usual responses, including emotional reactions. She or he shares this information with patients, families and other staff, helps to clarify misconceptions and prepare for anticipated reactions and problems, and knows sources of help and makes appropriate referral to community agencies and self-help groups.

Requesting Reassurance and Emotional Support from Family, Friends and Medical-Nursing Staff while Maintaining a Sense of Person Competence

Parents Anonymous is a self-help group of concerned parents who have abused or are afraid they might abuse their children.

A woman who is slowly dying requests that members of her family take turns in staying with her.

A young man came into the crisis center because he felt almost overwhelmed by the urge to jump off the bridge.

This coping skill maintains or restores hope with encouragement gained through reaching out to others and receiving responsive concern and help. The person combats helplessness in the current situation by asserting independence and mastery in other areas of personal competence. Worrying and uncertainty is lessened by sharing. If loss is imminent, the person experiences support by initiating the mourning process. The patient experiences encouragement from similarly affected patients or through being an active member of the health team in alliance against a difficult illness.

The nurse is aware of the many emotional reactions and needs for support by the patient, family and staff. She or he takes the initiative in encouraging the expression of feelings, responds appropriately, and provides opportunities for and encourages independent action to combat feelings of helplessness and maintain self-esteem.

Learning Illness-Related Procedures which Confirm Personal Ability and Effectiveness

The nurse taught a young mother the principles of behavior modification so that she could apply them sequentially in helping her child with Down's Syndrome to develop to maximal functioning.

The nurse taught a teenage boy with diabetes how to inject insulin, keep urine test charts, and regulate food intake so that he would be more independent of parental overprotection.

The nurse taught a young woman who hyperventilated a series of relaxation exercises. She instructed her in how to breathe in a paper bag to stop an attack rather than using a minor tranquilizer.

This coping skill maintains or restores hope with the sense of mastery and encouragement that some effective action can be learned. Information and practice of the procedure increases the reality base. Helplessness is decreased as both the patient and family experience a sense of pride in the accomplishments.

The nurse teaches the patient and family how to do the necessary procedures using the principles of learning and giving encouragement along the way. She or he is aware of the need for periodic follow-up and learning of new procedures when necessary and recognizes the importance of hope in motivation.

Setting Concrete Limited Goals

A child with terminal leukemia is given multiple short projects in the hospital school.

After open-heart surgery the patient has the goal of dangling before getting up out of bed and ambulating.

A "token economy" ward is set up in a large psychiatric hospital to provide an environment in which institutionalized patients can be encouraged to take care of themselves and the environment in a progressive way.

This coping skill maintains or restores hope with the encouragement gained by accomplishing set goals, which increases motivation to set new goals. Information about reality is gained as the person realizes that seemingly overwhelming problems can be broken down into small, manageable parts. Helplessness is decreased as the patient experiences the impact of actions on the outcomes. Instead of just worrying about something, action which results in success is taken.

The nurse is knowledgeable about the usual progression of a given illness and encourages the patient to exercise as much independence and control of his or her own care as possible. The nurse helps the patient to recognize the progress made and plan the sequence of goals which will lead to maximal functioning. She or he includes the family in setting and achieving goals. The nurse may plan the social and physical environment so that the patient is in contact with other patients in varying degrees of recovery and can compare progress and increase motivation.

Rehearsing Alternative Outcomes with Staff and Family

A teenage football player with a fractured leg argues effectively with his father about his plan to channel his energies into the debate team for the season.

After prolonged dialysis and two unsuccessful kidney transplants, an older man discusses with the staff his wish to be allowed to die.

After repeated unsuccessful trips back home after psychiatric hospitalizations, a young woman decides to live in a halfway house and uses the nursing staff to practice for her intake interview.

With this coping skill one maintains or restores hope by worrying about possible difficulties and reminding oneself of previous successes. By recognizing different options, the person feels encouraged and supported in meeting anticipated difficulties. Exploring alternatives helps in expanding the reality base on which to make decisions. Anticipatory action increases the sense of mastery and reduces helplessness. If death or another loss is imminent, this coping skill helps to initiate the mourning process for the patient, family and staff.

The nurse is aware of and responsive to the anticipated problems and helps the patient and family to talk about concerns and plans, suggesting additional alternatives and ideas from experience. The nurse may arrange for patients with similar conditions to meet in dyads or small groups. She or he is knowledgeable about the sequence of mourning and is prepared to help the patient, family and other staff in whatever stage they have reached. The nurse shares in the treatment plan with the rest of the staff in regard to alternatives.

Finding a General Purpose or Pattern of Meaning in the Course of Events of the Crisis, Illness, Treatment and Outcome

When all of the infants in a multiple birth died, the parents regarded it as an experience to learn from. They later adopted a baby. Subsequently, the woman risked becoming pregnant again and had a healthy boy.

The parents of a child receiving research protocols for leukemia found solace in thinking that even if their child died, perhaps the knowledge gained would save other children in the future.

After crashing his car while drunk, a man gave up drinking. He found spiritual meaning and a new support system through Alcoholics Anonymous.

Hope is maintained or restored with this coping skill by an increase in faith or belief in a divine purpose. The patient finds encouragement in the belief that suffering may have some meaning or help others. A deep, significant form of worrying may help to answer questions about the personal meaning of life and death. The patient, family and staff find mutual support in the process of rejoicing or mourning together.

The nurse recognizes the complexity of any given illness situation and respects how individuals differ in their responses. She or he provides contact for religious or spiritual counseling if desired; listens to the patient's philosophy of life and helps the patient make peace with self and the world; and helps the patient, family and other staff through the emotional experience of severe illness, recovery or death. The nurse applies the concept of hope to him or herself and turns to other people for understanding and solace to maintain hope in the meaning of the struggle between illness and health.

Where there's life, there's hope; where there's hope, there's life.

REFERENCES

1. Korner, I. N.: Hope as a method of coping. J. Consulting and Clinical Psychol. 34, 2:2-3, April 1970.
2. Stotland, E.: The Psychology of Hope. San Francisco, Jossey-Bass, 1969, p. 1.
3. Seligman, M. E. P.: Helplessness. San Francisco, Freeman, 1975, pp. 1-8; Jourard, S. M.: Suicide: an invitation to die. Am. J. Nurs. 70, 2:269-75, February 1970; Roberts, S. L.: Behavioral Concepts and the Critically Ill Patient. Englewood Cliffs, N.J., Prentice-Hall, 1976.
4. Fromm, E.: The Revolution of Hope. New York, Harper, 1968.
5. Kübler-Ross, E.: On Death and Dying, New York, Macmillan, 1969.
6. Davitz, J. R.: The Language of Emotion. New York, Academic Press, 1969, p. 86.
7. Vaillot, Sister M. C.: Hope: the restoration of being. Am. J. Nurs. 70, 2:271, February 1970.
8. Korner, Hope as a method of coping, p. 3.
9. Fromm, The Revolution of Hope, p. 11.
10. Ibid., p. 9.
11. Davitz, The Language of Emotion, pp. 116-17.
12. Erikson, E. H.: Childhood and Society. New York, Norton, 1963, pp. 147-251.
13. Fromm, The Revolution of Hope, pp. 19-20.
14. Schmale, A. H.: A genetic view of affects with special reference to the genesis of helplessness and hopelessness. *In*: The Psychoanalytic Study of the Child. New York, International Universities Press, 1964, pp. 287-310.
15. Seligman, Helplessness, p. 150.
16. Lynch, W. F.: Images of Hope. Baltimore, Helicon, 1965, p. 48.

17. Fromm, The Revolution of Hope, p. 13.
18. Ibid., p. 14.
19. Korner, Hope as a method of coping, p. 5.
20. Wright, B. A. and Shontz, F. C.: Process and tasks in hoping. Rehabilitation Literature. 29, 11:329-31, November 1968.
21. Moos, R. H., (ed.): Coping with Physical Illness. New York, Plenum, 1977, pp. 8-12.
22. Ibid., p. 11.
23. Motto, J. A.: Hope, suicide, and medical practice. JAMA. 234, 11:1150, December 15, 1975.
24. Ibid., p. 1150.
25. Drake, R. E. and Price, J. L.: Depression: adaptation to disruption and loss. Perspect. Psychiatr. Care. XIII, 4:163-69, 1975.
26. Beck, A. T., Kovacs, M., and Weissman, A.: Hopelessness and suicidal behavior. JAMA. 234, 11:1146-49, December 15, 1975.
27. Jourard, Suicide, pp. 269-73.
28. Stotland, The Psychology of Hope.
29. Moos, Coping with Physical Illness, pp. 12-15.

ADDITIONAL READINGS

Adams, C. L. and Proulx, J. R.: The role of the nurse in the maintenance and restoration of hope, and Poslusny, E. and Arroyo, M. K.: Bereavement and the nursing student. *In* Schoenberg, B., et al. (eds.): Bereavement: Its Psychosocial Aspects. New York, Columbia University Press, 1975, pp. 256-78.

Alvarez, A.: The Savage God: A Study of Suicide. New York, Random House, 1972.

Buehler, J. A.: What contributes to hope in the cancer patient? Am. J. Nurs., 75, 8:1353-56, August 1975.

Choron, J.: Suicide. New York, Scribner's, 1972.

Davitz, L. J. and Davitz, J. R.: How do nurses feel when patients suffer? Am. J. Nurs., 75, 9:1505-10, September 1975.

DeRosis, H. A. and Pellegrino, V. Y.: The Book of Hope: How Women Can Overcome Depression. New York, Macmillan, 1976.

Engel, G. L.: Psychological Development in Health and Disease. Philadelphia, Saunders, 1963.

Furman, E.: A Child's Parent Dies. New Haven, Yale University Press, 1974.

Kobler, A. L. and Stotland, E.: The End of Hope: A Social-clinical Study of Suicide. New York, Free Press of Glencoe, 1964.

Menninger, K. A.: Hope. Menninger Perspective. 4:4-11, 1975.

Neale, R. E.: The Art of Dying. New York, Harper, 1973.

Read, P. P.: Alive. New York, Avon, 1974.

Schoenberg, B., et al. (eds.): Loss and Grief: Psychological Management in Medical Practice. New York, Columbia University Press, 1970.

Stewart, W. K.: Hopelessness following illness in middle age. Psychosomatics. 18:29-32, 1977.

Weisman, A. D.: On Dying and Denying: A Psychiatric Study of Terminality. New York, Behavioral Publications, 1972.

Zderad, L. T. and Belcher, H. C.: Developing Behavioral Concepts in Nursing. Atlanta, Ga., Southern Regional Education Board, 1968.

12 HUMOR IN NURSING

Vera M. Robinson

ST. PETER'S HOSPITALS.
TEACHING DIVISION.
THE SHAFTESBURY HOSPITAL.
LONDON, W.C.2.

The talkative new graduate had bored us for most of the lunch hour with her ideas about "empathy" and "total patient care." Finally, Mrs. B., an old-timer snorted: "You and your empathy! Just how do you establish it with the patient?" "That's easy," said the neophyte airly, "Just put yourself in bed with him."[1]

Convinced of the value of humor, having expounded at length about the lack of it in nursing practice and nursing education, I found myself, like that talkative new graduate, "in bed" with a concept and faced with the reality of my desire to establish humor as having an important and unexploited place in nursing. Humor is a form of communication extensively used by human beings as a coping mechanism in a variety of situations, including times of illness and hospitalization. However, there has been little deliberate use of humor by health professionals as a tool in the helping process.

The concept of humor has been explored from as far back in time as humans could express themselves in writing and probably long before that. Humor has been discussed from the point of view of philosophers, psychologists, psychoanalysts, anthropologists, sociologists, physiologists, dramatists, poets, prose writers, satirists, comedians, educators, child development specialists, industrial management specialists and others ad infinitum. "Probably, no human reaction has given rise to so many conflicting opinions as those found in works dealing with laughter."[2]

A simple, universally accepted definition is as difficult to find as a universal theory of humor or a universal language. One cannot begin to study humor without encountering a myriad of related or integral ideas such as wit, laughter, joking, comedy, kidding, teasing, clowning, mimicking, satire and so on. Certainly, humor includes all of these.

Adding to the complexity of this elusive concept is the fact that, like the clock which stops when it is taken apart to see what makes it tick, humor loses its impact when it is analyzed. E. B. White says that humor "can be dissected, as a frog can, but the thing dies in the process and the innards are discouraging to any but the pure scientific mind."[3] Martin Grotjahn in *Beyond Laughter* apologized because his book was "not funny." Laughter, he says, "has a tendency to disappear when we focus our intellect on it and try to understand it." But, he goes on, "the hope remains that we may laugh even more merrily and with greater inner freedom when we understand laughter better."[4]

Spurred on to rise above the physical burden (the verbosity, theories and definition) in my pursuit of humor, I found myself hit with its emotional impact as well. My initial review of the literature revealed analyses of such devastating factors as fear, aggression, hostility, narcissism, sadism and masochism as the basis of humor. I was suddenly faced with a horrible thought. Had I simply been finding a permissible outlet for my own hostility in asserting that humor is healthy, has therapeutic value, and is an excellent catalyst in learning? For a time, I worried that my strong belief that humor and laughter can be used as a constructive force might not survive as I struggled in "that bed," fending off the grasping arms and groping hands of hostility and aggression.

Continuing my research brought back my perspective. Certainly one would agree that humor is a socially acceptable outlet for hostility and aggression, but, even in this context, it is still a constructive and useful mechanism. As a relief for tension and a way of coping with stress, it is a most beneficial agent. But beyond that, I have felt that the need to laugh and, thus, the need for humor is as basic as the need for love, security or trust, and it should be added to the list of basic needs. One of the infant's first reactions to people is the smile. We pay outrageous prices for comedians to entertain us. A sense of humor is valued as an admirable characteristic and a sign of maturity. No adult would really ever admit to having no sense of humor. Further reading reassured me.

> Laughter is a way of human communication which is essentially and exclusively human. It can be used to express an unending variety of emotions. It is based on guiltfree release of aggression and any release makes us perhaps a little better and more capable of understanding one another, ourselves and life. What is learned with laughter is learned well. Laughter gives freedom, and freedom gives laughter. He who understands the comic begins to understand humanity and the struggle for freedom and happiness.[5]

My interest in the concept of humor arose originally from two mental health concerns: one involved facilitating students' adaptation to the stresses encountered in nursing; the other, providing a therapeutic milieu within the hospital in which patients' ability to cope with the stresses of illness and hospitalization could be fostered. One of the mechanisms which has been observed in both situations is the use of humor.

There is an increasing emphasis on a more humanistic approach to the individual within the helping professions. We recognize each person as a psychosocial being with unique perceptions, motivations and behaviors. Within this humanistic framework of openness and warmth and caring, humor is a natural phenomenon.

> The time is ripe for health professionals to do more than just enjoy humor. We need to understand it. We need to begin to be able to laugh at ourselves, at life and at our establishments. And, we need to begin to help our students and patients to deal with their stresses, tensions and frustrations through the use of humor. We need to believe that humor is constructive and healthy; we must encourage its use as a coping mechanism, and cultivate its use as a viable tool in communication.[6]

If we accept the premise that all human behavior is purposeful, has meaning and can be understood, then it behooves us to look at humor in the same manner as we do other behaviors. What purpose does it serve? What meaning does it have for the individual? When is it a constructive element and when is it not? How can humor be developed and cultivated as a tool in communication and intervention? These are some of the questions which need to be answered in applying the concept of humor to nursing.

DEFINITION

The definitions of humor are many and varied, and some authors simply solve the problem by not defining it. The archaic definition of humor (umor) is "moisture, vapor." In medieval physiology, humor meant the four principal fluids of the body: blood, phlegm, cholor (yellow bile) and melancholy (black bile). When any of these fluids predominated, it determined man's health, temperament or mood. A just balance made a good compound called "good humor"; a preponderance of any one of the four made a bad compound called "ill humor." We still speak of a person's "good humor," implying a sense of well-being and readiness to laugh.

Most definitions also include the idea that it is the unexpected shock, the sudden twist, the incongruous, ludicrous note which creates the humor. Often humor points up a familiar dilemma or weakness which strikes home because it is common to all of us. Thus, humor has been defined as the frank enjoyment of the imperfect, which generates some physical response such as smiling or laughter. Often humor and laughter are used interchangeably.

A generic definition would avoid getting bogged down in an attempt to distinguish between these and other terms, such as wit, joking, comedy, and provide for the breadth and varieties of humor which can occur in a natural setting. Most humor in health settings is spontaneous or situational, often witticisms and pleasantries, rather than formal joke telling. Therefore, for the purpose of this discussion, humor will be defined as any communication which is perceived by any of the interacting parties as humorous and leads to laughing, smiling or a feeling of amusement. And both humor and laughter will be used in a generic sense to encompass all the other related words or terms.

THE NATURE OF HUMOR

Theories describing the nature of humor span philosophical, physiological, anthropological, sociological and psychological perspectives. Humor and laughter have been described as instincts, biological reflexes, social correctives and protections, agents of psychological liberation and comparable to play as growth and survival mechanisms.

William Fry in *Sweet Madness* calls humor a paradox of abstractions. He describes its relationship to play. Both involve smiling and laughter; both are found in interpersonal interaction communication; both are sensitive to what he calls the spontaneity-thoughtfulness balance. When we become too thoughtful or self-conscious about either play or humor, we lose it. There is a correlation between the development of humor and play from childhood through adulthood. Fry feels the transition from a child's humor to an adult form of humor requires some psychological level of maturation and achievement of the ability to abstract and conceptualize.[7]

Yet the element of childhood play persists even in adult humor. Freud speaks of the "infantile" factor in the comic who reduces him or herself to a child and makes us discover the child in us. The pleasure comes from being the onlooker and not the victim.[8] In the process of achieving the stability and security of adulthood, "we sacrifice spontaneity and genuineness," says Harvey Mindess.[9] Our sense of humor frees us from the constraints and realities of daily living.

With maturity, however, comes not only the comfort derived from laughing at the minor distresses of others, but also the ability to laugh at one's own minor misfortunes. This implies the attainment, to some degree, of the power of objectivity—of seeing ourselves as others see us. There develops also a "larger humour," says William McDougall,

> . . . which finds occasion for laughter in those defects and shortcomings which are common to all men; such humor, including in its objects the laugher himself, does not wound, as does the lower, simpler form of laughter; for it brings a bond of fellowship between him who laughs and all his fellows, inviting all men, without discriminations, to share in the genial exercise.[10]

Humor, Freud says, has something liberating about it. It has grandeur and elevation. The grandeur lies in the "triumph of narcissism, the victorious assertion of the ego's invulnerability." The main thing is the intention which humor carries out, whether acting in relation to the self or other people. It means, "Look! here is the world, which seems so dangerous! It is nothing but a game for children—just worth making a jest about."[11] Humor in our culture seems to range on a continuum from "laughing at" to "laughing with."

Many of the writings in this area are classics, accepted as partial answers to the nature of humor. Much of the past studies have been speculative or based on psychoanalytic theory. More recently, research outside of the psychoanalytic framework has opened new avenues related to cognitive, perceptual and social facets. "Our understanding remains in a highly fragmentary state, due to the continuing lack of any systematic empirical and theoretical attack on humor."[12]

THE PURPOSE OF HUMOR

Why do we need humor? Why do we laugh? These questions also have intrigued writers over the centuries, and the answers are again many and varied: so that we will not cry; for relief; to delight; to decrease social distance; to satisfy repressed impulses; to dissipate hostility; to assert superiority. For whatever reason, it becomes apparent that humor is a "pleasure upon which mankind pounces at the slightest excuse for indulging in it."[13] Humor appears to serve "a myriad of communicative functions." William Fry agrees with Freud that a joke has a host of "unconscious chords" which sound in the audience's mind no less loudly than does the explicit joke. This, he says, proves the vital link between humor and life. "By these bridges of the unconscious the stream between humor and life is crossed and re-crossed, and there is found to be ample traffic from Shore to Shore."[14]

Humor in Nursing Situations

Within the health setting, humor is usually an indirect form of communication. It is subordinated to the formal communication patterns of the hospital; when used, it is casual and generally inconspicuously blended into the flow of events. However, it serves a valuable purpose in "promoting the continued harmony of a social relation at the same time that important messages are conveyed."[15] It often has the overall effect of diminishing discomfort and managing some of the "delicate situations" which occur. One reason for this is that humor is a familiar pattern of communication which both nurses and patients bring with them into the health setting.

Three major functions of humor—communicative, social and psychological—are intertwined in health settings. The humor used in nursing situations predominantly serves:

1. to establish relationships.
2. to relieve anxiety, stress and tension.
3. to release anger, hostility and aggression in a socially acceptable way.
4. to avoid or deny feelings which are too painful and stressful to deal with at the time.
5. to facilitate the process of learning.

Any one, or any combination, of these purposes may be operating in any given humorous situation. As in all interactions, there are many factors which will affect the dynamics of the situation and many techniques of humor which can be used. However, of primary concern in evaluating the usefulness of the humor in a situation should be the needs which are being served rather than the type, technique or content of the humor. Humor is healthy when it deals with immediate issues and helps the individual handle realities. It becomes destructive and dysfunctional when it abets pathological denial of reality—when it becomes a means of running away from the difficulties of living rather than easing the way to dealing with them.

Establishing Relationships: "To laugh, or to occasion laughter through humor and wit, is to invite those present to come close . . . it aims at decreasing social distance."[16] Humor is used frequently in health settings to break the ice, to reduce fear of the unfamiliar and encourage the sense of trust, to establish a feeling of comaraderie and friendship. It says to the patient, colleague or student: "You can trust me. Relax, I am a friend. This isn't such a terrible place." It sets a tone for cohesiveness, team spirit, working together in a therapeutic atmosphere. Often humor takes the form of a witticism or pleasantry. Sometimes it consists of telling a joke, teasing or jocular talk, a practical joke or a situation joke which occurs spontaneously in the interaction.

Humor among colleagues relaxes the rigidity of the social structure without upsetting it. A group of beginning students were assigned to their first experience in the hospital. An x-ray orderly had at one time accidentally mispronounced the head nurse's name (which was Westrack) and continued this friendly interplay each time he came to the ward. With a blank innocent expression, he would say something like "Mrs. Beartrack" and she would groan. When this occurred on the students' first morning, it delighted them and helped to set a tone of warmth in which they, as low men on the totem pole in the hospital hierarchy, immediately felt comfortable.

In times of illness, strangers are suddenly thrown into very intimate and somber contacts. There is no time to build a relationship. Humor serves to facilitate the trust and cooperation which is needed and expected.

Patients on admission to the hospital, which is a strange and unknown environment, may joke with the nurses about all "the hotel service" they will be getting and the "pretty nurses" to take care of them. In some instances, the nurse can initiate such joking to set the tone for a more relaxed atmosphere, much as a dinner speaker does with a typical introductory joke. Sociologist Rose Laub Coser, who did a study of the social structure of a hospital ward, believes that the contribution humor makes to social economy within the institution of the hospital should be stressed. "In such a shifting and threatening milieu," she points out, "a story well told, which, in a few minutes, entertains, reassures, conveys information, releases tension, and draws people more closely together, may have more to contribute than carefully planned lectures and discussions toward the security of the frightened sick."[17]

Relief of Anxiety, Stress, Tension: Anxiety is perhaps one of the most common sources of discomfort which prompt the use of humor. Of course, anxiety is inherent in all the needs which humor might help to alleviate, but, in some situations, it is the predominant theme.

Humorous get-well cards and the myriad jokes and cartoons about illness, hospitals, doctors and nurses attest to patients' use of humor to attempt to deal with anxiety-provoking stressful situations.

In Coser's study of the hospital ward, she observed that there was much jocular talk among patients which consisted mainly of griping. This talk seemed to relate to three areas of anxiety: about self, about submission to a rigid authority structure, and about adjustment to a rigid routine.[18] Humor as a means of allaying anxiety and preserving the self against the pressure of routine and the patient's low status has a liberating effect and triumphs over weakness. The use of the jocular talk and particularly the jocular gripe transforms the individual complaint or experience into a shared or collective one. "It's better than hotel service. Where else can you get fresh ice water at 5:30 in the morning?" is a typical example of such a jocular gripe regarding a common annoyance to patients.

The intimate procedures to which the patient is subjected are also a subject for jokes. Humor seems to provide a way to manage anxiety, shame, embarrassment and social conflict.

Jokes about bedpans, bathrooms, enemas and so on are numerous.

> One student was told a joke by a patient about a nurse who worked in a hospital where the call lights above the doors were red when turned on. When the nurse went to take her driver's test, she went through a red light and her response to the policeman was, "Oh, I thought it was just another patient wanting a bedpan."

Bedpan humor raises the question of regression in the service of the ego. Under stress, primary drives, normally under control in the healthy individual, may take over and need to be channeled through a socially acceptable medium such as humor. In a study investigating the reflection of group anxiety in art, a collection of French political cartoons during the Franco-Prussian War (1870-71) was analyzed. When the war outlook seemed bleak, the cartoons showed a frank regression to oral, anal and sexual levels. As the war situation improved, the maturity level of the cartoons rose.[19]

In her study of a gynecological ward, Joan Emerson found it was usually the staff who initiated the jokes about the pelvic examination. It seemed to be "an institutionalized way the staff coaxed the patients to put up with affronts to their dignity."[20]

She also found a high incidence of joking behavior between male patients and female staff. Teasing and joking are closely related to flirting. In a provocative situation like the health setting where male-female roles are distorted, there is confusion and conflict as to appropriate behavior. Often, the male patient, placed in a dependent, powerless position in which his body image and masculinity are threatened, typically responds with sexually oriented jokes and joking. This type of humor, in which the patient relates to the nurse as man to woman rather than patient to authority figure, provides an avenue for asserting his masculinity. If he also makes the nurse embarrassed and uncomfortable, he asserts his superiority over the situation.

The nurse, who may react as a female and not recognize that the patient's behavior is defensive and useful to him, may wonder what she has done to encourage such a situation. Rather than becoming counterdefensive, she should assess the need behind the humor, respond with appropriate banter and then use this behavior as a cue to other impending threats to the patient's ego.

In their initial reactions to the "reality shocks" of nursing, students make frequent use of humor to relieve the anxiety and stress. The delightful old "Probie" cartoons in *RN* ("Quick, pick it up off the floor before it gets unsterile.") often pinpointed the stresses. As James Thurber once said, humor is often emotional chaos remembered in tranquility. In describing the process of reality shock which new graduates experience in their first work situations, Marlene Kramer states, "A beginning sense of humor is the first sign of the recovery phase. There is a lessening of tensions and an ability to see the amusing side of things. . . ."[21]

Because of the life and death struggle within the health setting, the type of humor often used is macabre, grim humor, similar to the black humor of fiction. This type of humor is called gallows humor, a term derived from Freud's famous story of the rogue being led to the gallows. It was a Monday, and the prisoner remarked, "Well, this week's beginning nicely."[22] Although pity is initiated for the condemned man, his stoic jibe releases the listener from having to suppress the painful emotion of pity to use the emotional energy to laugh.

This bravado in the face of death was described in *Experiment Perilous,* in which sociologist Rene Fox reports what happened on a small experimental metabolic ward. Because of the gravity of the diseases with which the physicians had to deal, under the constant threat of failure and death, and the problems and uncertainties involved, which could be coped with only by trial-and-error methods, the physicians evolved a highly patterned and intricate form of humor as a way of handling their stresses. As one physician said, "Our humour is a kind of protective device. If we were to talk seriously all the time and act like a bunch of Sir Galahads or something, we just couldn't take all this."[23] They joked about the uncertainties, about their inability to "cure" patients and about possible impending deaths; they made bets about the unknown.

This type of joking is so characteristic of physicians that it is generally referred to as "medical humor." In the earliest years of their medical training, physicians learn that an effective and appropriate way to handle their reactions to death and other stressful or emotionally provocative professional situations is to joke with their colleagues about them in a look-it-in-the-face-and-laugh manner. Other health professionals also utilize this type of humor in stress situations.

The hospital is a place in which staff must deal with problems (such as death) from which other people in society attempt to insulate themselves.[24] Humor neutralizes the significance of this emotionally tinged event. Although personnel joke among themselves, they rarely joke about death with a patient or visitors. Sometimes, however, a patient will initiate this type of humor, saying, for example, "How's my blood pressure? Do you think I'll live?" Another example is illustrated with this anecdote:

> The doctor was visiting his 90-year-old patient. She asked him, "Do you think I'll get well?" He answered sadly, "I hope so—but we doctors aren't magicians. We can't make our patients younger." Her eyes twinkled. "But, Doctor," she said, "I don't ask you to make me younger. I want you to help me get older."[25]

Patients on the metabolic ward which Fox studied also used a gallows type of humor. They wrote humorous "case histories" and "death reports" and told "death" jokes. "The value and usefulness of gallows humor for each individual, patient and staff, as a mechanism for coping, cannot be overlooked. . . . The recognition of whose needs are being met and when and in what situation seems to be the crucial factor."[26] Laughing at death, says G. Mikes, gives triple pleasure: the pleasure of the joke itself, the malicious joy of laughing at death's expense and the pleasure of taming and fraternizing with death.[27]

Another source of great anxiety to both patient and health team is the operating room, and here, too, humor is a frequently used mechanism for relieving tension. A cartoon which appeared in *The Saturday Evening Post* some years ago pictured an operating room with six gowned and masked persons standing around an empty operating room table, with the surgeon saying, "Come, come, now, one of you must be the patient."

In an operating room there is usually much jocular talk ("Do I have to work with you again?") and joke telling. Following an operation, during which the surgeon interspersed his discussion of the procedure to the student nurses observing it with several jokes, the surgeon commented: "Well, I guess you learned a few things today, including some new jokes."

The reaction of students to humor in this strained situation varies greatly, depending on their own anxiety, which may be increased rather than lessened if the humor disgusts or embarrasses them by being too macabre or risqué.

The following situation joke amused a group of students one day. It was used by the nursing instructor to relieve the tension of a student who had arrived late because of an accident with her car and had missed the surgery she was scheduled to observe. Instructor: "I'm so glad to see you. I heard you had an accident." Student: "I'm really sorry. I'm really sorry I'm late, but I'm so shook up." Instructor: "Well, that's all right. We'll just put you in the Recovery Room for today."

When anxiety or tension is too high, however, an attempt at humor may fall flat. The comic cannot be enjoyed when there is a "release of distressing affects," Freud says.[28] If the person is a victim of great pain or high anxiety, all his or her energy is needed to ward off the danger and the comic effect is lost. Anxiety must be mastered or controlled before reference to it may be enjoyed in the humorous situation.

Jacob Levine, in a study based on this premise, found that a joke seems funny only if it arouses anxiety and at the same time relieves it. He believes there are three types of reactions to a joke: (1) if it evokes no anxiety, the listener will be indifferent to it; (2) if it evokes anxiety and immediately dispels it, the listener will find it funny; (3) if it arouses anxiety without dissipating it, the listener will react with disgust, shame, embarrassment or horror.[29] When an elderly, dying patient moaned in pain, "Oh, God, dear God," an intern stepped behind a screen and said, "This is God. What do you want?" Everyone on the ward reacted with disgust rather than laughter because, for them, the anxiety was not relieved, although for the intern it was an attempt to relieve his feelings of helplessness in the situation.

Relieving Hostility and Aggression: Within the hospital society, there are many sources of frustration and anger, but, as in society in general, their outward expression is usually looked upon with disfavor. Civilization, says Freud, has caused repression of many basic impulses, and joking is a socially acceptable way of satisfying them. By making light of the forbidden impulse, the joke or cartoon releases the inner tension and permits momentary gratification. The unconscious source of the person's tension is so disguised in the joke that it is usually not disturbing. Because sex and aggression are basic instincts which create more conflict in our culture than almost any other, they seem to be the basis for much of the humor in this society.

The rigidity of hospital routines and their dehumanizing elements often make the patients angry. But they know that to be openly hostile is contrary to the "good" patient role and might alienate the staff upon whom they rely for care. Therefore, the jocular gripe provides an acceptable outlet for performing the function of complaint. The humor is a safety-valve. Comments like "Where else can you get ice water at 5:30 a.m." or "I'll have to go home to get a rest," are evidences of frustration. The patients' anger at their illness is also often revealed and dissipated through the use of humor: as with the patient who referred to his colostomy as "Old Stinky."

The staff within the health setting may also use humor as a way of handling their own reactions to the frustrations of the work situation, as in the following incident:

> A physician had ordered all stools of a patient who had been admitted for tests and observation to be saved. The nursing staff believed those which were filled with barium and the patient's enema returns were not valuable and disposed of them. The doctor, upset at this decision, rewrote the order to read, "Save everything that emits from the anal canal." The nurses then proceeded to send buckets of enema returns to the laboratory, and also took a large plastic bag used for linen, filled it with air, and labeled it "fresh flatus."

For the nurses who felt rebuffed that their judgment had not been accepted, this practical joke was an outlet for relieving their anger. As the word spread throughout the hospital, other personnel who laughed at the incident vicariously relieved some of their own pent-up frustration. Whether or not the physician involved wanted to "take a joke" like this one, the social pressure was on him to be a "good sport" and laugh with the others, which he did. Thus the mechanism served to restore communication in the physician-nurse relationship and to prevent either an outbreak of undisguised hostility or the bottling up of frustrations. Coser says that in a hospital the "give and take of support through humor helps the participants to live up to role expectations and to overcome the contradictions and ambiguities inherent in the complex social structure, and thereby to contribute to its maintenance."[30]

H. Kaplan and I. H. Boyd studied the social functions of humor on an open psychiatric ward established as a "therapeutic community" and observed patients' use of humor to express hostility.[31] When the humor was directed toward the staff, it served as a morale booster among the patients. When expressed toward "civilians," it functioned to decrease the distance and the difference between them. The expression of hostile humor toward other patients served to forestall deviant behavior by imposing a negative sanction. However, much of the humor directed by members of the therapeutic community toward other patients served to enhance the group's solidarity and comradeship, functioning almost as an initiation rite to their "in" group and providing members with support. Self-deprecating humor, on the other hand, was used either to deny the seriousness of a patient's illness or to "accommodate" the staff. However, it was felt that this self-ridicule permitted the person for the first time to take a detached view of him or herself and the problem; this recognition is the sine qua non of the therapeutic process.

William Fry describes the relationship not only between humor and play, but also between play and fighting, which he says may explain somewhat the frequent association of aggression and hostility with humor. Smiling and laughter are unconscious, nonverbal communication signals of aggressive-passive behaviors in the social hierarchy, with humor being the territory in which these interactions can be carried out.

Certain figures of speech in our language demonstrate these relationships: a disarming smile, a winning smile, weak with laughter, a triumphant laugh, "Smile when you say that" and the like. The joke teller is the dominant one; the joke is the weapon; laughter is the sign of victory. The audience is submissive; their laughter is the sign of their acceptance of defeat. "I give up," they say. In a joke orgy the pecking-order changes and the dominant role is passed on as each new joke is told.

It is difficult sometimes to determine, in play and fighting, the point at which one stops and the other begins, as in animal play, for example. The participants, however, must determine that they are playing, not fighting; therefore, they must set up a "play frame" which says "This is play, it is not real." There must be metacommunications, cues to convey the message that "This slap is in fun, not in anger," although the slap itself is real.

The same kind of metacommunication occurs in humor. It says "This is a joke, it is not for real." Thus the stage is set for the punch line, to which the surprised listener reacts with laughter.

The term "punch line" is related to fighting; in burlesque, it is called the "sock line." Its origin? From Punchinillo, the medieval Italian comedy figure. We all know of Punch and Judy puppet shows and *Punch,* the English humorous weekly. Probably all derive from Punchinillo which comes from the Italian word, polcino, for chicken. Thus Punch, the cocky rooster, an honored figure in the tradition of comedy, reveals on the stage some truths about ourselves, as represented by life in a barnyard.

What is the purpose, then, of the punch line? Fry says it is "to snatch some of the implicit materials" from innumerable themes within the joke and "project it into the workaday world" of reality.[32]

In *On Aggression,* Konrad Lorenz also deals with the relationship between aggression and humor. He believes that, along with knowledge, humor is one of civilization's great hopes for reducing the human aggressive drive to a tolerable level. He sees humor as exerting an influence on social behavior that is analogous to moral responsibility—it tends to make the world a more honest and, thus, a better place.

> Unlike enthusiasm, laughter—even at its most intense—is never in danger of regressing and causing the primal aggressive behavior to break through. Barking dogs may occasionally bite, but laughing men hardly ever shoot.[33]

Denial:

> And if I laugh at any mortal thing,
> 'Tis that I may not weep.
> Lord Byron

In many instances, humor is used to deny or avoid pain and distress. The "cut-up" who does not stop long enough to allow feelings often falls into this category. When the stress is too great, a person may use this mechanism in self-preservation until he or she is able to deal emotionally with the source of the stress. The nurse who jokes and laughs after a long, tiring night of emergencies and deaths or the patient, apprised of a lump in the breast, who begins joking about making a will are examples of people using humor to serve as denial of affect. After a near-fatal car accident, the young man who had been asleep in the back seat quipped, "First accident I've ever been in, and I had to sleep through it!"

Freud has said that in humor the ego refuses to be distressed by reality. In fact, the trauma becomes an occasion for it to gain pleasure. This rejection of reality and regression to the pleasure principle to ward off suffering are also characteristic of other more pathological methods used by the human mind, namely neurosis, psychoses, intoxication and so on. Humor, however, manages to achieve this escape effect "without overstepping the bounds of mental health."[34]

McDougall believes that laughter has "survival value." When we laugh, it is not that we are pleased, he says, but rather that the ridiculous situations would displease us, be painful or distressing, because mankind is endowed with primitive sympathetic tendencies. This emotional contagion is the cement of society, but it is also a great disadvantage in that we share the mishaps of others. This excess of sympathetic distress would destroy the individual if there were no antidote such as laughter.[35]

The humorous get-well cards on the market today may indicate our society's inability to handle the emotions inherent in illness, such as fear of death and loss of control. The funny card is a denial of real feelings, according to Catherine Norris, a "cover it up with a laugh" or an expression of helplessness, even though the person sending it is very concerned about the patient. It may be sending a message which says "I hope that you are not really ill, therefore, that this lighthearted card is appropriate. . . ."[36]

Humor in the Nursing Care Plan

The use of humor was incorporated into a written nursing care plan for an elderly widow who, following major surgery, had become depressed, lethargic and unwilling to participate in her own care. In a team conference, the nursing staff first recognized that, because she was without family and probably quite lonely, she needed to be shown a great deal of attention to feel someone cared. As the discussion proceeded, several cues led the staff to decide to try an approach of joking, teasing and humor with her, rather than solicitousness. For example:

> The student who had given the patient morning care after surgery had handed her a wet washcloth and said, "Would you like to wash off your face before breakfast?" The patient had replied very soberly, "No, I don't want to wash it off," as she took the cloth and washed. The student had not realized, until the same thing happened the next day, that the patient was teasing her.
>
> One of the graduate nurses had come to the room to take an apical pulse. The patient's roommate mentioned that the patient was an active member of the local Senior Citizen's Club and loved to play shuffleboard. The patient said, "I won't play anymore." The nurse tried to reassure her without success. After taking the apical pulse, the nurse remarked, "I can tell you're a shuffleboard player from your heartbeat." The patient looked surprised, then burst into laughter.

The team passed on their plan to personnel on the evening and night shifts who also used a joking approach with the patient throughout the next week. A nurse would tease her about running a race as she walked down the hall or about giving her a speeding ticket. When the patient grumbled "Is it?" to the head nurse's "Good morning" the head nurse threatened to hang her by her heels if she did not smile. The patient announced she would "cry like I did the first time I was hung by the heels," and then she laughed.

The patient began to respond to the extra attention and to participate more actively in her care. Her spirits improved and soon she was initiating the humor. By the end of the week, she was asking to go home.

The use of humor as a nursing intervention is in contrast to traditional psychiatric nursing approaches to the depressed patient. Why did it prove successful in this situation? There seemed to be two main factors: first, the lifestyle of the patient, and, second, the tone or climate of the ward.

The patient was described by a friend as the "cut-up" of the Senior Citizen's Club who had always had a "good sense of humor." Also, her depression was not so severe that all affect was frozen, and thus she was able to respond.[37] The additional attention she received, with the warmth and caring the humor conveyed, may have added to the success of the approach.

Humor was used extensively as a form of communication by the nursing team on this unit and set the tone for the patients to express their feelings in this way. The head nurse also used humor, joking and teasing with her patients as she made rounds. This seemed to be the most comfortable way for her to communicate. Through humor she was able to ascertain patients' needs, give them the feeling she was concerned about them, but reassure them that their being in the hospital was not so deadly serious an event.

The nursing team members also used humor to relieve their own anxieties and stresses. Besides the usual bantering and teasing, the blackboard in the locker room next to the nurse's station became a daily source of humor, with the graduates, student nurses and aides all contributing cartoons. One chalk drawing showed bedraggled, weary students on night duty with the dates of their service crossed off each morning and the instructor with wings and a jumpsuit hovering above. Another was of a student on "Preops" struggling with a syringe twice as big as herself with patients running in all directions and the student saying, "But it's only 1 cc. of each."

In summary, the use of humor on this ward was a therapeutic force. It created a warm climate and promoted good staff interpersonal relationships. The warmth was transmitted to the patients who, in turn, were able to use humor as a method of relieving the stresses of hospitalization. Yet the use of humor was controlled: the realistic needs of patients were not lost in the laughter, and the humor could be turned off when it was not effective.

Patient responses to humor must always be carefully evaluated. Not many unsuccessful jokes occur in hospitals, but, when they do occur, it is because "some implicit message which may be unsuitable for direct communication is stripped of its camouflage."[38]

> An enema was ordered for a young male patient who had had a hemorrhoidectomy and was going home. The nurse, who felt she had had a good relationship with him, thought she would tease him, and brought into the room a huge milk bucket and the largest piece of hose she could find. The patient took one look, ran to the bathroom, and refused to come out, apparently frightened and unable to see the joke.

The patient in this instance may have been reacting to the embarrassment of the intimate procedure or to the anticipation of pain. Very often the young to middle-age adult reacts to illness and hospitalization with a higher level of anxiety. To young, work-oriented members of society, illness may be so serious a threat that they find humor totally unacceptable and it falls flat. Conversely, the older patient who has faced many crises and, perhaps, has dealt with prospects of decreasing good health can take more in stride and needs the lightness of humor to get through the not-so-hopeful last years.

> A 70-year-old gentleman was having a Levin tube inserted. Finally, after much discomfort and gagging, it was in place. The patient lay against the pillows exhausted. The instructor said, "There, how's that? Better now?" He looked up, slowly grinned, and said "Oh, yes, it has a marvelous flavor."

Humor to Facilitate Learning

Humor in the learning situation can serve all the purposes described above—establishing warmth, relieving stress, releasing anger, avoiding feeling—and can also enhance the learning. "What is learned with laughter is learned well."[39]

In patient teaching, the use of humor facilitates the learning. The nurse who is able to relate appropriately humorous experiences while instructing a patient in some aspect of care helps the patient to laugh at uncertainties and anxieties.

> In teaching postcast care to a patient with an extensive leg cast, one nurse, in explaining how to manipulate with it, usually says, "And wait till you try to sit on the john!" This always gets a laugh. Then she goes on to explain how to support the leg when sitting.

The socialization of the student into the health profession begins the first day of classes. He or she learns very quickly that humor is one way to facilitate the process. However, there has been little attempt by educators to make conscious, deliberate use of humor in educational settings. There are four interrelated aspects to be considered:

1. enhancing the learning process itself.
2. facilitating the process of socialization into the profession.
3. teaching the concept of humor as a tool in communication and nursing interventions.
4. modeling the use of humor as a vehicle for facilitating the other three.[40]

For example, role playing in the classroom before the actual clinical experience helps to relieve the anxiety and make the anticipated situation less frightening. It is interesting that children in their play also seem to deal with anxiety-producing aspects of life—playing house, cops and robbers, cowboys and Indians. Dealing in advance with a serious situation in a play fashion says, "See, it's not such a frightening business."

When such procedures as admission and preoperative care were role played in a classroom, at first in a very negative way, the students laughed uproariously. When they were done again, this time in a positive manner, the class seemed to progress more comfortably and with much less anxiety.

Making use of situation humor in the classroom adds to an instructor's humanness. The instructor who can relate some of her or his own humorous experiences as a student or staff nurse helps the student, who usually has unrealistic expectations, to relax. It is easier as a student to laugh at your own mistakes if the teachers can laugh at theirs.

Students' imitations and mimicking of instructors and hospital staff, not only in private, but also at school parties with the objects of the humor present, aid in the socialization process and are a combination of affectionate teasing, expression of hostility and relief of tension. The student who can initiate humor comfortably with the faculty gives evidence of an interpersonal skill which will be reflected in the ability to relate to other people.

The planned use of humor in education is an art that can be cultivated by instructors. Techniques for creating humor have been described by many authors and can be added to one's writing, speaking or communication in the learning situation. The value of laughter in all of education has been aptly stated by Kenneth Eble in *The Perfect Education.*

> Learning begins in delight and flourishes in wonder. . . . Parents . . . must laugh greatly. For children, solemnity is like a whole pane of glass in an abandoned building. Solemnity invites shattering. . . . But why laughter? Because laughter is giving and recognizing. It forces a physical giving that releases for a moment the very self. And if we did not recognize some rugged corner of ourselves, some flawed reality, we would not laugh. Such giving is necessary to prepare the self to learn. . . . Parents can hardly do better than respond to their children's sense of absurdity, to let physical ticklings grow into wit, to let wit grow into a sense of the world as it is and as it should be. . . .
>
> Laughter makes parenthood bearable—and it creates the very air in which learning thrives. . . . Surely the thing that drives hundreds of bright, laughing college students out of the colleges of education is the solemnity of their utterances as well as their behavior. . . .
>
> Education . . . [should] keep us alive and hopeful . . . and lead us to laugh in the face of heaven or hell. For serious as our strivings are, they should never be so serious that we cannot lean back and laugh at the absurdity of our being and doing. Education should teach us to play the wise fool rather than turn us into the solemn ass.[41]

How often have we in nursing education commented on the students' decreasing involvement, the apathy which begins to set in by the second year, the fact that somehow, the young, eager, enthusiastic students we see as freshmen have disappeared by the time they are ready to graduate. Have we destroyed their motivation for learning and eagerness for nursing by our "solemnity" and adherence to the "seriousness" of this nursing business? Might not the cultivation of humor and laughter in the classroom enhance the learning, foster the student-teacher relationship and provide the vehicle for developing the students' ability to relate in a warm and "human" way with their patients and colleagues? Although we usually include in any list of characteristics essential for a nurse that of a sense of humor, do we do anything realistic to maintain or develop it? Or do we squelch it in the process of nursing education? Is humor the missing element in nursing?

> The perception of the Comic is a tie of sympathy with other men, a pledge of sanity. We must learn by laughter as well as by tears and terror. Ralph Waldo Emerson

CULTIVATING THE USE OF HUMOR AS A TOOL IN NURSING INTERVENTIONS

How does one learn to use humor constructively and effectively? Whether a sense of humor is inherited or acquired has long been a controversial issue. Certainly the ability to smile and laugh is innate, but, the ability to enjoy humor and create it varies widely in individuals. It is a myth that "one is born with it" and "you have it or you don't." Studies have shown that humor is a developmental process. The development of personality and a sense of humor seem to be closely related. Each person thus develops a unique sense of humor and style for creating humor.

Very little research has been done, however, on how humor develops and what facilitates it. As Mindess has said,

> Our sense of humor is, without a doubt, one of our most valuable faculties. Yet no one seems to know how to cultivate their own, or anybody else's, sense of humor.[42]

Mindess has suggested that, in adulthood, to cultivate and expand our sense of humor requires an attitude which allows us to see the absurdity in life, in events and situations, in others, and, above all in ourselves. How we express this attitude becomes an individual matter. This attitude frees us from conformity and the restrictions imposed on us in the process of growing up. It allows for the change and creativity and spontaneity needed to redevelop a sense of humor. However, like any other skill, humor must be practiced if it is to become an integral part of our communication pattern.

Elements and techniques for producing comedy have been suggested by many comedy writers and comedians. A guide developed by this writer, which incorporates many of these, includes analyzing and choosing your humorous style, collecting material as base-line data and creating your own humor through specific devices for modifying old jokes and humor or creating new ones, with suggestions for delivery and timing.[43] The guide can be used by care givers to facilitate the helping process as well as by the teacher to enhance the learning process.

Incorporating humor into the plan of care for our patients and clients employs the same problem-solving process utilized in planning other nursing interventions: making an assessment, identifying the problem, determining the mode of intervention and then evaluating the results.

There is almost no situation in which humor is not permissible. However, to be effective in that situation we must always be aware of the appropriateness of the humor and the receptiveness of the other person, as well as establishing the "joke-frame" so that the patient knows we are being humorous.

Assessment means "knowing your audience." Who are your patients? What cues do they give you that they use humor or would be receptive? What indications that they would not? Would their emotional level or physiological state be such that the humor would be perceived as irritating or noncaring? Analyze the problems or needs for which you would be utilizing the humor. Are the patients using humor? What messages are they conveying? Our planned humorous intervention then would be based on the data we collect about the patients, the situations and our own style. It may be a witticism, a teasing remark, a joke or even a funny anecdote that may have happened to someone in similar circumstances or with the same anxieties.

Once the interaction has occurred, evaluate it. Was it effective? If not, analyze why. Was it your technique, the content or was the patient not ready to accept your message?

Humor, as an indirect communication, usually serves its purpose without further intervention, since its function is to provide a mechanism for dealing with issues and conveying messages which might be unacceptable if stated directly. However, humor may also be used to open up a serious discussion. "A joke may serve as a trial balloon to invite a discussion of doubtful propriety."[44]

Humor may also be used as a pattern of communication in a long-term relationship to facilitate the therapeutic process.[45] Humor in psychotherapy has been a controversial issue, with classic psychoanalysts expressing doubts about its use, while the humanistic and existential therapists have incorporated humor into their practice as part of the process.[46]

Among the variables to be considered in the planned use of humor is the culture of the patient. Every culture has its practices and beliefs which influence illness and health care. Would the culture of the patient make a difference in the use of humor if the professional were not a member of that culture? Are there differences in the kinds of humor used by particular ethnic groups or cultures and how do they relate to health and health care practices? Definitive answers to these questions are not available; however, a small exploratory study of three cultures conducted by this writer suggests that there are differences.[47] Black-American, Spanish-American and Southwest Indian cultures were investigated. The differences in the use of humor were related to the cultural beliefs, beliefs about health, minority group status, degree of acculturation and socioeconomic status.

There are many other unanswered questions regarding humor and much more research to be done. However, we must begin to explore the use of this concept, to try out various approaches, to experiment.

> In the total plan for the care of our patient, humor is one communication tool, one mechanism for coping, one teaching methodology. It is useful and therapeutic in the right situation and the right time. As with anything else, a good thing can be overdone; a judicious amount is the right amount. If a drug is good, three times the dosage is not better. As with grief when there is a need for lightness and humor, so there will be times when humor will turn to tears, when laughter no longer suffices. What is important is to understand humor, to become skilled in recognizing when it is appropriate and beneficial and to encourage, not ignore it.[48]

In this time of technological advances, when patients often feel like extensions of machines, humor can be a means for retaining humanness in nursing, lessening the depersonalization and conveying our warmth, caring and respect.

Adlai Stevenson once paraphrased Socrates' famous statement, "The unexamined life is not worth living," with "Life without laughter is not worth examining."

REFERENCES

1. RN, May, 1964, p. 53.
2. Piddington, R.: The Psychology of Laughter: A Study in Social Adaptation. New York, Gamut Press, 1963, p. 9.
3. White, E. B.: Some remarks on humor. The second tree from the corner. *In* Enck, J. J., Forter, E. T., and Whitley, A.: The Comic in Theory and Practice. New York, Appleton-Century-Crofts, 1960, p. 102.
4. Grotjahn, M.: Beyond Laughter. New York, McGraw-Hill, 1957, p. vii.
5. Ibid., pp. viii-ix.
6. Robinson, V. M.: Humor and the Health Professions. Thorofare, N.J., Charles B. Slack, 1977, preface, p. v.
7. Fry, W. F. J.: Sweet Madness, A Study of Humor. Palo Alto, Calif., Pacific Books, 1963.

8. Freud, S.: Jokes and their relation to the unconscious. *In* Strachey, J. (ed.): The Complete Psychological Works of Sigmund Freud. Vol. 8. London, Hogarth Press, 1960, pp. 222-36.
9. Mindess, H.: Laughter and Liberation. Los Angeles, Nash, 1971, p. 23.
10. McDougall, W.: The instinct of laughter. *In*: An Introduction to Social Psychology. New York, Barnes and Noble, 1963, p. 395.
11. Freud, S.: Humor. *In* Strachey (ed.): The Complete Psychological Works of Sigmund Freud. Vol. 21, pp. 161-66.
12. Goldstein, J. H., McGhee, P. E.: The Psychology of Humor. Theoretical Perspectives and Empirical Issues. New York, Academic Press, 1972, p. xix.
13. Bergson, H.: Laughter, *In* Enck, Forter, and Whitley: The Comic in Theory and Practice. p. 58.
14. Fry, Sweet Madness, p. 67.
15. Emerson, J.: Social functions of humor in a hospital setting. Diss., University of California at Berkeley, 1963, p. 47.
16. Coser, R. L.: Some social functions of laughter. *In* Skipper, J. K., Jr., and Leonard, R. C. (eds.): Social Interaction and Patient Care. Philadelphia, Lippincott, 1965, p. 293.
17. Ibid., p. 304.
18. Ibid., p. 295.
19. Stuart, I. R.: Primary and secondary process as reflections of catastrophie: the political cartoon as an instrument of group emotional dynamics. J. Soc. Psychol. 64:231-39, December 1964.
20. Emerson, Social functions of humor, p. 238.
21. Kramer, M.: Reality Shock, Why Nurses Leave Nursing. Saint Louis, Mosby, 1974, p. 7.
22. Freud, Humor, p. 161; Jokes and their relation to the unconscious, p. 229.
23. Fox, R. C.: Experiment Perilous. Glencoe, Ill., The Free Press, 1959, pp. 76-77.
24. Emerson, Social functions of humor, p. 240.
25. Robinson, R.: More candles for her cake. RN. 27:57 August 1964.
26. Robinson, Humor and the Health Professions, p. 73.
27. Mikes, G.: Laughing Matter. New York, Library Press, 1971, p. 40.
28. Freud, Jokes and their relation to the unconscious, p. 228.
29. Levine, J.: Responses to humor. Sci. Amer. 194:31-35, February 1956.
30. Coser, R. L.: Laughter among colleagues. Psychiatry. 23:81-95, February 1960, p. 95.
31. Kaplan, H., and Boyd, I. H.: The social functions of humor on an open psychiatric ward. Psychiat. Q. 39:502-15, July 1965.
32. Fry, Sweet Madness, p. 152.
33. Lorenz, K.: On Aggression. New York, Harcourt, 1966, p. 294.
34. Freud, Humor, p. 163.
35. McDougall, The instinct of laughter, pp. 389-92.
36. Norris, C.: Greetings from the lonely crowd. Nurs. Forum. vols. 73-82, Winter 1961-62.
37. Nussbaum, K., and Michaux, W. W.: Response to humor in depression: a predictor and evaluator of patient chance. Psychiat. Q. 37:527-39, July 1963.
38. Emerson, Social functions of humor, p. 150.
39. Grotjahn, Beyond Laughter, p. ix.
40. Robinson, Humor and the Health Professions, p. 91.
41. Eble, K. E.: A Perfect Education. New York, Macmillan, 1966, pp. 3-4, 15, 214.
42. Mindess, Laughter and Liberation, p. 13.
43. Robinson, Humor and the Health Professions, pp. 146-61.
44. Emerson, J. P.: Negotiating the serious import of humor. Sociometry. 32:169-81, 1969.
45. Robinson, Humor and the Health Professions, pp. 173-74.
46. Ibid., pp. 74-89.
47. Ibid., pp. 102-29.
48. Ibid., p. 187.

ADDITIONAL READINGS

Adams, W. J.: The use of sexual humor in teaching human sexuality at the university level. Family Coordinator. 365-68, October 1974.

Berlyne, D. E.: Laughter, humor and play. *In* Lindsay, G. (ed.): Handbook of Social Psychology. Vol. 3. Cambridge, Mass.: Addison-Wesley, 1969, pp. 795-813.

Chapman, A. J. and Foot, H. C. (eds.): Humour and Laughter: Theory, Research and Applications. London, John Wiley, 1976.

Eastman, M.: The Enjoyment of Laughter. New York, Simon and Schuster, 1936.

Flugel, J. C.: Humor and laughter. *In* Lindsay (ed.): Handbook of Social Psychology, Vol. II, pp. 709-34.

Fox, R. C. and Swazey, J. P.: The Courage to Fail: A Social View of Organ Transplants and Dialysis. Chicago: University of Chicago Press, 1974.

Grotjahn, M.: Sexuality and humor—don't laugh. Psychol. Today. 51-53, July 1972.

Handleman, D. and Kapferer, B.: Forms of joking activity: a comparative approach. Am. Anthropologist. 74:484-517, 1972.

Koestler, A.: The Act of Creation. New York, Macmillan, 1964.

Kubie, L . S.: The destructive potential of humor in psychotherapy. Am. J. Psychiatry. 127:861-66, January 1971.

Levine, J.: Humor. *In* Sills, D. (ed.): International Encyclopedia of the Social Sciences. Vol. VII. New York, Macmillan, 1968, pp. 1-7.

McGhee, P. E.: Development of the humor response: a review of the literature. Psychol. Bull. 76:328-48, 1971.

Mendel, W. (ed.): A Celebration of Laughter. Los Angeles, Mara Books, 1970.

Murphy, B. and Pollio, H. R.: I'll laugh if you will. Psychol. Today. 106-9, December 1973.

Obrdlik, A. J.: Gallows humor—a sociological phenomenon. Am. J. Soc. 47:709-16, March 1942.

Orben, R.: The pied piper of humor. *In:* Talent. Cleveland, Ohio, International Platform Association, Spring 1972, pp. 34-36.

Poland, W. S.: The place of humor in psychotherapy. Am. J. Psychiatry. 128:635-37, November 1971.

O'Connell, W. E.: Freudian humor: the eupsychia of everyday life. *In* Chapman and Foot (eds.): Humor and Laughter, Chap. 14, pp. 313-29.

———: Humor for actualization and survival. *In* O'Connell, W. C. and Bright, M. B.: Natural High Primer. C icago, Alfred Adler Institute, 1977, pp. 147-55.

Roland, C. G.: Thoughts about medical writing. Can it be funny and medical? Anesthesia and Analgesia . . . Current Researches. 50, 2, March-April 1971.

Laughing Matter? A Symposium of Studies on Humor as Communication. J. Comm. 26, 3:102-204, Summer 1976.

Wessell, Sister M. L.: Use of humor by an immobilized adolescent girl during hospitalization. Maternal-Child Nurs. J. 4, 1:35-48, Spring 1975.

Wolfenstein, M.: Children's Humor. Glencoe, Ill., The Free Press, 1954.

13 DENIAL OF ILLNESS

Sister M. Martha Kiening

The impact of illness with its many implications for the sick person's ability to deal with a changed life situation is important in the effectiveness of nursing care. The threat to the self-system depends not only on the actual degree of physical disequilibrium brought about by the illness itself but, more important, on the alteration of the self-concept that takes place as a result of impaired physical functioning. One way an individual may deal with the stress produced by the threat to integrity is to deny the threat. Denial operates to allay anxiety by reducing the perception of the threat.

The concept of denial has been treated extensively in psychiatric literature. Recently, there has been increasing focus on denial as an adaptive maneuver used to reduce anxiety generated by crippling, disabling or socially unacceptable diseases. Several articles written by nurses demonstrate that the nursing profession is beginning to recognize the importance of denial as a nursing problem that sometimes seriously interferes with the patient's plan of care.[1] More recently, serious attempts have been made by clinical investigators to use a more precise approach to the appraisal of denying behavior in illness.[2] However, W. B. Miller and his coworkers report considerable discrepancy between denial of illness ratings, observer bias and physiological variables. Consequently, they concluded that a denial rating scale proved inadequate for their study.[3]

The tendency to deny the seriousness of an illness and its possible outcome for the individual has long been noted by health workers. Perhaps the earliest comments on this tendency were made by Benjamin Rush in his account of the 1793 yellow fever epidemic in Philadelphia. With something akin to wonder, he remarks that these patients, even in the advanced stages of the disease:

> . . . did not acknowledge that they had any other indisposition than a common cold. I was particularly struck with the self-deception in many persons who had nursed relatives who had died with yellow fever and who had been exposed to it in neighborhoods where it had prevailed for days and even weeks with great mortality. . . . Perhaps it would be proper to rank that self-deception with respect to the nature and danger of the disease which was so universal among the instances of derangement of mind.[4]

It may be said that all defenses operate to deny reality in one way or another. Such terms as dissociation, repression, selective inattention and suppression all concern unconscious denial of material into consciousness. Freud distinguishes between repression and denial when he says:

> If we wish to differentiate between what happens to the idea distinct from the affect we can restrict "repression" to relate to the affect; the correct word for what happens to the idea is then "denial."[5]

Denial is a defense mechanism operating outside of and beyond conscious awareness in the endeavor to resolve emotional conflict and to allay anxiety. It achieves its purpose by disowning, rejecting or ignoring one or more of the elements of the conflict. Obvious reality factors that the person finds painful or unpleasant are perceived as a threat to the self-structure and treated as if they did not exist. If the threat cannot be escaped or attacked, anxiety may be reduced and comfort reestablished by denying its existence. Reality is rejected or distorted and replaced by wish-fulfilling or "as-if" behavior. The person may explicitly deny verbally what is perceived or act as if the painful situation did not exist. Unpleasant and intolerable facts, wishes, thoughts and actions are disowned by an unconscious process of elimination.

Avery Weisman, in his work on dying and denying, carefully distinguishes between the fact and the process of denial. He sees the process as one in which there is:

1. acceptance of a primary, public field of perception.
2. repudiation of a portion of the shared meaning of that field.
3. replacement of the repudiated meaning with a more congenial version.
4. reorientation of the individual within the scope of the total meaning in order to accommodate the revised reality.

The fact of denial needs another person (or persons) who judge that denial of their shared reality has occurred.[6]

For the purposes of this discussion, denial is defined as the kind of behavior that indicates a failure to accept either an obvious fact or its significance to the individual involved in the situation. Operationally, we may say that denying behavior includes the following steps:

1. A reality situation exists.
2. The individual perceives or anticipates some element in the situation as threatening.
3. Anxiety occurs in response to the perceived threat.
4. Either the facts or their significance in the threat-producing situation are completely or partially disclaimed.
5. Psychological equilibrium is temporarily regained and maintained by ignoring or rejecting objective evidence connected with the threatening situation.

The denial, however, serves only to cover or minimize the anxiety-provoking aspects of the reality that constitutes the threat. So long as the person can maintain denial in the face of objective evidence, it serves as an effective protection against overwhelming anxiety. Its inconsistency with reality makes it a very brittle defense, however, and when it finally must come face to face with reality it may crumble, leaving the person defenseless. As reality begins to storm the bastion of denial, depression may result, possibly leading to personality disorganization or even suicide. More frequently, aspects of reality are admitted to consciousness gradually and disorganization is less profound.

Denial is one of the earliest and most primitive of the defense mechanisms and is thought to precede even the mechanism of repression in the developing infantile ego. Its earliest and most rudimentary manifestations may be seen in the very young infant who deals with disturbing external stimuli by closing the eyes, then by turning the head away. In this early stage, denial consists, perhaps, simply of a separation of that which is unpleasant or anxiety-producing from the rest of the emerging personality organization. By the time the infant begins to experience the early forms of anxiety, the mechanism of denial has been established and soon begins to operate automatically in the service of the ego. D. Miller classifies denial with the "first family" of defenses, all of which have four common features: (a) they seem applicable to every type of conflict, (b) their use requires no previous learning, (c) they distort reality markedly and (d) they are of little help in solving real social difficulties.[7]

Denial as a part of the normal developmental process is readily observed in the play of children when they use fantasy to live in a world of their own creation and unpleasant reality can be reversed or blotted out. The normal child, however, can readily abandon play and return to the everyday world on demand. Although vestiges of this mechanism linger even into mature adulthood, frank denial in the face of obvious reality in an adult is usually an indication of serious mental illness, particularly if it persists for any length of time.

Interruptions to health always pose some threat to the individual's life situation. Although the fear of death or disability looms as an important factor in the patient's response to the impact of illness, there are many other needs whose fulfillment is jeopardized by an alteration in physical or psychological well-being. Even a minor health problem calls for some readjustment in the self-concept of the person who previously saw him or herself as "whole" or "well" and is now faced with a change in body image, be it ever so slight. Pride, self-esteem, sense of achievement and power, self-identity and sexual identification are only a few of the self-attributes which undergo change as the individual is thrust away from wellness and mastery into illness and loss of control.

Denial of illness can, at times, seriously interfere with the treatment program. It may defeat the nurse's best efforts to establish a helping relationship with the patient. On the other hand it may, and often does, serve as a protection for the ego, preventing the person from becoming overwhelmed by anxiety and averting extensive emotional disorganization. If this defense is too forcibly undermined in an attempt to make the patient "deal with reality," he or she may become increasingly disorganized, and a severe depression may be the result. It is not uncommon, however, for denial to be so effective in relieving anxiety that it cannot be undermined easily. The denier may have explanations for any reality factors presented. The practitioner under such circumstances need not worry about precipitating a crisis by "saying the wrong thing." It is important, then, that the nurse learn to: (1) recognize the manifestations of denial, (2) be able to assess the degree to which it is impeding the patient's progress toward regained health, (3) understand the dynamics of the behavior, (4) try to determine the need which the denial is serving, and then (5) make a nursing decision that best serves the needs of the patient at this time. This decision must take into account the fact that ego support must be given high priority in the treatment goal. If the behavior by which the patient communicates distortions or rejection of reality is not understood, it is more likely to trigger anxiety, resentment and anger on the nurse's part, thus making it even more difficult for the patient to obtain the help needed at this time.

The range of behavior along the continuum of denial is wide. There are differences, both in the level of awareness at which denial operates and in the degree to which reality is excluded. Explicit verbal denial can be a symptom of severe emotional disturbance: the blind person who denies being unable to see, the paraplegic who insists that he or she can move the paralyzed arm or leg. This complete denial can only occur as a result of serious psychological disequilibrium; yet the vestiges of this primitive, automatic response to sudden threat remain even in the mature, normal adult. The shocked "Oh, no," "It can't be," "I can't believe it!" with which tragic news is often met is denial operating on a higher level of awareness and in a much shorter time-span, but completely shutting out the unwelcome fact. It is as if the ego needs to stand back in order to gain time to absorb a shattering emotional impact. Full realization and acceptance are never accomplished all at once.

A more common way of denying illness is by disowning or ignoring only certain aspects of it. This is typified by the coronary patient who experiences substernal pain but attributes it to something eaten or by the injured athlete who makes plans to play in the next big game in spite of rather extensive incapacitation. The ideals of health, beauty and eternal youth fostered in our society exploit the tendency to deny the realities of a changing body image concomitant with maturity and aging. Tenure, prestige and social advancement that come with increasing years are goals to strive for, but the physical marks of aging—grey hair, wrinkles and decreasing physical vitality—are aspects that are ignored, disowned, in short, denied—a denial actively encouraged in our contemporary culture. This same attitude of massive denial can be observed in the way our present-day society reacts to the whole area of death and dying. Death, the great reality of our human condition, is probably the one which is most actively denied in America today.

Some patients, while not denying explicitly, tend to minimize the illness or certain aspects of it. Expressions such as "It's not so bad," "It could be worse," "It will all turn out all right" may be used to minimize the entire unpleasant experience of the illness. Or certain symptoms and syndromes may be minimized, as in the case of Benjamin Rush's yellow fever patients who acknowledged the symptoms, but attributed them to a cold.

Where denial is explicitly verbalized, the evidence is clear and the nurse can validate the hypothesis that the patient is denying, simply by listening to what the patient says and then consulting obvious reality as seen by the nurse and consensually validated by others.

Behavioral clues to implicit denial may pose more of a problem for the nurse. Because they are often acted out, these clues may not be so easily recognized. Here again, the range of the behavior is wide—from the quiet, reticent, model patient whose understatement of needs may be so great that the medical staff and the family overlook the patient's real feelings and requirements to the hostile, "uncooperative" patient who flagrantly violates medical orders. Clues to denial may be picked up all along the continuum by the observant, knowledgeable nurse. How the nurse validates these clues and follows through on them will depend first on the nurse's astuteness, and then on the need they serve for the patient, the patient's tolerance for stress and, of course, the nurse's own feelings and degree of self-awareness and ability to cope with her or his feelings.

Patients with severe, long-term physical disability seem more prone to denial than do those with more acute illnesses. This is particularly true of the amputee, the cancer patient and patients who have suffered a myocardial infarction. Franz Reichman and N. Levy, reporting on a group of hemodialysis patients state, "We have not seen denial used as massively as by this group of patients, as a whole, in any other patient population with physical illness."[8] In any long-term physical disability, feelings of anxiety, depression and anger are normal. If they are not exhibited, one should suspect that denial is operating against the perceived threat. Here we may also mention chronic alcoholism in all its phases and stages. Denial of the extent of dependency on alcohol is a classic feature in the confirmed alcoholic. In this situation, denial not only perpetuates the destructive, addictive behavior but also prevents the victim from seeking and accepting needed help.

Manifestations of implicit denial may include missed clinic appointments, failure to carry out a prescribed treatment regimen, refusal of medications, selective inattention to the symptoms of the illness or a cheerfulness that seems inappropriate in the face of reality. There may be changes relating to attitudes about food, bowel and urinary function, physical contacts and sexual behavior. Humor is frequently employed as a denial mechanism. Some patients may use the second or third person when referring to the illness. A common form of implicit denial is the displacement of concern about the illness to another person or describing the illness in terms of what other people said or did: "The doctor said I had a stroke." Many people tend to reassure themselves by plunging into overactivity as if to convince themselves that the symptoms are an illusion or at least trivial. Some men see their masculinity threatened by illness and may engage in a dangerous denial of symptoms through overactivity.

Basic to any discussion of behavioral dynamics is the question: "What need is the behavior serving?" Denial has been classified as one of the major defense mechanisms and, as such, came to have a somewhat negative connotation. Recent literature, however, reflects a more positive view. Although most authorities agree that reinforcement of the denial is highly questionable therapeutically, there is a growing respect for the protection which this mechanism affords the ego in times of overwhelming emotional onslaught. All authorities consulted seem to agree that this defense should certainly not be directly attacked, and most seem to think that as the stress of the anxiety-producing situation is ameliorated, the person's need to deny will likewise decrease.

During the past decade, studies have focused repeatedly and with telling accuracy on the role of denial in death and dying. Elisabeth Kübler-Ross's extensive research has identified denial as the first stage in the process through which the dying person finally comes to an acceptance of the reality of impending death.[9] It is to be noted, however, that the denial factor operates in the service of the ego only by protecting it from the pain of anxiety which is generated by reality. It is important, therefore, to distinguish between acceptance of the reality of impending death and acceptance of death itself. It is quite possible to be clearly aware of the fact that death is inevitable but still wish to live rather than die. The decision of whether or not to tell the patient he or she is going to die poses difficulties not only for the physician and medical staff, but for the family as well. The extent of the patient's denial and how it is serving the need for comfort in this time of crisis are prime factors to be considered in the overall therapeutic approach. Patients need to be given an opportunity to be actively involved in the management of their own dying.

Present-day literature does seem to reflect a more balanced approach to the problem of understanding and support of the dying patient than only a few decades ago. Kübler-Ross maintains that patients need to be supported both verbally and nonverbally through all phases of the dying process.[10] If patients are permitted to be more involved in the management of their own dying as circumstances allow, the exigencies of reality will more readily and naturally begin to replace implacable denial. Among those who have reported extensive work with dying patients, B. G. Glaser and A. L. Strauss think it important to work realistically with the dying person, but also state that "staff members could do much to soften the disclosure, handle the depression so as to encourage acceptance and guide the patient into active preparation for death."[11] This latter position seems in accord with a philosophy that acknowledges the right of the individual to know whatever facts will enable him or her to make judgments and decisions based on reality and the individual's dignity as a human being.

Although much of our knowledge of defense mechanisms has come from work with the neurotic patient, these mechanisms are not pathogenic in themselves. Thus, denial is a normal way of dealing with anxiety; it may be thought of as coping behavior through which the adaptive process is brought about. In its externally directed aspect, coping behavior is judged for its social effectiveness; in its internal aspect adequacy is judged by the degree of comfort it effects. The mentally healthy individual can usually achieve the necessary balance between the reality of the illness and the proper amount of denial.

The process of adaptation varies with individuals, but there seems to be a general sequence of stages which most chronically ill patients go through over the months and years. Although the transition from one phase to another is a gradual process with no clearly perceptible divisions, it can be described as occurring more or less sequentially. S. Garrard and J. Richmond, in working with the parents of children with a chronic illness or handicap, have identified three phases in the sequence:

1. *A period of disorganization*
   a. Great anxiety is usually present. There are efforts to deny or minimize the impact in one way or another, but the defensive mechanisms are almost completely ineffective in coping with the stress.
2. *A period of reintegration*
   a. During this period, which usually coincides with the acute period of the illness, there is extensive use of defenses—in this case, extensive denial of the nature of the illness, its seriousness and its probable outcome.
   b. Denial is rarely effective in completely relieving distress. There is gradual acknowledgment of some of the more obvious aspects of reality about the illness.
3. *A period of mature adaptation*
   a. Most of the realities of the situation can be faced.
   b. There is an appropriate response to this confrontation with reality, such as seeking information about the factors relevant to the illness and assessments of the probable long-term limitations.
   c. This phase is usually characterized by periods of depression which may be looked upon as normal grief and mourning.
   d. Resolution of the conflict by the slow transition from a self-concept of physical vigor to one of physical limitations.[12]

Although phases 1 and 2 have been most extensively dealt with in the literature, the series of approximations and adaptive behavior that follows the initial phase may have been given less recognition than it deserves and may have more significant implications for the nurse. Phase 3 is, of course, the desirable goal in psychological management, and it is one that some persons never reach or attain only incompletely. It is while the patient is gradually coming to a realization of the changed life situation that the nurse's understanding, acceptance and support become increasingly important. An accurate assessment of the patient's anxiety level and appropriate nursing intervention (or nonintervention) may be crucial in helping him or her to regain emotional equilibrium and focus on the problem to be mastered.

Denial of illness, either explicit or implicit, is not confined to the person who is ill. It is a behavioral pattern commonly encountered in the family threatened by the illness of a member.

Extensive studies of denial by the family have been carried out by a number of investigators. R. Woodfall, in working with the families of mentally retarded children, reports behaviors in parents ranging from complete denial to denial of certain aspects of the problem.[13] The sense of failure generated by the production of a defective child, whom the parents see as a projection of themselves, may lead to attempts to minimize or disown the obvious signals of arrested development in the child's behavior. When there is complete denial, the parents are prevented from using available community services and thus providing the child with the necessary professional help. In cases of minimal denial, the parents may not accept certain aspects of the illness. They may have a more constructive approach toward treatment goals, but their goals tend to be limited because of their inability to acknowledge the full reality of the illness.

It may be said that denial is present to some extent in all parents of chronically ill children. This may be inferred from observations of such behavior as misunderstanding the physician's explanation, repetitious questions and "shopping around" for medical advice or treatment. Resentment, avoidance, seclusion and overprotection may be present especially in the parents of deaf, blind, mute or other severely handicapped children. Such reactions cause the parents to avoid teaching the children and to prevent them from learning the special skills they will need to cope with the real world.

T. A. Hollon, in his experience with patients on hemodialysis, found that family members as well as patients were prone to deny the illness and the concomitant emotional stress engendered.[14] Denial by families of cancer patients is common. Adela Baider, in an analysis of the interconnection between societal values and family structure, on the one hand, and the conception of death and dying, on the other, found denial to be a major defense mechanism employed by the family.[15] A. M. Goldstein and coworkers have recommended ways in which social workers can intervene in the family stress generated by chronic illness of a member.[16] Guidelines for helping families deal with the stress of chronically ill children have been offered by D. M. Kaplan and his associates. Again, denial is seen as an important factor to be recognized and dealt with.[17]

Denial may be employed by members of the helping professions as well as by patients and their families, and it is here, perhaps, that it has its greatest effect on the quality of care. Medical and nursing staff may actively foster and encourage denial in patients and families as a result of their own reactions of helplessness, frustration or anger in an emotionally charged situation. Professional literature seems to reflect increasing attention and concern in this area. P. R. Patterson points up the importance of respect for the defense of denial by the clinician.[18] L. E. Arnold, among others, has studied patterns of denial used by staff in working with suicidal and chronically ill patients. He notes that encouragement of denial for one's own convenience is culpable, but those around the patient need to make sure that they are considering the patient's need in their approach to his or her denial.[19] Reporting on her work with chronically ill children, Ruth Boyd contends that doctors seem to be more fearful of death than the dying themselves. She attributes this to the fact that conquering illness and death is a strong motivation for going into medicine.[20] Glaser and Strauss explore in some detail the many ways in which both the physician and the nursing staff attempt to deny or avoid the issue when it is known that a patient's illness is terminal. Observed behavior ranged from elaborate rituals for keeping patient and family unaware to elaborate games of mutual pretension in which both staff member and patient were aware, but neither wished to admit this openly to the other.[21]

In dealing with denial of illness as a nursing problem, the nurse needs to be able to assess, first, the extent to which the denial is harmful, and, then, the extent to which it is therapeutic for the patient. For example, the psychiatric patient who completely and actively denies the illness cannot benefit from a therapeutic program until this problem is recognized and at least partially resolved. In other circumstances, denial may be recognized as operating, but not as presenting a particular nursing problem at the time—in fact, it may be the emergency "brake" that prevents complete disorganization in the face of a crisis with which the person has not yet been able to cope. What is sometimes interpreted as pathology may be the valid use of a healthy protecting mechanism, or it may not even be denial at all, since many patients are very well aware of their illness and its implications, but choose consciously to face this alone rather than add to the stress and anxiety of other family members.

Confronting the patient with reality before he or she is ready for it will not serve any therapeutic purpose and will probably do more harm than good. Most patients will cling more tenaciously to those defenses which make the situation more comfortable for them. Patients undergoing the stress of acute physical illness, especially, are already in crisis and need support and understanding rather than psychic probing and confrontation. S. Applebaum observes that "insight into screened off aspects of one's self intensifies the conflicts which have necessitated the protective screening."[22]

Nurses are perhaps more intimately involved than any other person on the health team with patients' behavior and its effect on the success or failure of medical treatment. They are in a unique position, not only to observe denial of illness, but also to make the necessary nursing judgments and intervene therapeutically in reducing anxiety in assisting the patient and family to accept and deal with the painful reality factors that are being denied. However, before they can begin to be effective on any level with the persons denying illness, nurses must first be able to look at themselves and their own reactions. How they see the situation and what they do about it both will depend upon: (1) their own awareness of their feelings regarding the patients and their illness; (2) the coping patterns which they have developed as part of their behavior for meeting stress situations; (3) their perception of themselves in the professional role as a member of the treatment team; and (4) their relationships with the rest of the nursing staff and other members of the health team.

In a series of observations made by a group of faculty members in various clinical settings to which students were assigned for learning experiences, denial was found to be employed frequently by patients, family members and staff. In some of the following examples, nursing intervention was effective in reducing anxiety and reducing the need for denial; in others, it was only partially effective or not effective at all. The manifestations of denial ranged from a sudden reaction to increased anxiety or a well-entrenched pattern of pathological behavior.

In a sudden reaction, intervention may be effective or ineffective.

> A newly admitted patient was scheduled for a complete diagnostic study on the following morning. On the evening of his admission, the nursing aide approached the patient, saying: "Mr. A, you have been scheduled for an arteriogram in the morning. Has anyone told you what to expect?"
>
> Patient (angrily): "No, and I don't want to know. Why is everyone so anxious to give me all the information? I'm better off if I don't know what's going to happen."
>
> The aide excused herself and left the room.

A more sensitive appraisal of the patient's anxiety level might have elicited a less dramatic response from the patient. The failure to recognize the high anxiety level resulted in a nursing action which increased rather than reduced the anxiety and the nurse aide's attempt to be helpful precipitated the need to deny. A more therapeutic approach might have helped the patient to deal with the anxiety in a more constructive way.

The need for the nursing staff to carry out the therapeutic regimen in the best interests of the patient can sometimes present a dilemma. This is especially true when the patient's denial system is acted out by refusing to carry out the "doctor's orders." The following clinical example illustrates premature intervention into the denial, which resulted in complete conformity with the "orders" at the cost of a high level of apprehension and fear:

> A 38-year-old construction worker had been admitted the previous evening with "chest pain" which had been severe enough to warrant hospitalization for tests and observation. During the course of the morning, the nursing student who had been assigned to care for him reported that he would not stay in bed, no matter how much he was told that his doctor had "ordered" him to stay in bed. He seemed to enjoy the discomfiture of the nursing staff and laughed and joked at their concern. When the team leader came in, she found him again out of bed and stated:
>
> N.: Mr. F., did you know that the doctor wants you to stay in bed?
>
> P.: Oh yes, but there's no sense to that. I feel fine. Nothing is wrong with me.

N.: Oh, then how come you're in the hospital?
P.: Well, I just had a little stomach upset. I'm not sick.
N.: Mr. F., doctors don't send patients to the hospital just for a little stomach pain. What did your doctor tell you when he decided to send you to a hospital?
P.: Well—uh—he did mention it might have something to do with my heart, but that's crazy. It was just a stomach pain.
N.: It might not be as crazy as you think. Why do you suppose he ordered strict bed rest?
P.: It's OK. I'll stay in bed if you really think I should.

During the conversation, the patient's laughing, bantering attitude changed abruptly. A look of apprehension and anxiety replaced the smile. Later, the student asked the team leader: "What did you say to him. He sure is scared now. He's in bed and almost afraid to move." This patient, deprived of the shelter of his game and abruptly stripped of his defense of denial, which had been a tenuous one at best, had literally "no place to go" with his anxiety. It is well to point out here that denial is never suddenly relinquished once and for all. Fortunately for this patient's psychological equilibrium, we may suppose that some degree of denial again moved in to allay the anxiety and reestablish some degree of emotional comfort. Certainly, a more constructive approach might have been for the nurse to sit down with the patient and get him to talk about what happened to him. A simple observation, such as "You seem to find it hard to stay in bed, Mr. F.," might have given the patient the opportunity to tell his story and, hopefully, to express some of his anxiety. This might have been the beginning of getting the patient involved and responsible for his own care.

A middle-aged woman patient, scheduled for minor surgery in the morning, approached the nurse. Anxiety was obvious: the pallor, dry lips, the worried look on her face and the wringing of her hands as she spoke:

PATIENT: I'm so afraid I'll hemorrhage again. It's crazy to be so frightened, just crazy.
NURSE: You're afraid you will hemorrhage?
PATIENT: Oh, now you do frighten me . . . you think I can hemorrhage?
NURSE: But you said that at the beginning . . .
PATIENT: No. I didn't say that. Do you think I might have a cardiac arrest?

The nurse at this point decided to remain and listen. For half an hour she sat with the patient, permitting her to talk freely of her fears about the coming surgery. At the end of this time she appeared much calmer and mentioned a television show which she had planned to watch that evening. The nurse helped her select the channel and remained long enough to assure herself that the patient was involved in the program.

The nurse's intervention was based on accurate assessment of the patient's anxiety—the quick denial seemed to indicate the patient's extreme need for help in dealing with her anxiety at this time. It was neither necessary nor desirable to deal directly with the denial, since the real issue was not that the patient was using the mechanism but that anxiety had to be dealt with and reduced to manageable proportions if this patient was to successfully weather this particular crisis.

Denial is also used as an attempt to adjust to the threat of loss or change.

A former nursing supervisor, nearing 75 years of age, was retired when certain positions were restructured in her hospital. After retirement, she suffered what appeared to be a "little stroke." However, she was not incapacitated and she decided that she could do volunteer work regularly at the hospital. It soon became evident that this schedule was too strenuous for her, but she insisted that she could continue. When her relatives insisted that she discontinue this work she said: "I don't know why I am not allowed to do this. There is nothing wrong with me." When she was reminded that she had been ill: "I didn't have a stroke; and there is nothing wrong with me. The doctor said that he wanted me to keep busy." She engaged in many activities and went to many community affairs and events.

One of the nurses at the hospital, recognizing this behavior as part of the crisis of aging, found opportunities to engage in conversation with her. She attempted to emphasize the things the patient could still do well and to help her find less demanding activities in which she could still feel useful and productive.

Here again, a frontal attack on the denial might have resulted in even greater efforts on the part of the patient to retain the one mechanism which allayed anxiety and restored at least a measure of comfort and security. The nurse correctly assessed the behavior as indicating a need to feel wanted and productive and geared her efforts toward an attempt to work with the patient's strengths in a positive way. It is quite probable that the denial will recur if the patient is again in a position where her self-concept is threatened; or she may become depressed if the situation continues and her denial begins to lose its effectiveness over the long haul of adjusting to loss of self-esteem and usefulness.

The following situation illustrates how the nurse assisted a family member to begin to adjust to the loss of a loved one. It is important to note that the nurse's role was twofold: first, in assisting the mother to face reality and, perhaps more importantly, supporting her in the difficult period which immediately followed this realization.

The mother of an eight-year-old child who lay dying of a fatal illness, repeatedly turned to the nurse with such comments as "She is going to get well, isn't she?" The nurse met each question with a simple statement of fact: "She is very, very sick." Since the mother spoke English very poorly, a Spanish-speaking aide was found to explain to the mother in her own language that the little girl did not have much longer to live. After the aide left, the nurse remained in the room with the mother, offering support by her physical presence and empathic attitude. She permitted the mother to give as much physical care and comfort to the little girl as she wished.

Nursing intervention here was directed, first, toward relief of the mother's anxiety. The nurse's supportive attitude was one factor; establishing a more familiar psychological climate for the mother by providing someone who spoke her language was another. When denial was recognized, the need for it was accepted but it was not reinforced; the nurse pointed out reality by a simple statement of fact. Anxiety was then again anticipated and reduced by the helping relationship of the nurse and her coworker and by permitting the mother to become actively involved in a specific task directed toward the comfort and relief of her child.

An attractive woman in her late thirties was admitted for investigation of a lump in her breast. She denied concern by talking incessantly, joking and laughing with everyone who came into her room. The nurse, observing this behavior, tried first of all to adopt a quiet, accepting, listening attitude. She walked up and down the corridor with the patient as a means of helping reduce anxiety and making herself available. No attempt was made to comment on the patient's behavior or to explore her feelings about the forthcoming surgery. Although the nurse recognized the need for this, the patient was apparently not yet ready for such intervention.

In this case, further nursing intervention would have been for the nurse to plan frequent short contacts with the patient. During these periods the nurse would attempt to gain the patient's trust by establishing herself as an interested, helpful person, and would listen for cues that might indicate the patient's readiness to talk about herself, the forthcoming surgery and what it meant to her. This should be done before the operation, because a secondary reaction later might result in a depression and a more serious problem for the patient and her subsequent nursing care.

In working with the patient who seems to be using denial as a coping mechanism, the nurse must first determine:

1. how well defined the reality factors are.
2. what aspects of the patient's behavior are open to direct observation and can therefore be checked.
3. what protective function denial is serving at this time and how strong the patient's need for it is.
4. what other means are available to the patient for the reduction of anxiety at this time.

Particularly in making this last judgment, the nurse needs skill in carefully and continually assessing the patient's anxiety level and ability to tolerate the stress precipitating the denying behavior.

The nurse also needs to know and to be able to recognize the phases through which the individual passes while gradually working through the denial and again beginning to be able to deal with reality. This sensitivity to verbal clues that the patient is beginning to accept reality may be seen in the following example:

A patient on the psychiatric service had been informed that plans had been concluded for his transfer to another hospital nearer his own home. He had steadfastly refused to accept this in spite of specific information regarding these plans. During one interview with the nurse he stated:

"I'm glad you're taking notes about me. They might be valuable some time. Maybe you should send them to my doctor in L—."

NURSE: Then you will be seeing your doctor in L—?

PATIENT: Well, just in case he ever needs them. I'm going to stay here for a year and then I'll transfer to L—.

Although the patient evaded the issue as soon as he was confronted with it, denial was not as complete as it had been; he had been willing to admit one small aspect of reality, if only for a moment. The task of the nurse then became to focus more on this breakthrough and to aid him through the anxiety-laden period by her understanding, support and assistance in further exploring the reality of the situation and what it meant for him.

There are many unanswered questions concerning the abilities needed to intervene effectively in so complex a situation as denial often presents. Because denial operates to some degree in almost all patients, and because it can so often block the goals of nursing therapy, it would seem reasonable to expect that the professional nurse should be able to:

1. recognize behavioral cues that suggest that the person is denying some aspect of reality.
2. understand the need that denial helps meet for the person.
3. determine if the denial is interfering with treatment goals.
4. decide on appropriate action.
5. avoid reinforcing patterns of denial.
6. maintain a supportive, helping relationship as the patient begins to move toward a more reality-based orientation.

Accurate assessment of denial and other phenomena requires that the nurse have a relatively high level of self-understanding. Such understanding includes feelings about self and others, coping patterns, roles relative to other members of the treatment team and attitudes and values.

As a professional, the nurse needs continually to assess and to evaluate his or her own learning needs and to plan purposefully for professional growth. As personal knowledge and experience increase, the young graduate should, with further preparation, be able to work at ever deeper and more therapeutic levels with patients and families.

REFERENCES

1. American Nurses' Association: Nursing Approaches to Denial of Illness. Monograph No. 12. Report of the ANA Clinical Session, Detroit, 1962; King, J. M.: Denial, Am. J. Nurs. 66:1010-13, 1966; Wacker, M.: Analogy—weapon against denial. Am. J. Nurs. 74, 1:73-81, 1974.
2. Clum, G. A., and Clum, J. M.: Choice of defense mechanisms and their relationship to mood level. Psychological Reports. 32, 2:507-10, 1973; Houston, B. K.: Viability of coping strategies—denial and response to stress. J. Personality. 41, 1:50-58, 1973; Donaldson, P.: Denying death—a note regarding some ambiguities in the current discussion. Omega. 3, 4:285-90, 1972; Hackett, T. P., and Cassam, N. H.: White collar and blue collar responses to heart attack. J. Psychosomatic Research. 20, 2:85-95, 1976.
3. Miller, W. B., Rosenfeld, R.: Psychophysiological study of denial following acute myocardial infarction. J. Psychosomatic Research. 19, 1:43-53, 1975.
4. Schneck, J. S.: Benjamin Rush on denial of illness. Am. J. Psychiatry. 120:1129, 1964.
5. Freud, S.: Collected Papers. Vol. 5. Strachey, J. (ed.). New York, Basic Books, 1959, pp. 199-200.
6. Weisman, A.: On Dying and Denying. New York, Behavioral Publications, 1972, pp. 56-78.
7. Miller, D., and Swanson, B.: The study of conflict. *In* Jones, M. R. (ed.): Nebraska Symposium on Motivation. Lincoln, University of Nebraska Press, 1956, p. 163.
8. Reichman, F., and Levy, N.: Problems in adaptation to maintenance hemodialysis. Arch. Intern. Med. 130, 6:859-65, 1972, p. 862.
9. Kübler-Ross, E.: On Death and Dying. New York, Macmillan, 1969.

10. Ibid.
11. Glaser, B. G., and Strauss, A. L.: Awareness of Dying. Chicago, Aldine, 1965, p. 135.
12. Garrard, S., and Richmond, J.: Psychological aspects of the management of chronic disease and handicapping conditions of childhood. *In* Lief, H. I., Lief, V., and Lief, N. (eds.): The Psychological Basis of Medical Practice. New York, Harper, 1963, p. 391.
13. Woodfall, R.: The nurse, the mentally retarded child and his family. *In* American Nurses' Association: Nursing Approaches to Denial of Illness, p. 5.
14. Hollon, T. A.: Modified group therapy in the treatment of patients on chronic hemodialysis. Am. J. Psychotherapy. 26, 4:501-510, 1972.
15. Baider, A. L.: Family structure and the process of dying: a study of cancer patients and their family interaction. Dissertation Abstracts International. 34, 1:421 A, July 1973.
16. Goldstein, A. M., and Anderson, M. M.: A model for social work intervention in thanatology. Arch. Foundation of Thanatology. 5, 1:37, 1975.
17. Kaplan, D. M., Smith, A., Grobstein, R., and Fischman, S.: Family mediation of stress. Social Work. 18, 4:60-69, 1973.
18. Patterson, P. R., Denning, C., and Kutscher, A. H.: Psychosocial Aspects of Cystic Fibrosis. New York, Columbia University Press, 1973.
19. Arnold, L. E.: Suicide and denial in the management of Huntington's disease and other terminal, debilitating diseases. Arch. Foundation of Thanatology. 5, 4:430, 1975.
20. Boyd, R. R.: Developing new norms for parents of fatally ill children to facilitate coping: a group work experience and experiment. Arch. Foundation of Thanatology. 5, 1:101, 1975.
21. Glaser and Strauss, Awareness of Dying, p. 137.
22. Applebaum, S.: The dangerous edge of insight. Psychotherapy: Theory, Research and Practice. 13, 3:204, 1976.

ADDITIONAL READINGS

Abram, R. D.: Denial and depression in the terminal cancer patient. Psychiatric Q. 45:394-404, 1971.

Aguilera, D., and Messick, J.: Crisis Intervention: Theory and Practice. 2nd ed. St. Louis, Mosby, 1974.

Chafetz, M.E., Hertzman, M., and Berenson, D.: Alcoholism, a positive view. *In* Arieti, S. (ed.): American Handbook of Psychiatry. Vol. III. New York, Basic Books, 1974, p. 378.

Dayananda, Y. J.: The death of Ivan Ilych: a psychological study on death and dying. Literature and Psychology. 22, 4:191-98, 1972.

Froese, A. P., Cassem, N. H., Hackett, T. P., and Silverberg, E. L.: Galvanic skin potential as a predictor of mental status, anxiety, depression and denial in acute coronary patients. J. Psychosomatic Research. 19, 1:1-9, 1975.

Hackett, T. P., Cassem, N. H., and Silverberg, E. L.: Trajectories of anxiety and depression in denying and non-denying acute myocardial infarction patients during hospitalization. J. Psychosomatic Research. 18, 6:413-20, 1974.

Hagedorn, B., Jr.: Denial as a factor in patient reaction to the crisis of a myocardial infarction. Dissertation Abstracts International. 33, 4:1793 B, 1972.

Horowitz, M.: Stress-Response Syndromes. New York, Jason-Aronson, 1976.

Levine, J. and Zigler, E.: Denial and self—image in stroke, lung cancer and heart disease patients. J. Consulting and Clinical Psychol. 43, 6:751-57, 1975.

Maddux, J. F., and Desmond, D. P.: Reliability and validity of information from chronic heroin users. J. Psychiatric Research. 12, 2:87-95, 1975.

Rosillo, R. H., and Fogel, M. L.: Degree of disability and denial of illness rating scale—correlates of psychological variables and progress in physical rehabilitation: degree of disability and denial of illness. Arch. Phys. Med. Rehabil. 51:227-33, 1970.

Zarit, S. H., and Kahn, R. L.: Impairment and adaptation in chronic disabilities: spatial inattention. J. Nervous & Mental Disease. 159, 1:63-72, 1974.

14 PRIVACY

Dorothy W. Bloch

Entering a health care delivery system may provoke a multitude of thoughts within an individual. Of primary concern may well be thoughts of the meaning of the symptoms, the treatment course and prognosis. What a shock it is for the person in the admission process to suddenly be confronted with questions, routines and actions by others that seem to threaten his or her very being. Questions ranging from "Do you want a private room?" and "What kind of insurance policy do you have?" to "Do you have false teeth?" and "Have you had a bowel movement today?" may be asked of the newly admitted patient within the first hour after walking into the facility. For the individual who is not accustomed to sharing this type of information with strangers or even family members, these questions may invade private thoughts, feelings and behavior.

Our society has placed increasing emphasis on the concept of privacy for about the past 20 years. Newspapers, television programs and popular magazines have made the American public aware of the many ways in which one's privacy may be invaded. Familiar examples are the multitude of ingenious devices used to record conversations, the psychological tools and tests to measure personality traits and the huge data banks which may be tapped for information. With this sea of threats to privacy in all areas of daily living, there is a continuing necessity to explore the concept of privacy and how the patient's need for privacy is supported, encouraged, met or inhibited in the provision of health services and especially nursing.

THE MEANING OF PRIVACY

In order to approach the study of privacy from a consistent frame of reference, a definition to be used as a basis for the continuing discussion must be provided. Perusal of the literature to establish an acceptable definition of the term has resulted in several possibilities. The simplest definition is found in the title of Morris Ernst and Alan Schwartz's book, *Privacy—The Right to Be Let Alone.*[1] Alan Bates adds his definition of privacy as "a person's feeling that others should be excluded from something which is of concern to him and also a recognition that others have a right to do this."[2] Alan Westin, in his comprehensive classic on the importance of privacy as an essential in a free society, defines privacy as "the claim of individuals, groups, or institutions to determine for themselves when, how, and to what extent information about them is communicated to others."[3] Westin further elaborates on the relationship of the individual to a social group, stating that privacy is the temporary and voluntary withdrawal of an individual by physical or psychological measures.[4]

More recently, Eleanor Schuster has developed a definition of privacy based on ideas offered by hospitalized patients. Included in this empirically derived definition is reference to the person's autonomy or control to achieve a comfortable state of social retreat as well as the aspect of achieving a flexible boundary to maintain the state of privacy.[5]

From these several interpretations, a composite statement on privacy includes the following aspects:

1. the right of individuals or groups to exclude others from certain knowledges and information;
2. the awareness that others have the same privilege as the person desires for him or herself;
3. the factors of time, place, manner and amount of information, which may all be aspects to be considered;
4. the exclusion of oneself from others; this may be voluntary, temporary and achieved by physical or psychological means or both; and
5. the end goal of privacy is a state of comfort.

It should also be noted that writings concerned with privacy are not always found under that specific rubric. Among other terms with similar meaning are secrecy, confidentiality and solitude. Sociological concepts such as social distance and avoidance were also considered.

Although privacy can be understood as a variable pertaining to both individuals and groups, privacy will be explored primarily as a property or state of the individual. However, adaptation to group settings can easily be made.

Following this definition of privacy, questions regarding its importance, functions and universality may be asked. How necessary is privacy? Is privacy a universal human need? To what extent is privacy important? What factors contribute to an individual's or group's need for privacy? What situations produce a change in the degree of privacy desired? Is it possible to have too much privacy, as well as too little?

Functions of Privacy

As an approach to answering some of these questions, the functions which privacy may serve can be delineated. The four functions identified by Westin provide one means of explanation.[6]

The first function, personal autonomy, relates to the beliefs regarding the uniqueness of humans and their basic dignity and worth as individuals.

Separation from others in order to develop one's feelings, thoughts, beliefs and values is a prerequisite for achieving a sense of individuality. Thus, freedom from intrusion is valued for its own sake and meaning to the individual. To maintain individuality and autonomy, some information about oneself will not be shared with anyone else.

A model for describing interpersonal relationships in terms of zones, regions or circles of privacy leading to the core of inner-self has been conceptualized. The inner portion contains those secrets, thoughts and beliefs which are not shared with anyone or perhaps only in situations of extreme stress when the person must share for essential emotional relief. There are concentric rings to denote the decreasing privacy from the inner to the outer layers, which is casual communication, observable to all.

Erving Goffman, a theorist on face-to-face interaction, has described ways in which people present themselves to others with the aim of controlling others' impressions of them. An aspect of this would be the region in which the performance takes place. The "back region" thus becomes the term for the area which is out of bounds to the audience, and "backstage" behavior is the regressive, intimate behavior not presented to the audience.[7]

Potential threats to one's autonomy and thus one's privacy occur in situations in which others seek to enter the inner core and learn its secrets. Also threatening are those behaviors which move a person into the "back region."

Emotional release is the second function identified by Westin. Because modern society imposes stresses and strains on people, they need opportunities for privacy in order to find emotional release. Several authors have noted the special need to obtain relief from tension brought about by the multiplicity of roles a person plays. In a similar vein, Barry Schwartz points out that privacy permits secret consumption.[8] The adolescent may find occasions for smoking or drinking in private just as someone else uses the privacy of the office or home to read pornographic books while openly displaying copies of best sellers or professional journals.

Another aspect of this function is the "safety-valve" effect, which relieves emotional pressure. Examples are situations in which people express anger, tension or anxiety at some authority in the privacy of their home, office or intimate circle of friends. A further form of emotional release is the possibility of minor noncompliance with social norms or social etiquette made by privacy. Exceeding the speed limit on a deserted highway, padding expense account vouchers, belching or picking one's nose may all be instances of nonconforming behavior permitted by privacy. Of special importance to the health professionals are the releases in bodily and sexual functions and emotional expression in times of loss or sorrow.

The third function, self-evaluation, describes the process whereby one is able to integrate one's experiences and gain some meaningful perspective. Assessment of data and consideration of choices are best handled in private. Closely related behaviors are those of creative thinking, moral inventory taking and various forms of meditation in which awareness of outside stimuli is temporarily turned off.

Limited and protected communication is the fourth function of privacy. One aspect of this function is the opportunity for sharing confidences provided by privileged communication for such groups as physicians, clergy and attorneys established by social norms. Schwartz refers to the rules of privacy as assisting in the maintenance of status divisions. Further, the ability to invade another's privacy is reflective of one's status in the hierarchy, as is demonstrated in physician behaviors.[9] The second aspect of limited and protected communication sets boundaries or distances in interpersonal relationships, such as student-teacher and parent-child relationships.

Aspects of Privacy

Research by Schuster has led to the categorization of three aspects of privacy, in relation to the period of time involved.[10] The most transient form is called privacy of event, meaning privacy necessary for some particular action, like bathing or meditating. Through the use of physical or psychological boundaries, the person can be apart from others. Privacy of event, as described by Schuster, encompasses the two levels of privacy known as solitude and the creation of psychological barriers.[11] These mean, respectively, separation from the group and the deliberate choice made by an individual to limit communication with others.

A less transient form is privacy of lifestyle. Influenced by one's culture, this form refers to privacy afforded through one's dwelling, geographic location or family constellation. The equivalent level of privacy is intimacy, which refers to the individual's acting as part of a small unit that exercises seclusion.

A nontransient aspect, privacy of personality, refers to the abstract concepts of dignity and autonomy. Viewed as a relatively permanent trait of the personality, this form exists as an individual variable.

Anonymity is recognized as another level of privacy which affords the person in a public place freedom from being personally identified and supervised. Anonymity can be preserved with strangers and in the publication of ideas without a person's identification.

Variables Influencing Privacy

The number of variables which influence the development and expression of privacy is evident as the concept of privacy is explored. Three of these variables will be presented as examples of the multitude of factors which can be considered in examining one's state of privacy.

Cultural: Studies of cultures and subcultural groups by anthropologists have increased the understanding of the importance of cultural values and norms on one's behavior. Observations made of the differences among various cultures in the participation of the father in childbirth demonstrate the extent to which privacy is considered important for the mother. White, middle-class Americans are usually viewed as having rigid concerns about privacy, especially when the event concerns bathing, sexual acts and elimination. Madeleine Leininger reports an example of differences in expectations regarding privacy between a British nurse and her patients in an Iranian hospital. The nurse initiated structural changes in the large ward units to provide for patients' privacy. Resistance to these moves was expressed by Iranian nurses and patients who valued the greater opportunities to see, talk and learn from one another in the ward situation than in double- and single-patient rooms.[12]

Political Systems: The differences between the totalitarian state and the democratic system can illustrate the relationship between the political system and privacy. In the totalitarian state the governing body is allowed a high degree of secrecy, while disclosure and surveillance is the rule for individuals and groups. Because loyalty to the state is demanded, the person's privacy, autonomy and individualism are attacked as "immoral" and "antisocial." While eventually a totalitarian state may relax somewhat and thus afford more privacy to institutions such as the church and the arts, the balance favoring disclosure and surveillance is necessary for totalitarian political systems to function.[13]

By contrast, the democratic state favors publicity and open hearings and investigations of the government as a means of control. At the same time, privacy is encouraged for individuals and groups. Democratic societies support the idea that individuals should have interest areas apart from the political system; therefore, these interests are encouraged. Strong family systems, personal retreats, religious choice and a variety of group associations are all highly valued in democratic theory. Thus, the balanced state of privacy maintained in a democracy is one in which individual and group needs are protected by privacy, but governmental groups are usually open to investigation and disclosure. An exception to the disclosure of governmental offices is the high degree of secrecy permitted for the security systems, such as the military and the Central Intelligence Agency.

As an example of legislation to protect individuals in our democratic society, the Federal Privacy Act of 1974 was passed to regulate the information practices of federal agencies. Through this act, an individual has the rights to know what information is in his or her file and to obtain copies of and know who has seen the file.[14]

Socioeconomic Status: Another variable to be considered for its relation to privacy is socioeconomic status. Particularly in a society with variation in status, rights and privileges are delegated, depending on one's place in the hierarchy. Frequently observed is the extent to which privacy is "a luxury," "an object of exchange."[15] Consider the differences in degree of privacy which can be purchased in hotels, theaters, public restrooms, housing areas, hospitals and transportation systems.

Rules about the invasion of another's privacy also vary with status. The physician with high social status has the authority to overcome the usual barriers to privacy. Somewhat paradoxically, the servant or maid is also able to ignore some of the usual rules of privacy afforded to one of higher status. This deviation is allowed because of servants' special categorization as a "personless" class.

Universality of Privacy

Is privacy a universal human behavior? Although most people tend to think of the desire for privacy as strictly human, some interesting studies of animal behavior have increased the knowledge about privacy and seclusion as necessary components of all animal life.

Space: As stated in the definition, physical and psychological measures may be used to promote privacy. In his seminal work on space, *The Hidden Dimension,* Edward Hall presents his concept of "proxemics," the term he coined for the theories related to man's use of space.[16] From his description of territoriality and spacing mechanisms as utilized by animals, he developed similar ideas related to man's perception of space. Thus, according to Hall, man also uses rules of personal, intimate and social distance in his interpersonal relationships.

The utilization and meaning of an individual's personal space continue to be of interest as the human population increases and urban areas experience congestion and crowding. *Public Places and Private Spaces,* in addressing the field of environmental psychology, presents an analysis of our everyday environments. Variables such as rate of information, complexity, certainty and emotions are used to describe environments and project the degree of privacy afforded by them.[17]

Findings of empirical studies on the importance of individuals having their own private space are not conclusive. Jonathan Freedman reports no negative effects from high density crowding in living arrangements.[18] Hypothesizing that hospitalized patients would experience anxiety when their territories and personal spaces were invaded, Constance Allekian found that intrusions into the patient's area of the hospital room did provoke feelings of anxiety. However, invasion of the personal space or the four-foot area surrounding the patient's bed did not influence anxiety.[19]

Human Needs: While norms regarding privacy do vary among cultures and societies, within each there are rules to insure individual and group privacy. Within an individual's daily interactions with others, in small groups, as well as in larger collectivities, privacy is maintained to the extent that persons have been socialized into those norms. Rules exist concerning individuals relating to one another, development of family rules regarding communication patterns and customs providing privacy for certain events.

Counterforces to Privacy

In addition to factors operating to promote privacy, counterforces exist which act against the preservation of privacy. There is some indication that this tendency to invade the privacy of others may be a universal behavior. The trait of curiosity has been observed to begin in very young children and to continue throughout life. Gossip as a means of obtaining and communicating private information is a common behavior among many people. Observing others' behavior, making judgments and interpretations and forming opinions also allows for gaining information about others that is not voluntarily presented.

Along with this individual behavior is the group behavior of observation and surveillance by authorities to enforce the rules of the society. Socially accepted means of insuring rights of individuals and groups by invading one's privacy are established.

Balanced View of Privacy

In this chapter, primary focus has been given to the desirability of privacy to the individual. However, in viewing privacy realistically, the equally important needs for companionship, sharing and socialization must also be recognized. This balance of privacy and disclosure is achieved by changing experiences and opportunities as one moves through the states of privacy or finds satisfactions in interpersonal relationships with others. Privacy is not proposed as an ultimate state or even a state to be achieved solely as an end in itself. Rather, privacy is a way of achieving individual goals and adapting to the stimuli of interactions and the environment. As pointed out by Georg Simmel, information must be shared between people in a relationship to achieve social cohesion and interaction. An individual must know certain things about another person for the relationship to be established and maintained.[20]

Individuals seek to have privacy at the times they need solitude. However, too much or too little privacy can be inappropriate and cause an imbalance. The values of group participation have been recognized by many theorists in group dynamics and group therapy. The importance of group work and actions, as well as the benefits for the individual member, are among the advantages of group membership. On the other hand, the study of social isolation and sensory deprivation has added to the knowledge about the effects of this extreme degree of solitude. When an individual is isolated from others, emotional deterioration occurs similar to that produced by sensory deprivation. Thus, the individual must strive for the continuous adjustment between these counteracting needs of privacy and companionship. In a sense, this freedom of the individual to decide for him or herself pertains to the very meaning of the right of individual privacy.

PRIVACY AND NURSING

Since relatively little of the literature reviewed on the concept of privacy came from the health sciences or was in any way related to the utilization of privacy by health professionals, the intention of this portion of the chapter is to develop nursing application of these ideas. What knowledge of privacy is necessary in nursing intervention aimed at providing privacy for patients? What nursing situations are especially pertinent as examples of the need to preserve privacy? How does the nurse's knowledge of the patient's rights to privacy coexist with the nurse's concern for research or to share information with or about the patient?

The rights of patients have become of such concern that, in 1972, the American Hospital Association adopted a ten-point Patient's Bill of Rights. This document provides a much needed mechanism for protecting the rights of patients, including the right to privacy. Item 5 states in part that "the patient has the right to every consideration of his privacy concerning his own medical care program." In 6, confidentiality regarding communications and records is emphasized.[21]

Privacy for Patients

To introduce the relationship of privacy to nursing care, nursing situations will illustrate the functions of privacy cited previously. The needs for personal autonomy, emotional release, self-evaluation, and limited and protected communication are seen frequently by nurses as they interact with patients in a variety of nursing activities.

The importance of considering the patient's autonomy has often been suggested as an essential aspect of nursing care. Individualized or patient-centered care has been a popular expression in nursing for a number of years. This approach has been supported by some psychological theories presenting various layers or rings which denote the degrees of confidentiality of one's personality, including thoughts, desires and beliefs. As nurses develop interviewing skills, they have often been cautioned not to probe or ask penetrating questions that require the patient to reveal more than he or she desires. Sensitivity on the part of the nurse would aid in respecting the individual's right to privacy and at the same time provide for a therapeutic interview. Insuring privacy in the setting might be the approach when certain difficult and revealing topics are discussed or when the patient indicates a desire to exclude other patients from the information being shared with the nurse.

The admission process, including the nursing history, may be an example of a situation in which nurses have a responsibility to provide privacy for the patient and family as a means of respecting the worth and dignity of the individual. Some kinds of patient teaching might best be accomplished in a setting in which questions and answers can be freely explored without embarrassment.

Consider also the person with a terminal illness who needs first to keep this knowledge private. Exposing the patient's state of health to other patients might be an invasion of privacy and a threat to the patient's individual autonomy. Are there ways of protecting this patient's privacy which might be provided? Indeed, in certain situations maintaining privacy might be a very difficult task; however, specific places on the unit should be available for the times when physical seclusion is important.

In community health nursing, a nurse entering a home at unannounced times to assess the family and home could also be viewed as an intrusion. Consider the family whose lifestyle, child-care practices, health beliefs, food preferences and work motivation can all be revealed by a visit to the home. What information is necessary to the nurse as a care giver? And, further, which knowledges gained through home visits need to be communicated to other members of the health team, and which observations and interpretations should remain as confidential information?

A question which has been raised in psychiatric nursing is related to the use of therapeutic community concepts and especially the techniques of reality confrontation. A patient who has recently experienced a traumatic event may be encouraged to discuss this openly in a group situation with both other patients and staff. How does the group decide how much to allow or encourage the patient to reveal? There is a possibility that the patient will need assistance to protect his or her privacy to prevent feeling "overexposed" to the group later. On the other hand, the nurse who assumes that the patient is not ready to discuss the situation may be providing for unnecessary protection. Careful assessment and exploration of the patient's readiness and goals will need to be made to avoid false assumptions.

The second function served by privacy, emotional release, is undoubtedly a familiar one in nursing. It has been frequently said that illness or threat of illness produces stress in an individual. If privacy provides people with the opportunity to blow off steam or obtain emotional release, it would seem to be necessary for those experiencing the multiple stresses of illness. For example:

> A community health nurse is making a home visit to a new mother who has recently returned from the hospital. The infant has been diagnosed as having a congenital disorder. A neighbor who has arrived at the same time as the nurse sits down and gives no indication she plans to leave.

Since this is the first home visit to this mother and infant, the nurse might consider how she can intervene at this time of stress to provide the privacy needed for the mother to obtain emotional release she may need in discussing the baby's health. The nurse may need to make a rapid assessment to know if the presence of the neighbor will invade the privacy of the interview. If so, the nurse may need to assist the mother in asking the neighbor to return at some other time.

Physical separation or solitude is one way of excluding others for privacy. However, in the absence of this possibility, as in many hospital and clinic settings, psychological privacy can be achieved through the use of a soft voice, slow speech and well-chosen words. Consideration needs to be given to means of providing both physical and psychological privacy in the health agencies where nurses are with patients and families.

The patient's need for emotional support is frequently included as an accepted goal in nursing care plans. While the value of another person listening and caring is important, at times an individual may need privacy first or at subsequent intervals to gain more from the person providing the emotional support. In this situation, also, the desire for a balance between privacy and interaction with others has to be considered.

For the emotional expressions following death, families may need an opportunity to be alone with the deceased before being interrupted or involved by the personnel. They should be permitted the release of their tensions, anger, guilt or sadness through the provision of privacy. Some families may prefer to talk with others immediately, and then secure moments of privacy with the deceased, followed again by a desire to talk with staff. Providing a room where a family can be alone as desired will enable the family members to express emotions in private as they choose, without having to fit themselves into any routinized pattern of behavior.

Nurses deal with people frequently in need of assistance in relation to bodily functions. Within the American culture especially, privacy for the body and its functions, such as elimination, sleeping and sexual activities, has been accepted. Patients should be provided with access to the privacy measure of screens, curtains around the bed or a closed door. And when the door is closed, is the patient's privacy respected by the nurse knocking on the door prior to entering? Or does the nurse enter without asking for permission? And, when leaving the room, does the nurse ask the patient whether the door should be open or closed?

The third function of privacy, self-evaluation, can be viewed as a frequently occurring need as the person's illness, altered body image, pain and other symptoms are integrated and become meaningful and manageable to the person. The provision for privacy can allow for and encourage this reintegration. A woman told of the need for major surgery involving a change in body image, such as a bilateral mastectomy, may need some time to be alone to review the situation, study the possible alternatives of treatment available, consider the consequences and make some decisions. This desire of the patient to be alone does not preclude the nurse being helpful in the problem-solving process; but, as has been stated, balance between privacy and companionship is the desired optimum, with neither privacy nor social interaction being ends in themselves. Again, the nurse will necessarily need to determine which is wanted and needed by the patient.

Limited and protected communication, the fourth function of privacy, is familiar within health situations where certain information is privileged due to the norms and boundaries of that relationship. Nurses sometimes face a decision when the patient says, "I'd like to tell you, but I don't want my doctor to know." The nurse will need to assess the situation to determine if this is indeed a legitimate request for privacy or if the patient is really asking another question, such as, "How much do you share with others?" or "Do you care enough about me to help me by telling the physician I am in trouble?"

Within hospital settings particularly, maintaining privacy for one patient may necessitate impinging on other patients. In rooms with two or more patients, one patient may find that a roommate's questions or conversation is an invasion of privacy. If the offended patient is ambulatory, moving to another place on the unit may be the solution. Drawing the curtains can also convey the need to be alone. However, there may be occasions when some intervention by the nurse is needed to protect privacy needs.

In intensive care units, privacy afforded to patients may be at a minimum in order to insure constant surveillance of patient conditions. The personnel in these units need to give special recognition to providing privacy at critical times.

In health facilities where continuity of care is practiced, the need for interstaff and interagency communication is especially critical. Patients need to be helped to understand the necessity of communications and encouraged to share actively.

Protecting the patient's rights to privacy requires a special response from the ever-increasing numbers of nurses engaged in research. Through an agreement regarding the subject's consent to participate, the nurse-researcher agrees to maintain the confidentiality of the subject's responses. In addition, the respondent is guaranteed the opportunity to withdraw from the study at any time or to withhold any information considered by the subject an intrusion into private thoughts or behaviors.

As we consider providing privacy for patients, a possible conclusion, as noted before, is that a balanced position between privacy and interaction is necessary. In order to function as health professionals concerned with various needs of the patients, some intrusion into personal matters is necessary. Obtaining a nursing history, giving a bath, performing certain treatments and patient teaching all involve dealing with the person's body, private thoughts or confidential information. The balanced view will necessitate knowing which information should be kept confidential and not shared with other team members, or asking purposeful questions, not questions just to satisfy one's curiosity.

. . . and for Nurses

So far we have been talking about the patient's needs for privacy; however, the nurse's own privacy deserves some attention. As has been stated in many philosophies of nursing, nurses should be aware of their own behaviors, values, norms and expectations. This general statement would encompass privacy as well, with the need for nurses to be aware of their values regarding privacy. In what situations do they require privacy? Are nurses able to maintain a satisfactory balance between privacy and participation?

Although the intention of this chapter is to focus on nursing, brief mention should be made of the situations in which the nurse's privacy may be the issue because of threats coming from within the nursing experiences. Nurses, too, may be threatened by probing questions asked of them by patients or staff. Nurses may feel unable to express in public the emotional responses they experience when a patient leaves the facility, dies or is told of a terminal illness. One study confirmed this by reporting the tendency of medical personnel to isolate the fatally ill child.[22] What opportunities are there for the nurse to obtain physical or psychological separation from others? The dining room, treatment room, nursing office and lounge areas may be the places sought out for the privacy needed by nurses.

What Nurses Need to Know

What sort of knowledge does the nurse need as a basis for intervention aimed at privacy? If the model used to describe the nursing process involves the steps of assessment, planning, intervention and evaluation, the nurse may follow this process in utilizing her or his knowledge to meet the patient's need for privacy more effectively. An example:

> A nurse enters a patient's room and initiates a discussion with the patient about the surgery planned for the next day. The nurse proceeds to ascertain what the patient knows about the procedure and the expected outcomes from the surgery. Suddenly the patient says, "Leave me alone. I don't want to hear about it."

Based on this amount of data, the nurse must make some assessment of the interaction and plan and initiate a nursing action. The nurse must decide if the patient is testing, wants to be left alone or, rather, wants the nurse to stay.

Before nurses can consider the possibility of any patient's need for privacy, they must have some awareness of the functions privacy can serve for an individual. They also need to know some of the variables which influence one's views about privacy. What meaning might a private room have for someone who is usually surrounded by members of the family? How can privacy needs be met for the person who lives alone and now is expected to share a room with three other patients?

Other variables which might be significant and worth considering are related to cultural background, social class, age and religion. These and other factors may all influence a person's individual needs for privacy. Knowledge of growth and development would suggest to the nurse that a five-year-old boy may much more readily share personal information about himself and his family than a fifteen-year-old boy who is turning toward his peers as confidants rather than to adult authorities, such as the nurse. With these two boys, what differences need to be provided for privacy during visiting hours or telephone calls?

As nurses establish relationships with patients they are able to gain knowledge about those persons' individual means of expressing the need for privacy. Verbal and nonverbal behaviors become apparent, and certain facial expressions or bodily gestures may be the patient's way of asking to be left alone. Also, because privacy may be needed for emotional release, symptoms of stress may be clues to the need for privacy. When a patient starts to cry, is this a clue that he or she wishes to be left alone, or does the patient wish to talk about the stress?

As suggested earlier, the nurses' awareness of their own needs for privacy will be another knowledge useful for successful intervention. Recognition of their tendency to isolate themselves or, on the other hand, to reveal their inner thoughts to others will assist nurse's in becoming aware that other people may have similar or different privacy needs.

The nurse's understanding of privacy should also include the concept of the desired balance between privacy and participation. An unfounded assumption that a particular person needs privacy could lead the nurse to isolating that person. Therefore, the degree of privacy provided needs to be carefully determined and evaluated to prevent privacy becoming an end in itself.

In sum, the nurse can:

1. understand that individual needs for privacy vary;
2. be perceptive of signs that a person's privacy is being invaded;
3. ascertain which information and knowledge acquired from patients and families is confidential;
4. be aware of the functions which can be met by privacy;
5. maintain a balanced perspective regarding privacy;
6. accept that some invasion of privacy can not be prevented while providing nursing care; and
7. assist the patient in the use of boundaries—physical and psychological.

SPECULATIONS

This discussion of privacy and its relevance to nursing raises many questions and ideas. Additional speculation might lead to new knowledges about privacy and further guidelines for the nurse.

In thinking about the application of privacy to all age groups, one question which occurs is how does privacy and its meaning develop in children? Are there differences in the expressions of privacy in girls compared with boys? The influences of child-rearing practices on the continuation or extinction of privacy might be studied in this culture as well as in other cultures.

A question related to the nursing process is how the need for privacy may vary as the nurse and patient progress through the stages of their relationship. Also, how is this similar to or different from the group process and its influence on privacy?

While the purpose of this chapter has been essentially to focus on the importance of privacy, additional studies on the effects of varying degrees of privacy might be done. The possibility of too much privacy has been indicated in patients who have experienced long periods of isolation or seclusion. The knowledge gained by studies of sensory deprivation might be studied for its possible relationship to too much privacy. When there is too little privacy, what kinds of behavior are observed? Sensory overload data are a part of this phenomenon, and additional information could be gathered about "people overload" as seen in situations where individuals are kept together in groups with little or no opportunities for being alone.

Study of individual variables would also be useful in our understanding of privacy in order to meet the needs of patients. For example, is the use of a patient's first name an indication that his or her privacy is being invaded? Or is touching a person an invasion of privacy? Within each clinical specialty numerous examples occur which can be identified and studied by clinical nursing specialists.

Nursing care will be enhanced as research on the nursing process continues. It is hoped that additional studies on the concept of privacy and its relation to the health-illness continuum and especially to the practice of nursing will be made in the future. These knowledges might then add to the body of nursing science which will contribute to more effective nursing care.

REFERENCES

1. Ernst, M. L., and Schwartz, A. V.: Privacy—The Right to Be Let Alone. New York, Macmillan, 1962.
2. Bates, A. B.: Privacy—a useful concept. Social Forces. 5:429-34, May 1964.
3. Westin, A. F.: Privacy and Freedom. New York, Atheneum, 1967, p. 7.
4. Ibid.
5. Schuster, E. A.: Privacy, the patient and hospitalization. Social Sci. and Med. 10:245, May 1976.
6. Westin, Privacy and Freedom, pp. 32-39.
7. Goffman, E.: The Presentation of Self in Everyday Life. New York, Doubleday, 1959, pp. 106-40.
8. Schwartz, B.: The social psychology of privacy. Am. J. Soc. 73:745, May 1968.
9. Ibid., p. 743.
10. Schuster, Privacy, the patient and hospitalization, pp. 245-46.
11. Ibid.
12. Leininger, M.: Transcultural nursing: a promising subfield of study for nurses. *In* Reinhardt, A. M., and Quinn, M. D. (eds.): Current Practice in Family-Centered Community Nursing. St. Louis, Mosby, 1977, p. 41.
13. Westin, Privacy and Freedom, pp. 23-24.
14. Westin, A. F.: Legal measures as national levels to protect privacy and confidentiality. *In* Laske, E. M., and Bank, R. (eds.): Safeguarding Psychiatric Privacy: Computer Systems and Their Uses. New York, John Wiley, 1975, p. 377.
15. Schwartz, The social psychology of privacy, p. 743.
16. Hall, E. T.: The Hidden Dimension. New York, Doubleday, 1966.
17. Mehrabian, A.: Public Places and Private Spaces. New York, Basic Books, 1976.
18. Freedman, J. L.: Crowding and Behavior. New York, Viking Press, 1975.
19. Allekian, C.: Intrusions of territory and personal space: an anxiety-inducing factor for hospitalized persons—an exploratory study. Nurs. Res. 22:236-41, May-June 1973.
20. Simmel, G.: The Sociology of Georg Simmel. Trans. and ed. by Kurt H. Wolff. New York, The Free Press, 1950, p. 323.
21. Annas, G. J.: The Rights of Hospital Patients. New York, Avon Books, 1975, pp. 25-26.
22. Spinetta, J., Rigler, D., and Karon, M.: Personal space as a measure of a dying child's sense of isolation. J. Consulting and Clinical Psychol. 42:751-56, December 1974.

15 RELAXATION

Sandra S. Sweeney

Relaxation is one of the many concepts yet to be defined, developed and made operational by the scientific method to form an armamentarium of nursing interventions. Relaxation, like so many other concepts in nursing, seems to suffer from frequent utilization while remaining in need of definition and prescribed application.

The study of relaxation as a nursing concept has been an interesting research experience. Examination of the literature has disclosed a vast number of clinical studies employing some method of relaxation therapy as the independent variable. In general, the majority of studies reviewed utilized only deductive research methodologies. Catherine Norris's arguments for the need for nursing to develop its concepts through inductive inquiry served as the impetus for the study of relaxation undertaken by this investigator.[1]

In this chapter the investigator intends to provide the reader with the results of a beginning attempt to define and develop a concept of relaxation. Conceptual and operational definitions are suggested, the usefulness of relaxation as a nursing intervention is discussed and implications and recommendations for future research and nursing practice are presented.

A DEFINITION OF RELAXATION

How frequently have nurses and other health professionals offered the following words of advice to clients, coworkers, family members or friends?

> "Just relax now and this won't hurt at all."
> "Try to relax your muscles and you'll be much more comfortable."
> "Just take a deep breath and relax."
> "You're just going to have to learn how to relax more."

When nurses and other health professionals made suggestions similar to these, what mechanisms, techniques or interventions were employed to assist the individual(s) concerned to attain the desired behavioral change—that of

The author wishes to express her appreciation to the following Nursing V undergraduate nursing students at the University of Iowa for their assistance in collecting data for the inductive study on relaxation: Diane Connelly, Carol Heppelwhite, Mary Ann Nihart, Cathy Odgard and Ellen Wilson.

relaxation? It is interesting to note that, while relaxation is frequently recommended and prescribed for clients and others, nurses and other health professionals remain unable to define, recognize and evaluate it—let alone attempt to teach and assist individuals to master it. If relaxation is to be useful as a nursing intervention for solving specific client problems of either physiological or psychological origin, then its application as a nursing intervention must be tested and evaluated by means of the scientific method. This means that the concept of relaxation must be defined both conceptually and operationally.

Relaxation has been defined in both physiological and psychological contexts, but in making it operational physiological criteria have generally been used. E. Jacobson defines relaxation as "a muscular lengthening as it occurs within a common, natural, physiological process requiring internal energy expenditure and giving off heat."[2] Others have defined relaxation as a hypometabolic or hypothalamic response representing decreased sympathetic nervous system activity. This reduction results in decreased oxygen consumption, carbon dioxide production, respiration rate, cardiac rate, and arterial blood lactate, pH and base excess levels. Conversely, there is also an increased frequency and intensity of electroencephalographic alpha and theta waves, increased skin resistance, and some increased muscle blood flow.[3]

The preceding definitions emphasize the physiological component of relaxation. A distinction should be made between the relaxation theories and therapies with a physiological emphasis and those theories or practices that have evolved from meditative schools of thought. Meditative practices that approach relaxation as a "state" include Zen Buddhism, Yoga, Taoism, T'ai Chi Chu'uan' and Transcendental Meditation. Research evidence indicates that successful practice of these psychophysiologic techniques have produced the same hypometabolic-hypothalamic responses indicative of the "relaxation response" as the physiological approaches. Investigators have subsequently suggested these techniques as potential clinical interventions in disease states associated with increased sympathetic nervous system activity.[4] In general, however, the meditative techniques have been developed in different eras, for different philosophical or religious purposes, and with different assumptions about the nature of man.[5] Primarily because of these differences, this aspect of the relaxation process is considered beyond the focus of this chapter. These differences and constraints placed on application and utilization of these meditative practices by nurses combine to make them less feasible as nursing interventions. Therefore, they are not included in the following discussion of potential nursing interventions.

Polarized definitions emphasizing only the physiological or the psychological component of relaxation remain inadequate for a conceptual approach to the topic. Further, an attempt to define relaxation inductively suggests it is frequently described and defined by what it is not rather than by what it might be. For example, relaxation was frequently defined as an absence of tension, fatigue, muscular rigidity, insomnia, fear, anxiety and so forth.[6] Other more positive descriptions and definitions of relaxation as a concept included the presence of such things as rest, sleep, leisure, fun, vacation, play, being at ease, quiet, calm and doing nothing.[7] The preceding descriptions consist of behaviors which may be affected by both physiological and psychological factors and suggest, therefore, that conceptual and operational definitions must be broad enough to represent a synthesis of physical and behavioral dimensions at both levels.

For the purposes of this chapter, relaxation is conceptually defined by this investigator as follows:

> A positively perceived state or response by an individual in attaining relative freedom from tension, toil or strain. It may be psychological or physiological in origin. It is psychological in control. It is an active and conscious process and can be influenced by both internal and external stimuli. It is manifested by both psychological and physiological behavioral responses.

This conceptual definition can be operationalized in a variety of ways and by means of diverse degrees and combinations of subjectivity and objectivity. Beginning at the subjective end of the continuum, for instance, relaxation can be measured simply by recording a client's self-report. Admittedly, use of the self-report is subject to the effects of numerous extraneous variables, but nevertheless, it remains integral to evaluation of relaxation interventions. What the client experiences and feels must be considered, accepted and evaluated since only the client can reveal such data to another individual.

Proceeding toward the objective end of the continuum, one may utilize various tools designed to measure the degree of relaxation experienced by the client. These tools could include various paper and pencil tests, scales, questionnaires and other instruments. Moving further toward the objective end of the continuum, data may include specific physical behaviors that have been documented as accompanying the relaxation state or response. Empirical verification of this concept would center on quantifying and catagorizing observations of the degree of tension or relaxation evident in the client's muscular status, especially in facial muscles. The inference is that as the tension decreases, relaxation increases. Other quantifiable physical data would include blood pressure readings, cardiac rate and respiratory rate.

It is obvious, therefore, that the criteria used to operationalize the concept becomes increasingly physiological as an investigator moves toward the objective end of the continuum. One must recognize, however, that observer bias and instrument decay are inherent in the methodology of these types of data collection procedures.

The greatest degree of objectivity in measuring relaxation that can be obtained at this time requires instrumentation. Physiological recording on either electromyographic or electroencephalographic equipment can provide accurate, valid and reliable measurement of relaxed states or responses. It is possible to obtain and operate some of this equipment relatively inexpensively and with minimal investment of time and effort. Even so, skill is essential for interpreting the results, and this poses the greatest challenge for nurses at the present time.

The preceding examples of operationalization are not intended to be either mutually exclusive or exhaustive. Ideally some combination of these tools, instruments and instrumentation is necessary and essential for adequate research on relaxation and for insuring some degree of objectivity in analyzing the findings.

SIGNIFICANCE OF RELAXATION TO NURSING

How then, one might ask, does all of this affect the discipline of nursing? Relaxation is necessary and essential to maintain both physical and mental health. To date, there have been relatively few nursing studies that have dealt with the concept of relaxation as a therapy or relaxation training as a technique.[8] Nurses are in a unique position to pursue research dealing with this concept because of the extensive interaction, counseling and teaching opportunities inherent in professional nurse-client relationships. To assist clients to learn how to relax neither requires medical initiation nor invades the territorial rights of other health professionals. Relaxation is an adaptive, coping process which lends itself to nursing interventions designed to promote and enhance health and, ultimately, the quality of life. Given this potential significance for nursing which is yet to be tested, perhaps it would be helpful to abstract from a review of the literature selected historical aspects and trends in the development of relaxation and relaxation therapy as a therapeutic intervention.

REVIEW OF THE LITERATURE

Much has been written about "relaxation." The literature ranges from accounts reflecting personal opinion and experience[9] to highly sophisticated research protocols and studies, some examples of which are documented later in this chapter. The influence of rest as a therapeutic intervention can be found in written lecture notes as far back as 1879. John Hilton writes:

> Nature devotes her best efforts, during the period of rest and sleep, to repair those powers which may have suffered exhaustion, to renovate the bodily strength, and to restore the mental vigor . . . enabling him [man] to resume his labor in all the delightful vigor of a renewed existence. . . .[10]

> . . . All viscera . . . require the alternate condition of activity and rest to keep them vigorous and in health. If this condition be not observed or attended to, structural changes and deterioration of function are sure to follow. Indeed, in reference to the etiology of diseases of individual organs, it may be asserted that a large proportion of these diseases originates in circumstances which deprive the organ of that rest which Nature has rendered necessary for the performance of its healthy function.[11]

It is perhaps of some interest to note here that data from this writer's inductive study on relaxation indicated a "rest" function was attached to relaxation in health and a "reparative-recuperative" function in illness.[12] Close to 100 years have elapsed, the terminology has been altered, but the basic notions expressed by Hilton in 1879 remain remarkably appropriate.

Jacobson provided the basis for developing a research perspective on relaxation as early as 1908. Subsequent research on the topic did not expand its parameters to any great degree until after 1940, when J. Wolpe and others provided a new impetus by modifying and developing Jacobson's early relaxation techniques into revised protocols and subsequent studies.[13] Since that time, the increasing complexities associated with lifestyles of the post-World War II era have resulted in an ever-expanding arena in which research on relaxation therapies and techniques could flourish.

Jacobson developed his technique of progressive relaxation training as one method of treating clients with diagnoses of various anxiety or related emotional states or disorders resulting in muscular tension. In general, his technique involves the individual systematically and progressively tensing and releasing specific groups of muscles while learning to attend to and discriminate among the sensations associated with their tension and relaxation. Once learned and used successfully, the individual can use the technique to achieve a deep sense of relaxation.[14] Jacobson views anxiety as a response to some perceived threat which activates the autonomic nervous system, thus producing increased muscle tension. Tension is viewed as a universal experience resulting from the interrelatedness of physiological and psychological systems. Progressive muscle relaxation forces the client to focus on discriminating among specific sensations that accompany muscular activities and combine to mediate excessive tension and produce reductions in perceived anxiety and tension on a subjective basis.[15] Most of Jacobson's work employed a one-to-one working relationship with clients, utilized 15 different muscle groupings and required a lengthy training period.

Wolpe modified Jacobson's early work and subsequently developed a more efficient relaxation program which decreased the training time considerably. Wolpe also altered the direction and emphases of relaxation training as a treatment; that is, he applied relaxation training as a counterconditioning reflex and emphasized the conditions causing the pressure of anxiety rather than the anxiety response per se.[16]

Since Wolpe's work, others have continued to modify, develop and test various approaches and methods of progressive relaxation. Jacobson himself has modified and expanded upon his earlier techniques. Since his early work focusing on the method of progressive relaxation, Jacobson has enlarged his therapeutic techniques to include the notion of "self-operations control." This latter element emphasizes the role and responsibility of the individual client in achieving a state of relaxation. That is, the individual client is expected to function somewhat independently of the therapist by assuming an active role in determining how, when and where he or she will relax.[17] This has become an important variable in considering and predicting the success of relaxation as an intervention. This point will be elaborated later in this chapter.

D. A. Bernstein and T. D. Borkovec have published a manual in which they provide a concise but comprehensive synopsis of relaxation research in general, as well as specific information and protocols outlining their own research efforts. Bernstein and Borkovec propose the following model to explain the relationship between psychological and physiological variables and the effects of relaxation training:

> Relaxation training has been found to reduce subjective tension and affect a variety of other physiological processes. Research has as yet produced few answers to this question. . . . Current thinking emphasizes the role of the reticular formation [a diffuse nervous tissue located in the central nervous system] in mediating the interaction among these three aspects [voluntary muscle activity, internal autonomic activity and mental behavior]. This is a model we can use to understand the relaxation effect. Decreased autonomic arousal could in this way be caused by the thing a person consciously thinks (cognition) and through decreased skeletal activity. Similarly, subjective feelings of anxiety may be eliminated by inherent suggestions or removal of the autonomic and skeletal components of these feelings.[18]

They have modified Jacobson's earlier techniques in several ways. For example, they utilize briefer training sessions (about 30 minutes in length) and focus on training and relaxing 16 specific groups of muscles. Their manual is an important contribution to the relaxation research literature. The sharing of their protocol, program and recorded training sessions assists other researchers in the field to overcome some of the methodological problems of standardization and bias so implicit in one-to-one training sessions.[19]

The ongoing and evolutionary research process in relaxation training has produced three major trends at the present time. These trends are toward:

1. more specification in protocols and more efficient training conditions and programs;
2. developing additional valid and reliable measurements of the physiological effects of relaxation; and
3. being more specific in the delineation of those behavioral problems most conducive to treatment by relaxation training.[20]

These trends must continue to be developed, pursued and communicated to others in order to provide direction for future research studies utilizing relaxation training as an independent variable. It is only by continued efforts in these areas that a substantive body of knowledge will be accumulated and application to clients with predictable results achieved.

RELAXATION THERAPY AND TECHNIQUES AS NURSING INTERVENTIONS

Nursing is in a unique position to initiate and pursue research studies focusing on the continued development of relaxation as a concept and relaxation techniques as an independent variable. Nursing should give serious consideration to the contributions it can make to the evolving body of relaxation knowledge, in general, and to the systematic examination of the usefulness of this knowledge as a nursing intervention in the care of selected patients, in particular. Nursing studies in either of these areas have been meager thus far; however, the potential for application of relaxation research suggests this area of study could provide ample opportunity for many nursing studies.

An extensive review of literature is beyond the scope of this chapter. However, when examining the literature, it did seem appropriate to select studies that would summarize some of what is known about relaxation, illustrate examples of clinical applications nurses could use to test relaxation therapy and techniques as interventions, and provide some recommendations and implications for further study based on previous research findings.

Inductively, research is still needed to identify the phenomenon of relaxation per se and to establish the parameters of its use. Questions of what creates or promotes a state of relaxation in another individual remain unanswered. Once this information can be identified, the nursing process can be utilized to assess, diagnose and intervene with a specific prescribed technique for clients needing assistance in learning how to relax and alleviate tension. What properties, if any, does relaxation possess? What precedes and follows relaxation?[21] There is a great amount of information on relaxation still not known, which must be explored, identified and articulated before or along with the establishment of propositions, interrelationships and theories derived from predominantly deductive studies.

Most, if not all, of the published research reviewed for this chapter used the deductive method of reasoning. Anxiety and its relationship to relaxation therapy and techniques remains a major source for the development and implementation of research studies. Relaxation therapy and techniques have been reported as successful interventions in studies dealing with treatment of acute, chronic, state and trait anxiety reactions. These studies examined the aspect of relaxation therapy used for anxiety associated with activities such as test taking, presenting material at conferences, visits to the dentist and as the primary complaint in a variety of psychiatric disorders.[22] Certainly nurses could begin to systematically test nursing interventions based on relaxation therapy with client anxiety. Assuming a relationship does exist between the concepts of anxiety and relaxation, nursing studies could focus on relaxation therapy with clients awaiting surgical operations or procedures, diagnostic procedures such as endoscopic examinations, radiographic tests such as myelograms, angiograms, lymphagraphy and so forth. Studies could also focus on the effects of relaxation therapy on the anxiety that accompanies and is so frequently associated with pain. The interrelationship among the concepts of anxiety, tension and pain, and, therefore, relaxation training and the relief of one or all of these symptoms, provides several foci for studying the complexities involved in each concept and creates a challenging assignment for developing techniques for intervention. Because anxiety exists in so many of life's experiences, it lends itself well to nursing research studies dealing with coping processes and strategies. If one task of nursing is to assist clients to adapt to their environment, then assisting individuals to cope with the anxiety that accompanies life experiences, whether in illness or health, is an appropriate area for nurses to identify and in which to test interventions which accomplish that goal. Relaxation techniques are specific interventions nurses can use to assist clients to improve their ability to cope with that illusive symptom—anxiety.

While anxiety which frequently accompanies pain provides opportunities for generating nursing studies, so also does the phenomenon of pain itself and its relationship to relaxation. A. K. Jacox used progressive relaxation training as an intervention in a recent nursing study which attempted to identify methods by which nurses could alleviate pain associated with three specific groups of clients. The groups consisted of individuals categorized according to the pain associated with (1) rheumatoid arthritis; (2) selected diagnoses of cancer; and (3) the postoperative phase of two elective surgical procedures.[23]

A tension-pain-tension cycle may develop in individuals experiencing pain and can become a self-fulfilling prophecy unless interrupted. Relaxation therapy and techniques would appear to be feasible methods by which one could reduce muscular tension and, therefore, pain. Research reports in this area, however, reflect inconsistent findings and suggest a need for further investigations. M. J. Bobey, for example, suggests relaxation techniques are the most effective to deal with a painful stressor.[24] Final results of Jacox's research are yet to be published; however, preliminary findings seem to indicate that the relaxation intervention was of limited usefulness in alleviating pain in all of the groups tested.[25] Clinical application of relaxation therapy and techniques as nursing interventions may be useful in relieving certain types of muscular tension and subsequent pain. Groups for which clinical application of these therapies are appropriate have yet to be identified. Relaxation has been advocated, however, as a means of mitigating muscular tension associated with labor in order to decrease the pain and discomfort of the child-bearing process.[26] Other applications need to be conceived, developed and tested.

Relaxation therapy and techniques may also provide useful nursing interventions for clients experiencing muscular aches, sprains or strains. Clients experiencing chronic low back pain, for example, may achieve some relief and satisfaction from an alternative approach such as relaxation therapy. H. Gottlieb and his associates have initiated a comprehensive low back pain management program which incorporates relaxation therapy and techniques as one facet of the therapeutic modalities. The report indicates a high level of success, with 79 percent of the clients being discharged from the program with unimpaired physical functioning levels and 81 percent having attained successful levels of vocational restoration.[27] Muscular aches and strains frequently accompany common experiences such as nervous tension, automobile accidents, overexertion of muscle groups or clinical disorders. Relaxation therapy and techniques may provide measurable relief for clients with these conditions as either a curative or preventive form of therapy. T. Howard employed relaxation as a means of reducing muscle cramping experienced by patients undergoing hemodialysis. There was evidence to support the hypothesized relationship between the technique of progressive relaxation and a decreased incidence of muscle cramping during dialysis treatments.[28]

Hypertension and selected aspects of cardiovascular dysfunction are other areas in which clinical application of relaxation therapy and techniques have potential as nursing interventions. H. L. Deabler has evidence to indicate that eliciting the relaxation response tends to lower both the systolic and diastolic blood pressures when the technique of progressive muscular relaxation is employed in both drug and nondrug groups of hypertensive subjects.[29] H. Benson et al. report similar findings and suggest further:

> The results of these investigations demonstrate that the regular elicitation of the relaxation response may have usefulness in the management of both untreated and pharmacologically treated hypertensive patients. The relaxation response may lower blood pressure by the same means as some antihypertensive drugs which interrupt sympathetic nervous system activity . . . it is unlikely that the regular elicitation of the relaxation response will be adequate therapy for severe or moderate hypertension; it might act synergistically with antihypertensive drugs to lower blood pressure, and may lead to the use of fewer drugs or a lesser dosage. In the case of borderline hypertension, the regular elicitation of the relaxation response may be of great value since it has no pharmacologic side effects and might possibly supplant the use of drugs.[30]

Hypertension is a chronic condition occurring in clients with whom nurses come in frequent contact. Nurses provide counseling, drug and diet information and formal or informal instruction covering many aspects of hypertension to clients in institutions, clinics, homes and various other settings. Relaxation therapy and techniques may offer yet other methods of assisting clients to influence and reduce their hypertensive state. A note of caution should perhaps be interjected at this time. P. P. Hauri concurs that relaxation training methods are effective in decreasing hypertension, but suggests that the halo effect may be creating a spurious influence on the results of some of the hypertensive studies. He states that clients "seem to enroll in such studies when their blood pressure is high," and questions whether the mere fact that they are actively "doing something about their hypertension might relieve much of their anxiety and in itself lower the blood pressure."[31] While Hauri points specifically to the hypertensive studies, his comments could apply to any study utilizing relaxation therapy and techniques and should be taken into consideration when designing the research study.

The effect of relaxation therapy and techniques on the occurrence and treatment of tension and migraine headaches reveals data that could be useful to nurses whose clients experience such conditions. In general, relaxation seems to generate more favorable results for headaches caused by tension than for migraine headaches. T. H. Budzynski reports success and favorable results with biofeedback and relaxation training techniques on clients suffering from tension headaches,[32] and Hauri proposes that the preceding combination of treatments should be the treatment of choice for headaches caused by tension.[33] As mentioned earlier, however, most writers do not advocate relaxation therapy as training techniques for treating migraine headaches. Some research reports indicate that the relaxation response was of limited usefulness in treating migraine headaches.[34] Other studies report relaxation therapy was helpful in reducing the prodromal tension preceding the onset of a migraine headache, but of limited or no value once the headache had progressed to the point of pain.[35]

Clients suffering from tension or migraine headaches comprise another sample in which nurses could intervene utilizing relaxation therapy and techniques. Clients whose headaches are caused by tension may obtain significant relief from learning and implementing relaxation techniques successfully. Migraine headache victims might be able to prevent the painful stage from developing if they can successfully interrupt the migraine cycle in the early prodromal stage. Relaxation therapy and techniques could provide migraine headache clients with a means of control, coping and possible prevention of a most unpleasant and disabling disease condition.

The notion of self-control was alluded to earlier in the chapter and deserves additional attention at this time. There has been a recent surge of interest in combining relaxation therapy and techniques with behavioral self-control. The client, not the experimenter, determines whether or not relaxation therapy and techniques are successful. The client must be responsive toward learning the relaxation technique, practicing it and ultimately initiating it whenever it is needed to alleviate a specific problem. This means, then, that once the technique is learned, the client remains in control of the complete relaxation experience. This is not true of the initial phase of relaxation therapy, however, and successful learning of specific techniques requires the client to relinquish an element of control to the experimental procedure itself. The client must be able to follow the directions implicit in the relaxation program and yield his or her mindset to receiving and following specific instructions and attending to and discriminating among the specific sensations of tension and relaxation. Successful relaxation remains the responsibility of the client. Just as with meditation practices, the client must be able to identify when it is needed, initiate the process and then actively participate in and cooperate with it.

Capitalizing on the notion of behavioral self-control, several studies have utilized the relaxation response as a means of controlling behavior, such as decreasing alcohol, drug and cigarette usage,[36] and weight control.[37] These changing client behaviors are additional examples of potential clinical applications in which nurses could intervene with relaxation therapies. Innumerable other situations provide researchable opportunities for nurses to use relaxation therapy and techniques. Clients who are experiencing insomnia, nervousness, fear, apprehension and so forth are all potential benefactors of relaxation therapy.

RELAXATION THERAPY AND TECHNIQUES—WHAT ARE THEY?

Relaxation therapy began as a technique of progressive contraction and relaxation exercises for a specific number of muscle groupings. This method, although modified, remains the primary technique used today. Investigators can follow procedures and directions of Jacobson, Bernstein and Borkovec or of A. Lazarus in devising their own approach or intervention. The procedures vary somewhat in the number of muscle groups utilized, the setting and strategy employed to instruct the client, and the duration of each relaxation session. Specific instructions regarding their protocols are published and readily accessible.[38]

In more recent literature relaxation therapy generally refers to a comprehensive program that includes a broad range of therapeutic modalities directed toward client intervention. It can involve counseling programs, medication regimens, relaxation techniques, physical and vocational-occupational rehabilitation and attempts to reeducate clients toward relaxation, recreation and socialization processes.[39] Relaxation techniques, on the other hand, usually refer to a specific phase or intervention, such as Jacobson's progressive muscle training program or biofeedback procedures. The distinction between relaxation therapy and relaxation techniques, therefore, concerns the comprehensiveness of the approach being employed and does not indicate that the processes or procedures are separate.

The setting in which relaxation therapy and techniques are employed should be quiet and relatively free from external distractions. This can be accomplished in a variety of ways: having a private room, drawing curtains or screens around a chair, bed or recliner, closing a door and so forth. The goal, obviously, is to decrease extraneous stimulation.

Strategies used to teach relaxation techniques utilize one-to-one therapy sessions in which the experimenter gives the specific directions for contraction and relaxation of muscle groups; or the experimenter may use the less personal but more standardized approach of audio-tape recordings to provide the directions for the client. The client's use of headsets or earphones for listening to audio-tape recordings is helpful in reducing external stimulation in potentially distracting environments such as hospitals. Biofeedback procedures involve direct client interaction with mechanical equipment. Group relaxation sessions may also be utilized as a strategy.

The duration of relaxation therapy and the length of individual relaxation technique sessions will depend, to a large extent, on the therapist and choice of technique being used. Individual sessions for learning the technique of progressive muscle relaxation can last from a minimum of 15 to 30 minutes up to a maximum of three hours. Most sessions utilized in research studies have been approximately 30 minutes. In addition to each relaxation technique instruction session, however, the client is expected to incorporate and actively participate in several independent practice sessions each day. Once the technique is learned, the client is assisted in identifying when relaxation is needed and directed to initiate the technique as a preventive control of his or her own behavior.

Caution is needed when undertaking relaxation as a nursing intervention. As with the administration of any other procedure, drug or aspect of client care, the nurse must be knowledgeable about the care being given. So, too, the nurse contemplating the utilization of relaxation therapy and techniques as interventions in either specific client situations or as independent variables of research projects must be responsible for and accountable to those clients. He or she must possess the necessary knowledge to insure competent and safe implementation of the relaxation therapy and technique chosen as an intervention. Relaxation therapies and techniques can be hazardous when they are improperly administered. Therefore, nurses must exercise caution and insure adequate preparation and knowledge prior to undertaking these procedures as interventions.

SUMMARY

In summary, who among us is not affected by some type or degree of tension? Who among us could not benefit from learning how to relax and reassess the effects that tension can have on our minds and bodies over prolonged periods of time? For those from whom tension has already exacted a toll, evidenced by physiological or psychological dysfunction, discomfort or disorder, perhaps relaxation therapy and techniques will provide an alternative to maintaining the status quo. Nurses are in a unique position because of the number of interaction, counseling and teaching opportunities in professional nurse-client relationships to promote research involving relaxation interventions which assist clients to cope with their environments and improve the quality of their lives.

REFERENCES

1. Norris, C.: The Methodology of Concept Formation. Lecture at University of Iowa, Iowa City, Iowa. November 3, 4, 1976.
2. Jacobson, E.: Tension in Medicine. Springfield, Ill., Thomas, 1967, p. 7.
3. Wallace, R. K., Benson, H., and Wilson, A. F.: A wakeful hypometabolic state. Am. J. Physiology. 221:795, 1971; Beary, J. F., Benson, H., and Klemchuk, H. P.: A simple psychophysiologic technique which elicits the hypometabolic changes of the relaxation response. Psychosomatic Med. 36, 2:115, March-April 1974; Benson, H., Greenwood, M. M., and Klemchuk, K. H.: The relaxation response: psychophysiologic aspects and clinical applications. Int. J. Psychiatry in Med. 6, 1/2:87, 88, 1975.
4. Goleman, D. J., and Schwartz, G. E.: Meditation as an intervention in stress reactivity. J. Consulting and Clinical Psychol. 44, 5:456, 461, 1976; Orme-Johnson, D. W.: Autonomic stability and transcendental meditation. Psychosomatic Med. 35, 4:348, July-August 1973; Beary, Benson, and Klemchuk: A simple psychophysiologic technique, pp. 115, 119.
5. Shapiro, D. H., and Zifferblatt, S. M.: Zen meditation and behavioral self-control. Am. Psychol. 520, July 1976.
6. Sweeney, S. S.: A concept of relaxation. Unpublished research data, University of Iowa, Iowa City, Iowa, 1977.
7. Ibid.
8. Aiken, L., and Heinrichs, T.: Systematic relaxation as a nursing intervention technique with open heart surgery patients. Nurs. Res. 20:212-17, May-June 1971; Howard, T.: Cramping, relaxation, and hemodialysis. Dissertation Abstracts International. 32:4860, 1972; Jacox, A. K.: Pain Alleviation through Nursing Intervention: Final Report. U.S.P.H.S. Research Grant NU-00-467-3, 1976.
9. Fink, D. H.: Release from Nervous Tension. New York, Simon and Schuster, 1943; Rathbone, J. L.: Teach Yourself to Relax. Englewood Cliffs, N.J., Prentice-Hall, 1957.
10. Hilton, J.: On Rest and Pain. 2nd ed. Jacobson, W. H. A. (ed.). New York, W. Wood, 1879, p. 2.

11. Ibid., p. 7.
12. Sweeney, A concept of relaxation.
13. Bernstein, D. A., and Borkovec, T. D.: Progressive Relaxation Training: A Manual for the Helping Professions. Champaign, Ill., Research Press, 1973, p. 3.
14. Jacobson, E.: Progressive Relaxation. Chicago, University of Chicago Press, 1938; Jacobson, E.: Anxiety and Tension Control. Philadelphia, Lippincott, 1964, pp. 28-65; Jacobson, Tension in Medicine, pp. 132-34.
15. Jacobson, Anxiety and Tension Control, preface.
16. Wolpe, J.: Psychotherapy by Reciprocal Inhibition. Stanford, Stanford University Press, 1958; Bernstein and Borkovec, Progressive Relaxation Training, pp. 3-4.
17. Jacobson, Anxiety and Tension Control, pp. 36-41.
18. Bernstein and Borkovec, Progressive Relaxation Training, p. 57.
19. Ibid., pp. 11-55.
20. Ibid., p. 4.
21. Norris, The Methodology of Concept Formation.
22. Townsend, R. E., House, J. F., and Addario, D.: A comparison of feedback—mediated relaxation and group therapy in the treatment of chronic anxiety. Am. J. Psychiatry. 132, 6:598-601, June 1975; Daniels, L. K.: The treatment of psychophysiological disorders and severe anxiety by behavior therapy, hypnosis and transcendental meditation. Am. J. Clin. Hypn. 17, 4:267-69, April 1975; Jacobson, E.: Modern Treatment of Tense Patients. Springfield, Ill., Thomas, 1970; Johnson, D., and Spielberger, C.: The effect of relaxation training and the passage of time in measure of state-and-trait anxiety. J. Clin. Psychol. 24:20-23, 1968; Canter, A., Kondo, C. Y., and Knott, J. R.: A comparison of EMG feedback and progressive muscle training in anxiety neurosis. Br. J. Psychiatry. 127:470-77, 1975.
23. Jacox, Pain Alleviation through Nursing Intervention, p. 1.
24. Bobey, M. J., and Davidson, P. D.: Psychological factors affecting pain tolerance. J. Psychosom. Res. 14:376, 1970.
25. Jacox, Pain Alleviation through Nursing Intervention, p. 8.
26. Field, P. A.: Relief of pain in labor. *In* Pain: A Source Book for Nurses and Other Health Professionals. Boston, Little, Brown, 1977, p. 428.
27. Gottlieb, H., et al.: Comprehensive rehabilitation of patients having chronic low back pain. Arch. Phys. Med. Rehabil. 58, 3:101, 107, 1977.
28. Howard, Cramping, relaxation, and hemodialysis.
29. Deabler, H. L., Fidel, E., Dillenkoffer, R. L., and Elder, S. T.: The use of relaxation and hypnosis in lowering high blood pressure. Am. J. Clin. Hypn. 16, 2:75, October 1973.
30. Benson, Greenwood, Klemchuk, The relaxation response, p. 92.
31. Hauri, P. P.: Biofeedback and self-control of physiological functions: clinical applications. Int. J. Psychiatry in Med. 6, 1/2:261, 1976.
32. Budzynski, T. H., Stayva, J. M., Adler, C. S., and Mullaney, D. J.: EMG biofeedback and tension headache: a controlled outcome study. Psychosomatic Med. 35, 6:484-96, November-December 1973.
33. Hauri, Biofeedback and self-control, p. 259.
34. Andreychuk, T., and Skriver, C.: Hypnosis and biofeedback in the treatment of a migraine headache. Int. J. Clin. Exp. Hypn. 23, 3:180, 181, 1975; Benson, H., Klemchuk, H. P., and Graham, J. R.: The usefulness of the relaxation response in the therapy of headache. Headache. 51, April 1974.
35. Stambaugh, E. E., and House, A. E.: Multimodality treatment of migraine headache: a case study utilizing biofeedback, relaxation, autogenic and hypnotic treatments. Am. J. Clin. Hypn. 19, 4:240, April 1977; Mitch, P. S., McGrady, A., and Jannone, A.: Autogenic feedback training in migraine: a treatment report. Headache. 269, January 1976.
36. Benson, H. and Wallace, R. K.: Decreased drug abuse with transcendental meditation: a study of 1,862 subjects. *In* Drug Abuse Proceedings of the International Conference. Zarafonetis, C. J. D. (ed.). Philadelphia, Lea & Febiger, 1972, pp. 369-76.
37. Ferster, C. B., Nurnberger, J. I., and Levitt, E. B.: The control of eating. J. Mathematics. 1:87-109, 1962.
38. Jacobson, E.: Anxiety and Tension Control; Bernstein, and Borkovec, Progressive Relaxation Training; Lazarus, A.: Audio Relaxation Tape Cassettes—Daily Living: Coping with Tensions and Anxieties. Chicago, Instructional Dynamics, 1970.
39. Gottlieb et al., Comprehensive rehabilitation of Patients, p. 101.

Section IV

Example of Applying Concepts from a Theory to Nursing: Transactional Analysis Concepts

INTRODUCTION

In previous chapters, the authors have taken eclectic approaches to developing the specific concepts and applying them to nursing practice. Some authors have combined developmental theory with sociological or psychological constructs to fully develop their content. In contrast, Silvia Lange takes a theory (transactional analysis) and shows how it provides an appropriate framework for assessing nurse-client communications/interactions and devising appropriate strategies for nursing intervention. Continuous evaluation is an integral part of transactional analysis and clues discovered from such evaluation may lead to revisions in nursing actions.

Lange introduces structural analysis of the personality as a basic concept of transactional analysis. She notes the existence of three ego states in each personality (Parent, Child, Adult) and suggests that the Parent ego state is divided into the Nurturing Parent and the Critical Parent; that the Child ego state is divided into the Adapted Child and the Natural or Free Child; and that the Adult stage is undivided in its realistic appraisal of the social and physical environment.

The chart of cues for each of these ego states lists words, voice, tone, body language, attitudes and situations applicable to that particular ego state. This chart should prove useful not only in clinical situations but also in the development of research protocols for the testing of the theory and its implications for nursing practice.

Lange notes the usefulness of egograms in analyzing both individual and typical categorical classifications of individuals. These analyses may then be used to suggest appropriate interventions to alter the communicative and interactive climates. Using the diagram to study the interaction of the ego states within an individual and the interplay between interactants is suggested as a graphic form of interpretation.

In applying the concept of ego states to the nursing situation, Lange suggests it may be hypothesized that there are normally recurrent shifts between ego states because of illness. Such shifts may elicit concomitant alterations in the caring personnel's ego states presented to the patient. Testing these hypotheses to identify specific situations in which particular ego states occur in either patient or personnel would strengthen nursing's body of knowledge.

After discussing transactional analysis proper, Lange notes the importance and classification of types of stroking. She defines a stroke as any act, verbal or nonverbal, which implies recognition of another. This discussion of stroking and its application to nursing practice implicitly offers many hypotheses for testing, formally and informally. Nursing studies of physical contact between nurse and patient would be strengthened in future projects by testing within the transactional analysis theory framework. Equally desirable would be the study of the efficacy of Parental or Adult ego state communications in specific nurse-patient situations.

Similarly, Lange's discussion of the ways to structure time (withdrawal, rituals, activities, pastimes, games and intimacy) is highly suggestive of testable hypotheses. The testing of her pragmatic observations about situations in which a particular structuring of time is probable could lead to proof or disproof of certain constructs of this theory.

Comments comparable to those above can be made of the discussions of basic life positions and scripts. The discovery of relationships between particular life positions and certain diseases or the finding of relationships between age, parental injunctions, contemporaries' injunctions or specific illness behavior and a life script would be of immense importance to the everyday practice of nursing.

Some suggestions for the testing of transactional analysis theory have been elicited from Lange's discussion of the theory and its utility to nursing. The perceptive reader will identify many more, not only from the presentation of the theory, but also from Lange's examples and applications to the nursing situation.

16 TRANSACTIONAL ANALYSIS AND NURSING

Silvia Prodan Lange

Communication and interpersonal relations are two vital concomitants of the nursing process. The basic nursing unit consists of two persons, the patient and the nurse. In this interpersonal relationship, the two individuals bring their past experiences and expectations to the present situation and attempt to find ways to express, understand and act on them.

The nursing profession has accepted the responsibility of providing comprehensive care, which includes understanding human behavior of patients and using this understanding for therapeutic results. F. H. Sanford stated:

> If medical care is to be truly comprehensive, and truly humane, there cannot be treatment of mere cases or mere symptoms. There must be treatment of people—whole, complicated people, weak and strong and courageous and frightened and cantankerously individual and mousily conformist people. . . . It is the nurse who must carry the therapeutic light in this very human side of medical care. It is the human skills—skills based on both knowledge and on personal attributes—which give the nurse a highly unique therapeutic function, the true significance of which has very probably not yet been fully appreciated.[1]

The body of knowledge about human behavior has expanded explosively in this century. Schools of nursing have utilized concepts from psychiatry, psychology, sociology and anthropology to better understand patients, colleagues and the nursing situation. The writings of Sigmund Freud, Harry Stack Sullivan, Erik Erikson, Carl Rogers, A. H. Maslow, J. Reusch, and B. F. Skinner have presented theories and information about psychodynamics, psychopathology, communication and behavioral change, all of which are useful in nursing.

In the 1950s Eric Berne introduced the initial concepts of transactional analysis (TA). *A transaction is the unit of social action between people. It consists of a single stimulus and a single response, verbal or nonverbal.* Each party gains something from it which is why he or she engages in the exchange. *TA is the study and treatment of the communication process—the ongoing transactions between people.*

Transactional analysis is both (1) a theoretical framework to explain personality development and human behavior and (2) a specific method of psychotherapy. Since the original work, Berne and others have developed and expanded theory and practice. This approach has gained acceptance among professional psychotherapists as an effective treatment method.

Transactional analysis is also applicable in settings other than traditional mental health services. Workers have used these concepts in situations such as education, probation, marital counseling, prison, welfare agencies, medicine and nursing. Transactional Analysis has been used to improve interpersonal relations in business and management. Basic concepts have been introduced into the curricula of elementary and secondary schools as well as colleges. The purpose is to understand human behavior, improve communication and prevent or detect early mental health problems.

The general public has verified interest in transactional analysis by support of such books as *Games People Play, I'm O.K./You're O.K., Born to Win,* and *Scripts People Live.* These books present the basic concepts of transactional analysis in terms that are easily understood; the jargon is deceptively simple at times.

The purpose of this chapter is to relate transactional analysis to nursing situations to better understand the communication network. Transactional analysis provides the nurse with conceptual guidelines to plan, carry out and evaluate interpersonal interventions.

Through study of this chapter, the reader should be able to define, describe and apply to nursing situations the following TA concepts: ego states, transactional analysis proper, strokes, time structure, basic life positions and scripts. The theory and techniques of transactional analysis as a form of psychotherapy are only covered in the suggested readings.

Although recognizing the sexist implications, the author will use the feminine pronouns for the "nurse" and the masculine pronouns for the "patient" or "physician" for the sake of clarity.

EGO STATES

Definitions

A basic concept of transactional analysis is structural analysis of the personality. Structural analysis is the identification of the specific ego state in operation. *An ego state is a consistent pattern of feelings and experiences directly related to a corresponding consistent pattern of behaviors.* There are three broad observable patterns of thinking, feeling and behaving that are part of everyone's personality. These parts are called the Parent ego state, the Adult ego state, and the Child ego state. (The capital letters distinguish between references to the ego state and to the chronological age or role of the person.)

These three ego states develop sequentially and are subject to modification throughout life. Theorists differ on the specific times in early childhood that the states emerge. The Child ego state is present at birth and becomes more differentiated through socialization. The Adult ego state emerges as the older infant separates himself from his mother and begins to figure out cause and effect relationships. The Parent ego state forms when the child begins to understand and respond to language and social rules.

In discussing the work of Penfield, T. A. Harris concluded that the brain functions as a high-fidelity (video-tape) recorder that stores up all the material of which a person is consciously aware.[2] The memory and associated feelings are available for replay under certain circumstances at any time. An ego state is "produced by the playback of recorded data of events in the past, involving real people, real times, real places, real decisions, and real feelings."[3]

A person is in only one ego state at a time, although rapid shifts take place. The specific ego state is identified through gestures, posture, voice tone, choice of words, subjective feelings and the situation.

Parent Ego State: The Parent ego state is borrowed from parental figures and divided into the Nurturing Parent and the Critical Parent (labeled by some as the Punitive, Prejudicial or Disciplining Parent). It reflects the ideas, feelings and behavior of one's own parents, particularly as expressed during the first eight years of life. It can be identified when one's language, intonation, attitudes, posture and mannerisms are similar to one or both parents.

> In the Parent are recorded all the admonitions and rules and laws that the child heard from his parents and saw in their living. They range all the way from the earliest parental communications, interpreted nonverbally through tone of voice, facial expression, cuddling, or noncuddling, to the more elaborate verbal rules and regulations espoused by the parents as the little person became able to understand words. In this set of recordings are the thousands of "no's" directed at the toddler, the repeated "don'ts" that bombarded him, the looks of pain and horror in Mother's face when his clumsiness brought shame on the family in the form of Aunt Ethel's broken antique vase.[4]

The Parent ego state is necessary when the time to raise children comes. It also makes many automatic responses concerning ethics, manners and how things "should" be done. The Parent ego state refers to both (1) the nurturing, sympathetic, reassuring, caring and caring for part of the personality and (2) the critical, opinionated, prejudiced, authoritarian and judgmental part.

Adult Ego State: The Adult ego state is adapted to current reality. When functioning, it identifies Parent prejudices and archaic childhood attitudes. It is that part of the personality which is engaged primarily in objective data processing and computing. It deals with facts and verifiable information.

The Adult ego state operates on what works, what is most efficient and what will solve the problem. An important function of the Adult is to make decisions based on the computation of information from the Parent, Child, previous data in the Adult and external reality factors.

Child Ego State: The Child ego state represents the continuation of feelings, thoughts and actions from chronological childhood. It is divided into two parts. The Adapted Child ego state operates under the influence of parental directives even though the person is "grown-up" in years. The Natural or Free Child is spontaneous, expressive and creative.

This ego state represents and duplicates the ways in which the young child experienced his world. Powerful emotions reside in the Child and are expressed in reaction to past reality or present situations. Many times a person finds himself feeling and reacting as a child with frustration, rejection, des-

Table 4
Descriptions of Ego States

Ego State	Words	Voice Tone	Body Language	Attitude	Situations
Critical Parent (CP)	You should/n't Don't Ought/n't Nice/bad Disgusting Shameful You are: stupid naughty lazy ugly a brat Shhhhhhh!!!! Clichés Stereotypes	Loud Controlling Threatening Boring Sneering Condescending Critical Disgusted Blustery Mean	Pursed lips Pointed finger Crossed arms Hands on hips Tongue-clucking Scowl Eyes rolled up Frown Head shaking: No, no! Eyes narrowed	Disapproving Moralistic Judgmental Authoritarian Hostile Rigid Admonishing Demands respect Righteous indignation *Always* right! *Never* wrong!	Child-rearing Politics Courtroom Philosophy Religion Marriage Sex (bad) School Supervising Critiquing
Nurturing Parent (NP)	Don't worry You're OK Come on, now Try Don't be afraid I care I'll help you You are: good talented beautiful adorable cute lovable an angel Good!	Reassuring Soothing Coaxing Encouraging Sympathetic Supportive Concerned Syrupy Cooing Lullabying Soft	Pat on head, back Cuddling Hugging Holding Rocking Arms outstretched Smile Head shaking: Yes, yes! Throwing a kiss	Loving Caring Understanding Giving Encouraging Compassionate Protective	Child-rearing Taking care of: self others pets plants Sickness Food Religion Marriage Emergencies

Adult (A)	Who? What? When? Where? How? How much? Possible Efficient Objective Factual Informative Constructive Alternative It seems to me . . . Relevant	Appropriate Audible Modulated Unemotional Level Steady Clear Paced well	Attentive Alert Congruent Relaxed Straightforward Poised Absence of Parent or Child behaviors	Reality-testing Flexible Investigative Alert Confident Open Calm Interested	Work Budget: time money Counting Decision making Planning School Refereeing Machinery operating Science Detective work Emergencies
Natural or Free Child (FC)	Wow! Wheeee! Yes! No! I want I Need I wish Yuk! Let's play I LOVE you!	Giggling Animated Expressive Laughing Crying Raging Fun-teasing High-pitched Rapid	Spontaneous Free Squirming Showing off Winking Bright eyes Mobile mouth Goo-goo eyes Muscles in motion Jumping up and down Hugs Tears	Curious Admiring Joyful Excited Impulsive Uninhibited Contagious Fun Sexy	Play Sports Parties Dancing Art Recreation Sex (good) Sensuality Entertainment Amusement park Food
Adapted Child (AC)	I can't! I won't You can't make me I dunno Anything you say	Mumbling Sullen Repetitive Rebellious Angry	Pouting face Slumped Raising hand to speak Nose-thumbing	Helpless Compliant Rebellious Vengeful Guilty	Parent/Child School Sickness Work Marriage

Table 4 (Cont.)

Ego State	Words	Voice Tone	Body Language	Attitude	Situations
Adapted Child (AC) (Cont.)	Please? I guess I don't know Do it for me You'll be sorry Yes, sir No, ma'am Obscenities Swearing Muteness No! Yes?	Annoying Sweet Fearful Whining Taunting Mean-teasing Loud/soft Fast/slow Unctuous Apologetic	The finger Blushing Trembling Averted gaze Rigid posture Mannerisms Tics Forlorn look	Ashamed Demanding Dependent Attention-seeking Obedient Seductive Coy	Crime Drug/alcohol abuse Violence Sex (bad) Competition

Ego states are identified by a variety of cues. This chart is a guide of observable behaviors and the situations in which they often occur.

Two other ways to identify what ego state is operating are the reactions of other people *and* subjective feelings. *Parent ego state often elicits either Adapted Child or Parent responses; Free Child stimulates the Child in others or hooks the Critical Parent. The Adult ego state is often responded to by the Adult in another.*

One's subjective feelings help to identify particular ego states, especially when combined with the above observable behaviors. Feelings of anger, rejection, disappointment, expectation, rage, helplessness, shame, guilt, pleasure, pride, approval and disapproval are from either the Parent or the Child. By definition, the Adult ego state does not experience emotion but can process information from the others. Some people confuse this to mean that the adult, the grown-up person, does not have feelings. This is not true, desired or possible.

pair, rage and inadequacy. In the Natural Child are the qualities of excitement, curiosity, sensual and sexual enjoyment. This is a person's zest.

The Adapted Child is the result of the ways in which the little person learned to get along with parents and other significant people, including siblings. Adaptation (or adjustment) includes lifelong patterns of rebellion or compliance. Common Adapted Child behaviors are temper tantrums, withdrawal, sickness, helplessness, submission, anger and fears.

All five ego states are functional. Some behaviors which differentiate positive and negative aspects are:

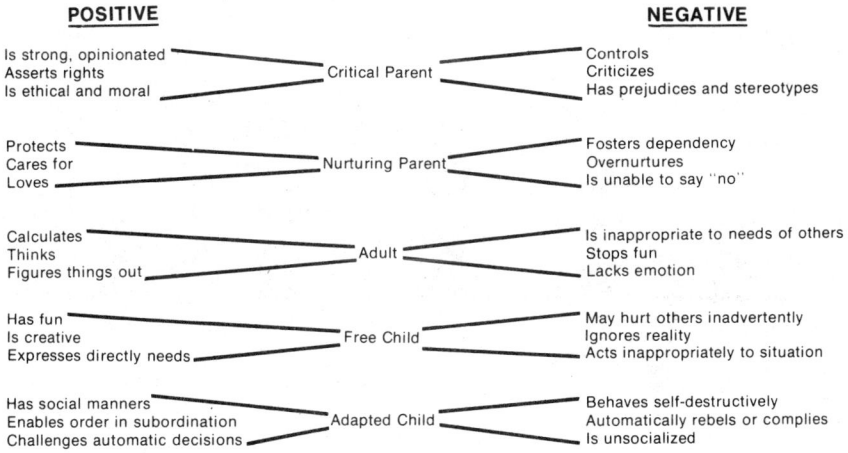

Figure 16-1

Ego states shift regularly and rapidly in ongoing transactions. However, there are patterns which describe a person's habitual behavior over time. *An egogram is the visual representation of how an individual appears to others.* It shows the relatively stable relationships between Critical Parent, Nurturing Parent, Adult, Free Child and Adapted Child. The graphs stand for the amount of psychic energy invested in the different ego states. John Dusay hypothesized that a certain amount of psychic energy is available for the combined ego states.[5] A shift in one will result in a shift in one or more of the others. It is easier to raise an ego state than to lower a high one. For example, if a person raises his Adult through increased thinking and problem-solving, he will probably take energy away from a high Critical Parent or Adapted Child. Raising Free Child through play often reduces Adapted Child.

There is nothing intrinsically good or bad about any of the ego states. They reflect the individual's basic personality. Difficulties arise when the person is dissatisfied with himself or in significant conflict with those around him. The egogram is a guide to desired change.

Following are illustrations of egograms:

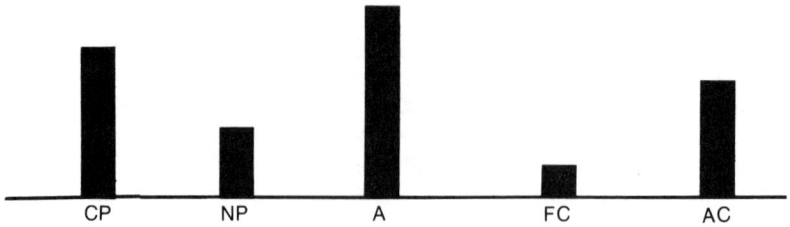

Brilliant but tempermental surgeon

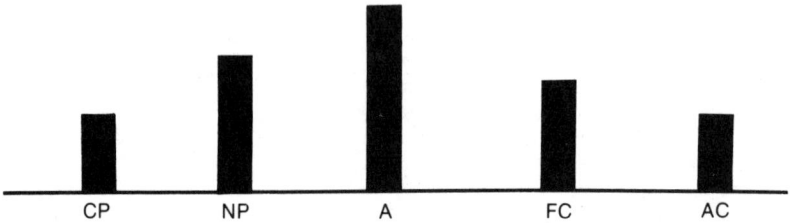

SuperNurse

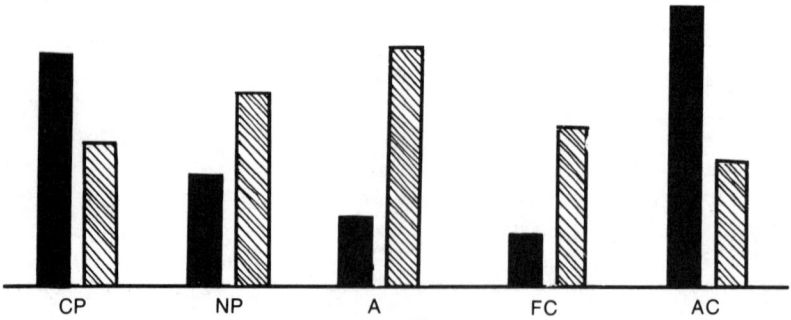

Depressed patient before psychotherapy (solid) and after successful treatment (striped)

Figure 16-2

A well functioning person is adaptable and flexible. He is able to use his Parent, Adult and Child ego states and respond to these in other people. In such a person the three ego states are separate and discrete, as represented in Figure 16-3.

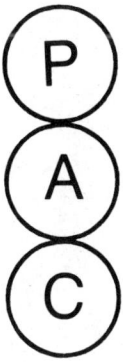

Figure 16-3

The two types of ego state pathology are contamination and exclusion. In contamination there is an intrusion of the Parent, the Child ego state or both into the Adult ego state. This results in prejudices (Parent contaminated Adult), phobias and delusions (Child contaminated Adult), and mixed parental messages and child fears (Double contaminated Adult).

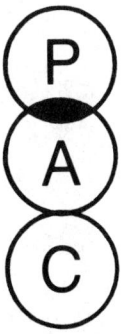

Parent Contaminated Adult

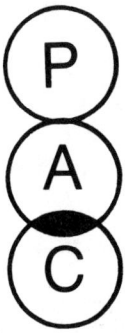

Child Contaminated Adult

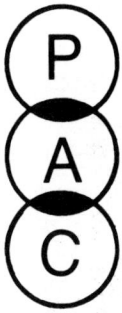

Double Contamination

Figure 16-4. *Contamination*

Exclusion as ego state pathology is divided into two types—the excluding ego state and the excluded ego state. One or more ego states is not operational. The excluding ego state takes domination over the other two. It is constant and rigid.

The excluding Parent ego state is seen in some judges, policemen and professional helpers. The excluding Adult results in a "computer personality"—the individual who thinks a lot and is not much fun to be around. The excluding Child plays a great deal, entertains and thinks and evaluates little. Clowns, comedians and some confused people with psychotic behavior show this type of pathology.

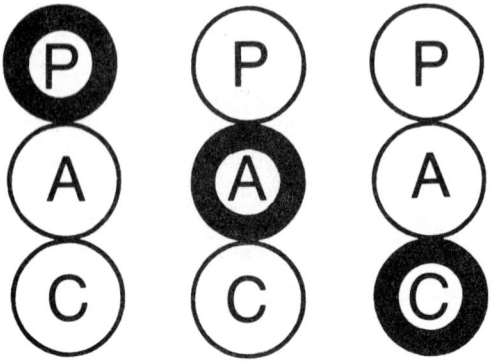

Figure 16-5. *Exclusions*

The second type of exclusion pathology is the excluded ego state. Two ego states are functional but the third is excluded. A person may exclude his confused, crazy Child while maintaining Adult and Parent ego states. An excluded Parent results in clever, well-thought out, manipulative behavior with little conscience or concern for others. When the Adult ego state is excluded by the Parent and Child, the resulting state is psychosis because of the inability to test reality. This is seen in schizophrenic reactions, psychotic depressions and drug-induced conditions.

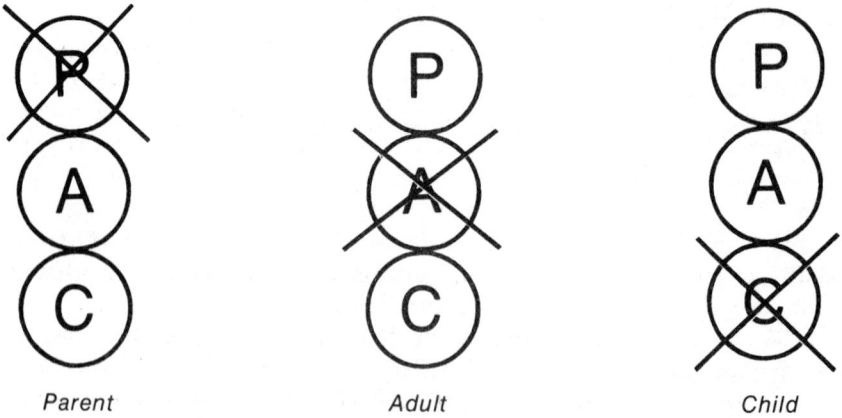

Figure 16-6. *Excluded: Parent, Adult, Child*

One task of transactional analysis as psychotherapy is to recognize and deal with contaminations and exclusions of ego states.

Application of the Concept of Ego States to Nursing Situations

The identification of ego states (structural analysis) provides a useful tool for understanding behavior in nursing settings. Under the stress of illness, the behavior of the patient with his family often indicates that the executive control has shifted from the Adult ego state to either the Parent or Child ego. This is expressed in behavior described as helpless, fearful, hostile, demanding, resistive, submissive, critical, manipulative and sexually provocative. Other people respond to these behaviors with tolerance or rejection.

A certain amount of regression (activation of Child ego state) is common in all illnesses. This precipitates the need for more nurturing. The Child is more clearly experienced and expressed. Many times the patient is quite aware of this shift and, through his critical Parent ego state, stands in judgment of himself. This is seen when a man cries out in pain or despair and then is deeply ashamed of his lack of control. He may apologize profusely for "being a baby."

A person may come to the attention of medical or psychiatric staff through actions which are labeled "acting out"—alcoholism, delinquency, drug abuse, violence, suicide attempts and deviant sexual behavior. These behaviors reflect the Adapted Child in action, often in rebellion against the internal or external Critical Parent.

The critical aspects of the Parent also can be directed toward oneself. When a person condemns himself as being inadequate, a failure or a coward, it is in response to earlier messages from his parents. This is a common experience of people who are depressed. A competent nurse who is continually dissatisfied with her performance despite reassurance from others shows the impact of her Critical Parent on her Adapted Child.

Patients often relate to staff as if the latter were parents or similar authority figures. This is related to early parenting, cultural expectations and the behavior of some doctors and nurses. The term "mother surrogate" describes the specific nurturing activities that nurses perform. Feeding, bathing, soothing, reassuring, protecting and encouraging are all Nurturing Parent actions.

Many people are attracted to nursing because of the nurturing part of their Parent—the desire to care for and be of help to others. In the process of nursing education, the student acquires knowledge and information (in the Adult ego state) to accomplish this purpose on more than a sympathetic, intuitive level. She develops "an educated heart."

In TA terms the statement that the nurse should not be judgmental means that she should not let her own Critical Parent pass open judgment on how the patient chooses to live his life. Even if her background, morals and religious beliefs are much different from those of the patient, she can respect his individuality and dignity. She examines her preconceived ideas, stereotypes and prejudices about people and illness to decontaminate her Adult and update her Parent.

When a person becomes physically or emotionally ill, he often retreats from the use of his Adult ego state. He temporarily surrenders decision making and problem solving to the medical/nursing staff and his family. When a person is extremely anxious, his Adult is generally decommissioned. He misinterprets information about treatment, surgery or routines. In denying illness, the person will not allow his Adult to process data accurately. Modern concepts of nursing include the expectation that the patient is a partner in his treatment. Whenever possible, the nurse encourages him to use his Adult ego state to exercise responsibility and control over his care and make decisions about his life.

The nurse uses her Adult ego state to determine the patient's needs. She decides whether he needs her to nurture him or whether she should refrain from direct help. She can view with objectivity the behavior which represents the Adapted Child ego state—uncooperativeness, demandingness, manipulation and hypochondriasis. She tries to understand how these behaviors meet the needs of the patient at this present time. She refrains from labeling him as childish or immature. Working from this basis, she can help the patient to develop more satisfying and more satisfactory ways of achieving attention and strokes. She attends to the Free Child by providing biological comfort and responding to feelings of fear, grief and anger.

The nurse also pays attention to her own Adapted Child so she can handle her feelings appropriately. She uses this information to understand herself better and deal with the situation in the present and not from her own past. At times she may need help from coworkers and supervisors to sort out feelings of anger, frustration, guilt, shame, resentment, inadequacy and envy.

If the nurse feels very critical and judgmental toward a patient or staff member, she examines her Parent ego state. Are her personal biases and beliefs being challenged or threatened? Or does her reaction come from her Child who feels put down, helpless, not OK and inadequate to cope? If she feels extremely protective and nurturing, she evaluates whether the patient really needs that degree of mothering.

The nurse uses the egogram to get a clearer picture of the various ego states in herself, her patients, other staff members and the total ward. One psychiatric unit graphed their collective egogram, shown in Figure 16-7.

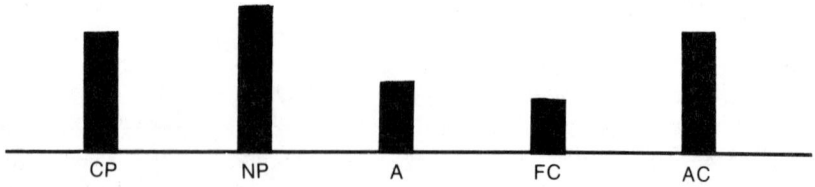

Figure 16-7

As a group, they decided to make changes in the treatment program to raise Free Child (dance group and more outings) and Adult (more decision-making power to patient government). This resulted in lowering both Critical Parent and Adaptive Child responses in both the staff and patients.

TRANSACTIONAL ANALYSIS PROPER

Definition

While this whole system is called transactional analysis, one particular part of it is called transactional analysis proper—the analysis of a single transaction with the transactional diagram. A transaction is a stimulus from one person and the response from another. This may be through words, gestures, body language, action or any other form of communication.

In interpersonal situations, these transactions occur quickly with many possible outcomes. Transactional analysis proper identifies from which ego state the stimulus originated and toward which ego state in the other person that it was directed. The response is analyzed the same way.

The three kinds of transactions are (1) complementary, (2) crossed and (3) ulterior. These are defined below and diagramed with illustrations in the next section.

A complementary transaction is one in which the ego state addressed is the ego state which responds. Lines drawn on the transactional diagram are parallel. As long as the lines remain parallel, the communication goes on indefinitely. There are nine possible types of complementary transactions between the two person's Parent, Adult and Child.

A crossed transaction is one in which (a) the response comes from an ego state different from the one addressed or (b) the response is directed toward an ego state different from the one giving the original stimulus. On the diagram, the vectors are crossed. In either case, communication stops or shifts to a discussion of the relationship of the persons.

An ulterior transaction is a complex communication exchange between two people which appears to be one thing but is actually another. The social level is the façade, the accepted message; the psychological level is the true message. The psychological level may not be recognized by either party. The professional salesman and confidence man deliberately use ulterior transactions to make a living.

Illustrations of Transactional Analysis Proper

In a transaction, the original stimulus can come from the Parent, Adult or Child ego state of the sender and is directed toward one of the three ego states in the other person. When the ego state addressed responds to the original ego state, the transaction is complementary. The nine possible combinations are diagramed in Figure 16-8.

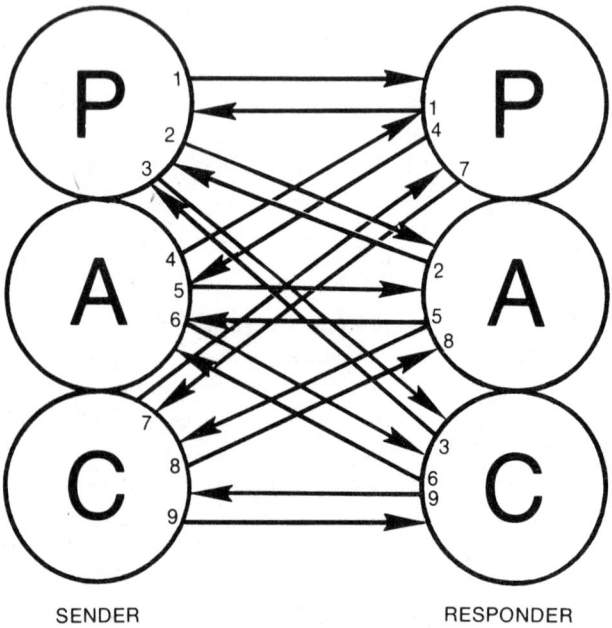

Figure 16-8. *Possible Transactions*

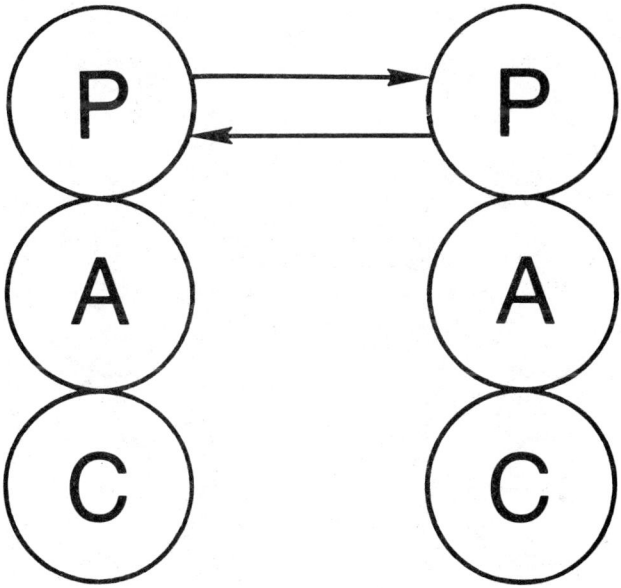

Figure 16-9. *Parent-Parent Complementary Transactions*

Stimulus— *Patient: The cost of hospitalization is outrageous these days!*
Response— *Roommate: Yes, and you don't get the good old bedside nurse these days.*

Stimulus— *Nurse: I told her the medicine was for her own good, but she just wouldn't listen to reason.*
Response— *Doctor: I'll give her a good talking to.*

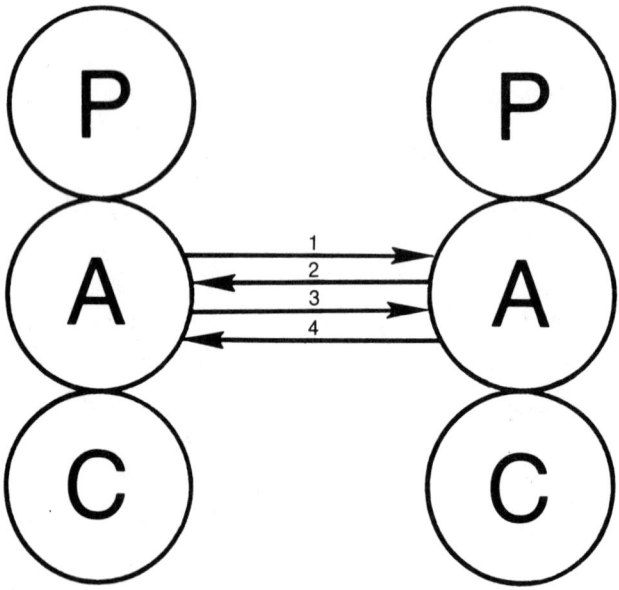

Figure 16-10. *Adult-Adult Complementary Transactions*

1. Stimulus— *Patient: I can't get to sleep.*
2. Response— *Nurse (New Stimulus): Are you thinking about something that's keeping you awake?*
3. Response— *Patient (New Stimulus): Yes. Just when am I scheduled for surgery tomorrow?*
4. Response— *Nurse (New Stimulus): 8:30* A.M. *I'll be giving you a sleeping pill later on. I have some time to listen if you'd like to talk about some of your concerns.*

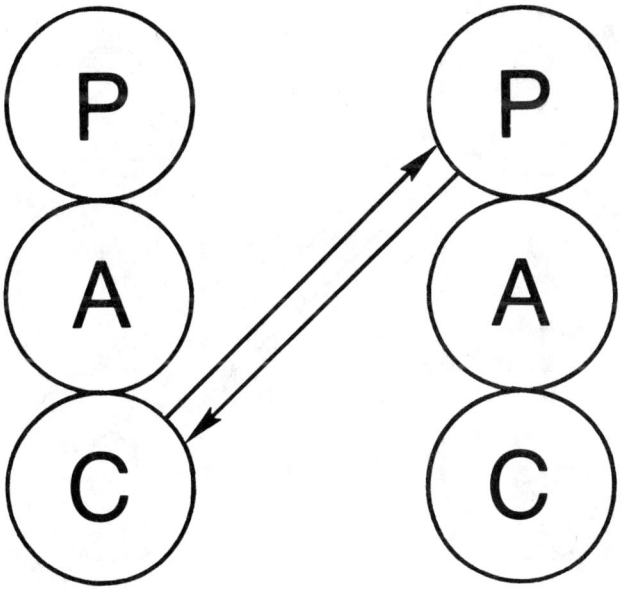

Figure 16-11. *Child-Parent Complementary Transactions*

Stimulus— *Patient: Nurse, please help me. It hurts so much.*
Response— *Nurse: Hold on. I'll get your medication.*

Stimulus— *Patient: (Crying and not able to say anything.)*
Response— *Nurse: You're really upset now. I'll just stay here with you.*

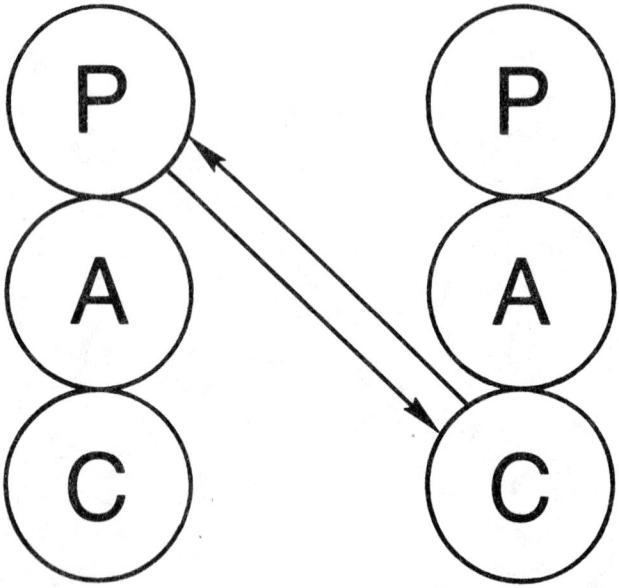

Figure 16-12. *Parent-Child Complementary Transactions*

Stimulus— *Nurse: What are you doing up? You know you're supposed to be in bed!*
Response— *Patient: Oops, I'm sorry. Please don't tell the doctor on me.*

Stimulus— *Doctor: How come you nurses can't follow a simple order?*
Response— *Nurse: (Clenched teeth) Sorry, sir.*

In these examples (Figures 16-9 to 16-12), the communication could go on indefinitely as long as the ego states do not shift. The vectors remain parallel.

Crossed transactions occur when the vectors on the diagram intersect. At this point the two people either stop communicating or shift their focus to their relationship rather than the original topic. Some examples follow.

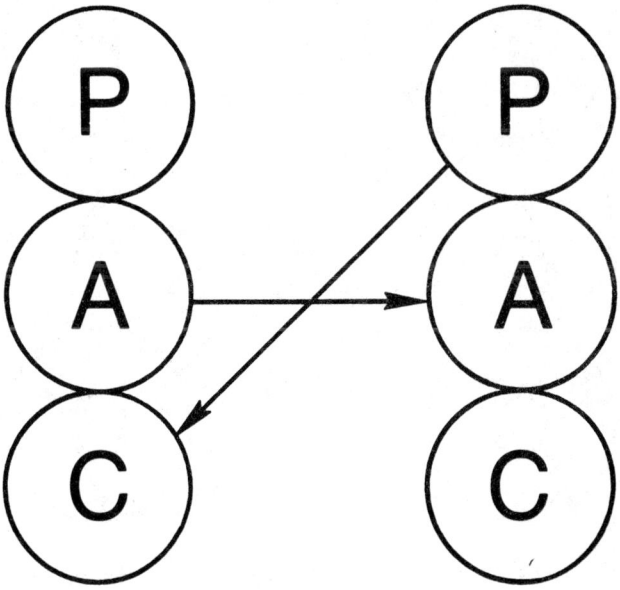

Figure 16-13. *Crossed Transaction*

Stimulus— *Nurse: I can help you with your morning care now.*
Response— *Patient: It's about time!*

The nurse gives information (what and when) from her Adult directed to the patient's Adult ego state; the patient responds from Critical Parent directed toward the nurse's Child. Now the situation shifts to one in which the bath may be given in mutually uncomfortable silence or the nurse may begin to defend her time schedule while the patient expresses feelings of irritation and neglect.

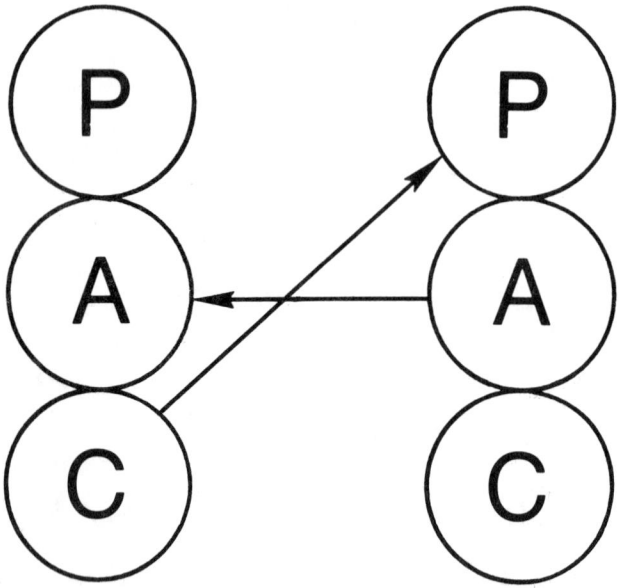

Figure 16-14. *Crossed Transaction*

Stimulus— *Patient: I'm signing out of this hospital and you can't stop me!*
Response— *Nurse: First, I'd like to know what is upsetting you. Maybe we can work it out.*

By crossing the transaction, the nurse interrupts the communication. The patient may continue to attempt to provoke a parental response, may stomp out of the hospital anyway, or may shift to his Adult ego state to problem-solve in response to the nurse's Adult invitation.

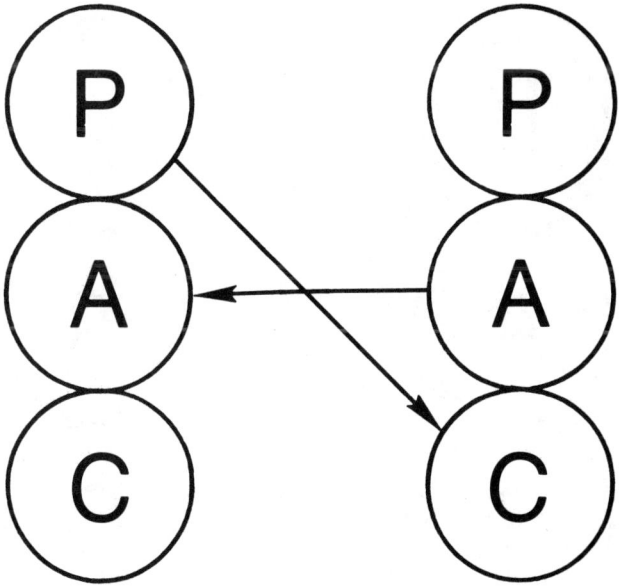

Figure 16-15. *Crossed Transaction*

Stimulus— *Nurse: Time to take your medicine. You'll feel better soon.*
Response— *Patient: It makes me sick if I take it before meals. Just leave it here.*

In this crossed transaction, the Nurturing Parent in the nurse is attempting to "take care of" the sick Child of the patient. The patient gives new information from his Adult ego state. Now the nurse must use her clinical judgment in processing this data or they will bicker about the hospital policy about leaving medicine at the bedside.

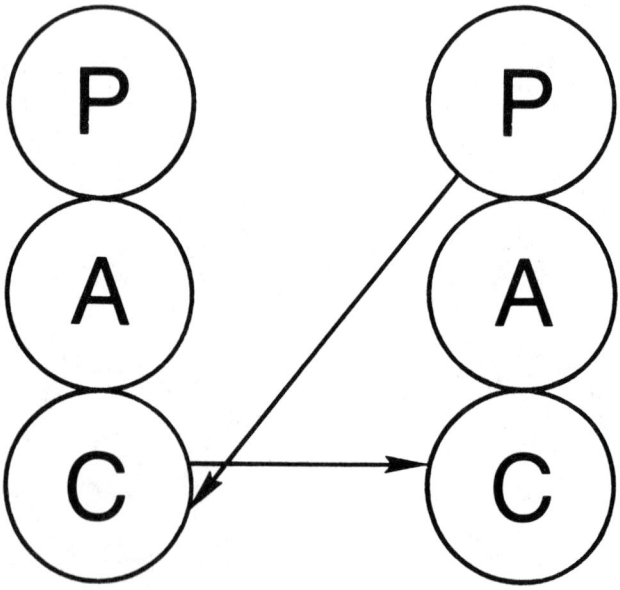

Figure 16-16. *Crossed Transaction*

Stimulus— *Resident: Hey! Let's go for coffee!*
Response— *Nurse: (Harried) Are you goofing off* again?

The resident is in his Child ego state and invites the Child in the nurse out to play. She responds from her Parent ego state, crossing the transaction. The situation shifts from coffee to criticism. Chances are, he will not ask her again.

Complex, ulterior transactions are represented by parallel, multiple lines on the diagram. The solid lines are the social level of the message; the dotted lines show the true, psychological message. There are two types of ulterior transactions: angular and duplex.

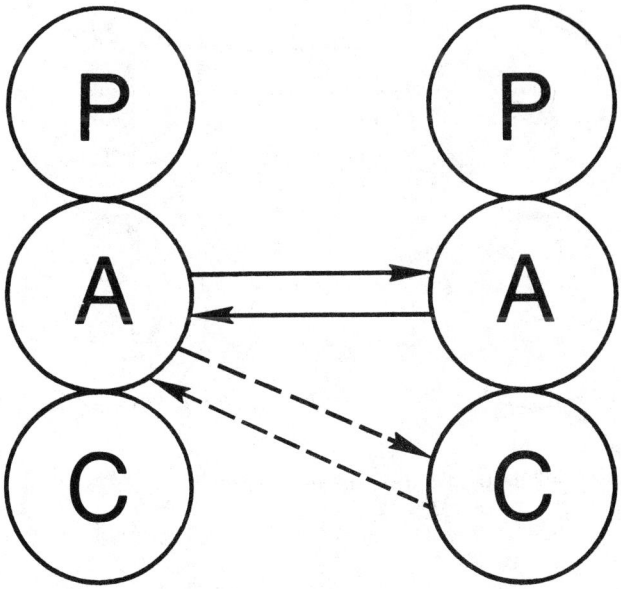

Figure 16-17. *Ulterior Transaction—Angular*

Salesperson: *That dress looks lovely on you, but let me show you something in your price range.*
Shopper: *Never mind. I'll charge it.*

In this transaction the interaction is Adult to Adult on a social level. On the psychological level, however, the salesperson (from her Adult ego state) directs her comment to the shopper's Child ego state with the subtle message, "You're too poor (or don't deserve) to have really nice things." The shopper reacts from her Child ego state with an unspoken, "Oh, yeah? You can't tell me how to spend my money. Besides, charging things doesn't really count." The transaction is called angular because the stimulus ego state is the same in both level's of communication, but it is directed toward two different ego states in the other person.

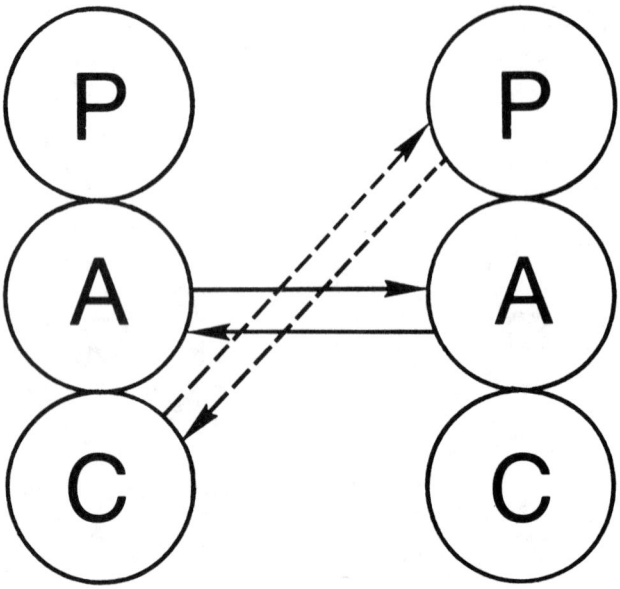

Figure 16-18. *Ulterior Transactions—Duplex*

Student: (Original Stimulus) *I'm really having trouble studying. Any suggestions?*
Teacher: *(First response which provides additional stimulus) How about setting aside a specific time and place?*
Student: *I've tried that but my roommate keeps interrupting me.*
Teacher: *You could go to the library.*
Student: *That's a good idea, but it's not safe to be out after dark.*
Teacher: *Ask a friend along.*
Student: *I'd like to, but I'm afraid that would be an imposition.*
Teacher: *Have you tried getting up early while your roommate's still asleep?*
Student: *Well, some people could do that, but I'm a night person.*
Teacher: *(Exasperated) Well, What are you going to do to study better?*
Student: *As a matter of fact, I've decided to drop out of school and work.*

In this transaction the social level is Adult to Adult, with an apparent exchange of information. The psychological level is Child to Parent, with the student asking the question from her Child ego state and the teacher trying to give advice from her Parent ego state. The payoffs are the student's sense of triumph in frustrating the teacher and the teacher's feeling of righteous indignation that "You can't tell kids anything nowadays." The game is called, "Why don't You . . .?/Yes, But. . . . " The transaction is called duplex because there are two separate sets of ego states being used on the two levels of communication.

Application of TA Proper to Nursing Situations

Transactional analysis proper is a tool for understanding communication. The use of each of the nurse's ego states directed toward each of the patient's ego states is appropriate at different times. When the patient is frightened, overwhelmed or approaching lack of control (in Child), the nurse intervenes with Parent or Adult. She soothes, reassures, directs, reinforces controls and gives necessary information.

Crying is a Child ego state behavior with many possible meanings, including interpersonal messages. A patient may be encouraged to cry by providing a noncritical (Nurturing Parent) listener and conveying, verbally and nonverbally, that he does not have to hold back feelings. At other times the nurse helps to interrupt the crying if it is becoming increasingly upsetting to the patient or is being used to manipulate others.

The nurse uses her Adult ego state directed to the other's Adult to problem-solve. She helps the person to describe, clarify and observe the world around him as well as his internal state. She helps him to consider alternatives and outcomes.

To build a strong Adult ego state, the nurse follows these suggestions by Harris:

1. Learn to recognize your Child, its vulnerabilities, its fears, its principal method of expressing these feelings.
2. Learn to recognize your Parent, its admonitions, injunctions, fixed positions, and principal ways of expressing these admonitions, injunctions, and positions.
3. Be sensitive to the Child in others, talk to that Child, stroke that Child, protect that Child, and appreciate its need for creative expression as well as the NOT OK burden it carries about.
4. Count to ten, if necessary, in order to give the Adult time to process the data coming into the computer, to sort out Parent and Child from reality.
5. When in doubt, leave it out. You can't be attacked for what you didn't say.
6. Work out a system of values. You can't make decisions without an ethical framework.[6]

To increase her level of self-awareness and effectiveness, the nurse evaluates her transactions with patients and coworkers. Ego states can be consciously altered when a person becomes aware that the way he is reacting and responding to other people is not accomplishing what he wants. The following examples illustrate how this can be done in a nursing situation.

"I felt so sorry for her when she begged me not to make her deep breathe and cough. But I knew she had to, so I insisted. I got real firm." The nursing student used her Adult ego state to recognize her Nurturing Parent response to the patient's frightened, hurt Adapted Child. She then shifted to Critical Parent to help the patient do something that was in her best interest.

When a patient developed a pressure sore, the doctor loudly criticized the nursing care. The head nurse burst into tears. He apologized profusely for upsetting her, but privately decided to send his patients to another floor when possible. Later, the nurse recognized her pattern of being oversensitive to the Critical Parent in others and her avoidance or lessening of their criticism by crying in the Adapted Child ego state. She used her Adult to determine how the pressure sores developed. She consciously used her Critical Parent to supervise her staff, which had become lax. Together, they mobilized their Adult ego states to work out preventive procedures. With her Adult, the head nurse realized that morale on the ward had been slipping, so she began to give positive strokes to her staff from her Nurturing Parent and Adult.

A nurses' aide had been continually calling in sick or coming in late. The charge nurse felt very angry and critical toward her because of the burden she placed on the rest of the staff. She felt like losing her temper, but, after recognizing this as her Critical Parent ego state which would probably only hook the aide's Adapted Child, she asked for a conference. Instead of continuing her rebellious behavior, the aide discussed her problems at home. They talked Adult to Adult and decided on reasonable expectations and limits.

Mr. Smith is considered a "problem patient" by all the staff. He is uncooperative, surly and resistive to care. He rejects attempts to help him and then complains to the supervisor that he is being neglected. At a conference, the staff expressed their feelings of anger, despair, frustration, indignation and hopelessness. The staff, hooked by his alternating Critical Parent and Adapted Child behaviors, had reciprocated. They decided to shift to either Adult or Nurturing Parent ego states and discussed how to do this in his treatment. After one orderly found that fishing was a common interest, he and Mr. Smith were heard laughing as they swapped stories about the "one that got away." Both their Free Child ego states were "hooked"!

To meet patient needs, the nurse must be aware of her own, too, and alter her behavior appropriately. This is one of the expectations for the professional nurse and is part of what is meant by the therapeutic use of the self.

The transactional diagram is useful when communication breaks down. The nurse should follow these general guidelines:

1. Use Adult to evaluate needs of the patient and the reality of the situation.
2. Recognize her own Parent and Child ego states.
3. Decide if and when expressions of these are appropriate.
4. Carry out deliberate nursing action based on available information.

STROKES

Definition

From birth to death, human beings have basic needs for sensory stimulation, attention and recognition. *A stroke is any act, verbal or nonverbal, which implies recognition of another's presence.* Stroking generally occurs between people, although pets and self-stroking (warm bath, food, good memories) are sources of satisfaction, also.

Strokes are necessary for developing and maintaining physical and emotional equilibrium. During the first year of life, the infant needs physical stimulation. This need is met by holding, feeding, caressing, jiggling, kissing and diapering.

There is a biological base for this need. Laboratory animals demonstrate physical, emotional and social pathology if proper mothering is disrupted experimentally. R. Spitz noted the high mortality rate in infants brought up in orphan asylums where their physical needs were met hygienically but without human warmth and relatedness through touch.[7] These babies seemed to give up the will to live and succumbed easily to disease or wasted away. The need for strokes—verbal and nonverbal—continues throughout life.

Description of Strokes

"Different strokes for different folks" means that there are many different ways in which people need recognition and stimulation. Early stroking is primarily physical. As the baby learns the social interaction of the smile, he shifts to more abstract stroking through action and language. In addition to the need for sensory stimulation, he develops the hunger for recognition. Strokes prove to a person that he exists.

To tell a six-month-old baby that you love him, you must hold and pet him. You can blow a kiss to a two-year-old. With an adult, you can sit across the room and signal with a smiling wink or write a love letter.

A child will tolerate almost any reaction from parents except being continually ignored, neglected and treated with indifference. If he cannot get noticed and recognized for his positive behavior, he will resort to other means—temper tantrums beyond age four, stealing, sulking, provoking, fighting, getting sick, failing in school and always being afraid. For survival, negative responses are better than none at all. Patterns of getting recognition through different kinds of strokes become part of each person's basic personality. Exchanging strokes is a vital human activity.

Strokes are classified as positive and negative. A positive stroke generally results in a good feeling and carries the message, "You're OK with me." Examples of positive strokes are: a smile, a pat on the back, a hug, praise, a present, compliments, an invitation to a party, a pay raise and a friendly "hello."

Negative strokes, direct or subtle, result in uncomfortable, unpleasant feelings. The person feels put-down and criticized. Some examples of negative strokes are insults, scowls, slaps, being fired, cursed at, snubbed and given a "left-handed compliment." Claude Steiner called positive strokes "warm fuzzies" and negative strokes "cold pricklies."[8]

Both positive and negative strokes can be unconditional or conditional. Unconditional strokes are given for simply being; conditional strokes are for being a certain way or doing something.

Positive unconditional stroke: "I love you just because you're you."
Positive conditional stroke: "You wrote a good paper. It's worth an A."

Negative conditional stroke: "I don't like you when you're late to meet me."
Negative unconditional stroke: "I just can't stand you. Get out of my life!"

Conditional strokes, positive and negative, are used to affect the behavior of other people, especially during child-rearing. When used appropriately and consistently, they are part of the socialization process which teaches the child how to get along with others. People who feel basically good about themselves seek out positive strokes; those who have learned to interact primarily with negative strokes tend to perpetuate their life patterns by eliciting negative strokes from others. One interpersonal game with this behavior is called "Kick Me."

There are five tasks of stroking that an individual does to keep in good physical and psychological equilibrium. These are:

Asking for strokes: Identify the type, quality and number of strokes which are important to you. Ask the person that you want them from. Have enough people in your life so that if one refuses a specific stroke, you can get it from another. Don't try to get "blood from a turnip." Recognize your need for both physical and verbal strokes and seek them out.

Receiving strokes: Accept positive strokes and own them rather than shrugging them off. Enjoy the hug. Say "thank you" to the compliment rather than diluting it with some apology. Don't feel you have to automatically pay a person back for the stroke he gives you.

Giving strokes: Look for and recognize the good and valued aspects of others. Volunteer strokes or respond when a person asks for a stroke you can give. Be sensitive to the special strokes that mean a great deal to the individual. Remember that genuine unconditional positive strokes are the most powerful. Monitor your giving of negative strokes.

Refusing strokes: If a person gives you a stroke, positive or negative, that you do not want, be free to decline it. This can be refused directly or by not feeling bad in response to a negative stroke. Let the other person know what kind of strokes you want and need instead of the unwanted stroke.

Stroking yourself: Figure out how you can be good and nurturing to yourself and do it. Decline to negatively stroke yourself. Remember and record positive strokes that you have gotten in the past. Let others see how OK you are and tell them about the OK things that you do.

Application of the Concept of Strokes to Nursing Situations

The concept of strokes has many applications in nursing settings. It helps to explain aspects of growth and development, change in behavior under stress of illness, therapeutic interventions and job satisfaction.

The ways in which a child is stroked in early childhood has a lasting effect on his personality. Mothers need help in learning effective means of child-rearing. The nurse in maternal/child, public health and school settings can use the concept of strokes to teach families how to get along better with each other. Children with behavior disorders are often inadvertently stroked for and encouraged in negative behavior. They need their strengths and assets to be reinforced through stroking.

On Pediatric wards children use all sorts of behavior to cope with the fears and threats of illness and separation from parents. Nursing staff may unwittingly strengthen difficulties with eating, sleeping, medication and disruptive behavior by strokes for these behaviors. A sick child needs warm fuzzies from his parents and the staff for his courage and coping under extreme stress.

Because indifference is the least tolerated attitude, children sometimes provoke their parents into scolding, spanking or otherwise punishing them. Both the child and the parents need help in developing new ways of relating. The way the parents were raised and stroked is the way they will probably raise their children. A tragic example of this is the fact that many battering parents were battered and abused children themselves.

The need for strokes varies in individuals. Some need a great many to keep going; others get along with a selected few. Illness generally disrupts the usual means of obtaining recognition and gratification. Anxiety, preoccupation with the body and the egocentricity of illness increases the need for strokes, particularly physical ones.

The "demanding" patient is generally signaling desperately that he needs attention (strokes). If the nurse anticipates the requests of such a patient, she spends time with him rather than ignoring him or responding grudgingly. The frequency and extent of his demands will generally decrease.

Physical care, given in the form of a bedbath or backrub, may provide a sense of being cared for because it revives earlier relationships and the pleasure of being physically stroked. Spending time with and listening to a person is a form of stroking.

Along with the need for recognition, there remains a need for continual sensory input to maintain psychosocial and physical equilibrium. Controlled experiments in sensory deprivation confirm this as well as the anxiety, discomfort and distorted perceptions of reality which have been experienced by patients in isolation, extensive body casts and respirators. The patient being monitored in intensive care units experiences excessive though necessary sensory stroking which may result in temporary disorientation.

The nurse who works in psychiatric/mental health settings can use the concept of strokes to understand the behavior of patients and staff. A deficit of positive strokes and surplus of negative strokes leads to depression. The nurse can intervene by helping the patient to change the way he gets himself stroked. No limits on warm fuzzies!

The theory and therapy of behavior modification can be understood as a means of regulating the stroke balance. When positive and desired behaviors are reinforced by strokes, the person changes his behavior. The reverse is also true. Institutionalization is the end product of stroking for compliance, lack of initiative and submission. Token economy wards aim to reverse this process.

In any setting the nurse must evaluate her own needs for recognition and strokes. To whom does she look as her major sources of satisfaction, appreciation and gratification? Because of their own increased needs, patients are often not able to give many positive strokes.

Staff members become unhappy and disgruntled when a patient seems unappreciative—"You can't do anything to please her"; "She never says thanks"; and "He won't *let* you help him." When feelings like these predominate, the staff generally withdraws from the unrewarding patient, leaving him with his own pattern (often lifelong) of unsatisfactory interpersonal relationships.

Periodic evaluation and supervision as well as acknowledgment by coworkers and the medical staff can meet the nurse's need for recognition. The nurse strokes her staff positively to recognize their worth and to appreciate their hard work. This helps to maintain morale even under demanding and difficult conditions.

TIME STRUCTURE

Definition

To a large extent, a person gains recognition and satisfies his hunger for stimuli through the ways he structures his time. Eric Berne defines time structure as the six possible ways of spending time.[9] These are: withdrawal, rituals, activities, pastimes, games and intimacy.

Withdrawal: Withdrawal refers to solitary behavior, with or without the presence of other people. A person may withdraw into preoccupation or fantasy while ignoring others. He retreats to privacy, isolation or sleep. The person may be actively involved in doing something by himself, but more often he turns his energies inward. There is little interpersonal risk or reward in withdrawal. Sometimes in this state the person remembers prior experiences, getting either positive or negative strokes.

Rituals: A ritual is a socially programed, stereotyped, predictable exchange of transactions. It is routine, relatively automatic and safe. A ritual serves the purpose of decreasing continual decision making in situations that occur frequently. There is little commitment to the other person involved, but there is pleasure derived from the feeling of being recognized and in step. The greeting ritual is pleasant but superficial stroking. But it is disconcerting to have your "hello" ignored or to have the other person respond to "How are you?" with an account of how they are feeling. Manners, social events, holidays, many religious events and customs are rituals.

Activities: Activities are generally synonomous with work and productivity whether at a job, at home, in hobbies or recreation. An activity is goal oriented and has to do with external reality. It can be recognized by a completed project, a pay check or a tangible accomplishment. Activities usually produce important satisfactions of both interpersonal and financial needs. They lead to feelings of accomplishment, self-worth, respectability and mastery. The risks and rewards regarding potential stroking are greater in activities than in rituals or withdrawal.

Pastimes: Pastimes refer to the matrix of superficial, social exchanges, verbal and nonverbal, which convey the message to people that they are recognized and reacted to. Pastimes take the form of social conversation or chitchat, recreation and entertainment. They are not goal oriented. The expression "killing time" fits into this category; the cocktail party is the arena for passing time. Topics include the weather, cars, sports, travel, diets and kids.

Pastimes may be a way to get through the day or to get to know others better in a nonthreatening, noncommittal way and, "on a larger scale, until bed-time, until vacation-time, until school starts, until a cure is forthcoming, until some form of charisma, rescue, or death arrives."[10] It is out of pastimes that people develop common interests and move toward friendship and deeper involvement.

Games: The concept of games is a cornerstone of transactional analysis. Berne defined a game as:

> . . . an ongoing series of complementary ulterior transactions progressing to a well-defined, predictable outcome . . . a recurring set of transactions, often repetitious, superficially plausible, with a concealed motivation; or, more colloquially, a series of moves with a snare, or "gimmick."[11]

Games have colloquial names which crisply convey the essence of the interpersonal maneuvers involved: If It Weren't for You; Uproar; Do Me Something; Why Don't You? Yes, But; and I Was Only Trying to Help.[12]

Because many people are afraid of intimacy and the other ways of structuring time are not satisfying enough, they settle for interpersonal games. Although games bring compromise, misery, disappointment or ultimate disaster, they also provide the following:

1. time structure;
2. means to get strokes—positive and negative;
3. avoidance of frightening intimacy;
4. maintenance of basic life position toward the self, others and the world;
5. furthering of one's life script;
6. making life predictable by finding other people who will respond in a familiar way.

Stephen Karpman described the "drama triangle" which illustrates the switch that occurs in the roles of game players.[13] The Victim sets himself up to be attacked, picked on, and saved. The Persecutor is the "heavy" who is overly strict, judgmental, attacking and punishing. The Rescuer, while appearing to be helpful, keeps others unnecessarily dependent on him. The drama occurs when the players suddenly switch roles: the Rescuer becomes the Victim and the Victim becomes the Persecutor. This takes place on the stage, in books, television and, most of all, in real life.

Intimacy: Intimacy is the game-free exchange of open, honest feelings and thoughts. It has to do with love, trust and vulnerability. It is possible in the absence of fear and exploitation. In this culture, intimacy is often rare and frightening. Many people, when they were small, learned that it was not safe to be open, expressive and responsive to the needs and wants of the self and others. That is why many people use the other modes of time structure to ward off the anxiety of being vulnerable. The deepest form of intimacy combines both physical and emotional aspects of sharing with another person, though one aspect may be present without the other.

Application of the Concept of Time Structure to Nursing Situations

The concept of time structure is applicable to all persons. Some specific examples in nursing situations include the following:

Withdrawal: Patients with significant physical illness structure much of their time in withdrawal. A certain amount of this accompanies physical malfunction and is useful in allowing the patient to regress, to let others care for him and to facilitate rest and recovery. However, if the person fantasizes a great deal about his physical condition, impending surgery or uncertain future, he may become increasingly anxious and depressed. Talking about these matters with another person moves the patient out of withdrawal and provides ventilation and reality testing.

If a person is not able to withdraw into sleep for an extended period of time, he becomes disorganized and distressed. This is seen in both general and psychiatric units. Resumption of a normal sleep pattern is an indication of successful treatment.

People withdraw from painful reality and stressful interpersonal relations by using alcohol and drugs. These are forms of self-stroking which often cut one off from others. Withdrawal through use of drugs or alcohol provides a temporary solution which may ultimately be physically, emotionally and socially destructive.

Some types of mental illness are characterized by profound withdrawal to the degree of stupor and muteness. This is seen in some types of psychotic depression and schizophrenic reactions. An essential part of treatment is interrupting the withdrawal by a combination of means, the most important being caring persons.

Rituals: Rituals are useful in a nursing setting, but they can also interfere with effectiveness unless they are continually reevaluated. All institutions have routines to accomplish frequently performed tasks. The purpose of the procedure book is to standardize routines for greater efficiency. Nurses should be flexible and cognizant of the need to alter routines and rituals in line with patients' needs.

The nurse, in doing such things as taking TPRs, passing bedpans and giving the morning bath, should take into consideration the patient for whom the ritual is being done. Certain routines of the hospital should be explained to the patient to make him less anxious by knowing what to expect next.

Patients, like most people, have developed their personal rituals. Illness and hospitalization interrupts them. Excessive behavior around rituals, orderliness and cleanliness is described as obsessive-compulsive. A patient may insist on having his bedside table a certain way or having his morning care done in a specific manner. Deviation from the ritual results in increased anxiety. With this patient, it is generally helpful if the nurse allows him time and opportunity to control his environment and care as much as possible. Ritualized behavior often takes up a great deal of time to prevent the person from having "time" for more threatening interpersonal or social involvement.

The human tendency to establish rituals may be used in helping patients learn how to give their own treatments, such as insulin injections or colostomy care. The disorganized person who has no routines (such as the getting-up-in-the-morning routine) needs help in establishing rituals as a means to structure time. The harried housewife/mother may need guidance in either increasing or decreasing her use of rituals.

Activities: Illness interferes with a person's ability to function and to work. The consequences of serious illness or injury may necessitate major changes in the patient's usual productive patterns. Even when acutely ill, he may feel anxious, useless and insignificant because he is not working. A sick mother may feel guilty over temporarily abandoning her family responsibilities. Even when quite ill, some patients are helped if they are allowed to maintain some family or job responsibilities. This reduces anxiety and maintains self-esteem. The nurse also helps the patient when she conveys the message that "getting well is a major activity and a full-time job at this time."

Pastimes: After the crisis of acute illness is over, the patient is left with a great deal of time to be passed until his convalescence is over. The nurse is challenged to provide a therapeutic environment in which this can be done effectively and satisfactorily. She can do this by encouraging patients to socialize with each other, arranging the environment for socialization and recreation and referring patients for diversional occupational therapy.

Generally, the conversation that a nurse has with a patient should be more than social chitchat because the patient often has vital concerns about his life. When a nurse pastimes a great deal in her exchanges with a patient, it is often because she is uncomfortable, unaware or unprepared to communicate therapeutically. She can learn to be more comfortable, recognize cues to patients' distress and communicate in a meaningful way. Transactional analysis offers methods to do so.

In extended care or psychiatric facilities, exchanges of social pleasantries are part of the therapeutic program. Many patients need help learning how to socialize through pastiming. The nursing staff offers models and a practice arena.

Games: When a person becomes a patient, he brings his characteristic games with him and seeks out new players. He may put himself in a treatment situation through such games as Alcoholic, Addict, Uproar, Kick Me and Look How Hard I Tried (often part of psychosomatic illness). Other games common in clinical work are: Ain't It Awful; Gee, You're Wonderful; Doctor/Nurse; How Do You Get Out of Here; and Wooden Leg.

The nurse may inadvertently get caught up in a game situation with a patient, family or fellow staff member. She finds herself in the drama triangle as either the Rescuer, Persecutor or Victim. Nurses are often cast (or cast themselves) in the role of Rescuer, which is different from being a helper. As Rescuer, she eventually becomes frustrated and shifts to the Persecutor position when the ungrateful Victim refuses to "shape up." Or, as the Rescuer, she ends up feeling the Victim after pouring so much time, interest and energy into the treatment of a patient who rejects (persecutes) her.

As the nurse becomes more familiar with game theory, she recognizes ongoing patterns of the patient and his family. She evaluates the degree of destructiveness and encourages psychiatric referral when indicated.

The nurse can also be more aware of the interpersonal games that she plays with patients, coworkers and the medical staff. All people play games to some degree. Although games serve many interpersonal functions, there are more effective and direct ways to communicate. Some clinical games are: I Was Only Trying to Help; Do Me Something; Let's You and Him Fight; and If It Weren't for You (Him, Her, Them).

Intimacy: One of the greatest opportunities in nursing is participation in the intimacy of other people's lives. These are profound moments of need, hope, joy and sorrow. The professional nurse accepts the awesome responsibility of entering into and meeting the needs of the patient. Sometimes this means just being there—the held hand, the concerned smile, the willingness to listen to hurt, anger and fear. These are all moments of treasured and unusual intimacy for both persons. The nurse may experience and express deep, meaningful feelings with patients and families. This can be very supportive. Yet some consider this "unprofessional," "too involved" and "losing objectivity." When describing their reaction to the death of a loved person, a family commented (positively) that *even* the nurse cried. How many nursing students and nurses have gone to the linen closet or restroom to hide their feelings from the very people who need them the most?

In addition to her own involvement, the nurse should be aware of the patient's need for intimacy with his family. She should structure the environment to make privacy available at visiting hours, especially during terminal illness and at the time of death. She should be aware that patterns of intimacy—emotional and sexual—may be disturbed by illness, prognosis and treatment procedures, especially major surgery. Alert to these possibilities, she is better able to help the patient express his problems, come to a solution or be referred to appropriate resources.

Summary

When a person becomes ill or comes into a treatment setting, his usual patterns of structuring time shift. Hospital routines which structure time for the whole unit may interfere markedly with an individual's choice. The nurse, after identifying the particular ways in which the patient structures time, can help him to find more effective and satisfying ways if needed.

Predischarge planning takes time structure into consideration. The nurse can use the concept of time structure to evaluate her own behavior in terms of the balance between withdrawal, rituals, activities, pastimes, games and intimacy as she plans and participates in her professional and personal life.

BASIC LIFE POSITIONS

Definition

A person's basic life position refers to his orientation toward himself and other people. It is also called the existential position—how the person views himself in the world. His basic position influences how the person thinks, feels, acts and relates to other people. Basic life positions are formed early in life as the result of how the child was treated. Through life, a person may shift his basic position in either a positive or negative direction.

Description of Basic Life Positions

In TA terms, the word "OK" means regarding people as basically good, worthwhile and lovable. An individual is valuable, attractive, intelligent and competent simply because he is. "Not OK" is the feeling that these qualities are lacking or that one is or other people are "lazy, crazy, stupid, ugly and bad."

The four basic life positions are:

1. I'm OK—You're OK.
2. I'm not OK— You are OK.
3. I'm OK—You're not OK.
4. I'm not OK—You're not OK.

It is speculated that the infant originally feels "I'm OK—You're OK" as his physical and emotional needs are met through adequate mothering. If he is fed, snuggled and kept warm and dry by a relatively anxiety-free mothering person, he experiences feelings which result in basic trust. He feels good about himself and others. He experiences confidence and feels encouraged to get along with the business of life. This is the winning position.

However, if the little person is neglected, abused or treated inconsistently, he may shift to one of the other positions. The optimistic view is that through corrective emotional experiences, he can shift back into the "I'm OK—You're OK" position.

Almost all people have some not-OK feelings about themselves. These stem from the period when the child realizes his relative smallness, powerlessness and inadequacy compared with his BIG, POWERFUL PARENTS and the confusing WORLD around him. A person who shifts into the basic life position of I'm not OK—You are OK often feels inadequate, ugly, worthless, guilty, helpless and pessimistically unhappy. This is why it is called the depressed position. Those operating from this position use withdrawal a great deal and generally try to get away from other people, problems and life.

The position of I'm OK—You're not OK is called the paranoid or criminal position because the individual distrusts and is suspicious of the actions and motives of other people. His slogan is, "Look out for number one because no one else will." The person operating from this position will be exploitive, manipulative, hostile and violent toward others. His general tendency is to get rid of by assault, divorce, murder, desertion and rejection.

The fourth position of I'm not OK—You're not OK represents an attitude of despair, isolation and futility. If the small child decides on this position, a life of hopeless withdrawal or eventual suicide may result. This comes about through gross physical and emotional abuse and neglect. A person may shift into this position because of early childhood experiences or traumatic injuries such as stroke, spinal cord impairment or rape. The person in this position experiences extreme helplessness and hopelessness and is generally going nowhere, except to an early death.

Application of the Concept of Basic Life Positions to Nursing

It is important to identify the basic life positions from which a patient, family or nursing staff are operating. Too often, health professionals maintain an unspoken "We're OK—You're not OK" attitude toward patients and families. The expression "accepting the patient" describes an attitude of the nurse who truly experiences others as OK despite socially stigmatized conditions, such as drug addiction, mental illness, alcoholism, homosexuality, abortion, mental retardation, age, minority status and poverty. A problem in treating the terminally ill or dying patient is that the staff may adopt a not-OK position toward him out of their own frustration, fears and discouragement. They may essentially desert the patient just when he needs human contact most desperately.

The nurse may use the concept of basic life positions in health counseling with families. She can help teach parents how to treat their growing children and each other in loving ways which will foster the basic position of I'm OK—You're OK. This is particularly important in working with people from minority groups. One of the most destructive aspects of prejudice is that the discriminated-against person may begin to accept the negative beliefs and biases about him. He experiences deep shame for himself and rage toward others.

An important thing to keep in mind is that people can and do shift positions of OKness and not-OKness. The nurse can help the patient maintain or regain the first position by regarding him as basically OK and helping him to take an active part in his own care so that he can "get on with it."

SCRIPT

Definition

The concept of script provides a means of understanding complex human behavior over time. *A script is a life plan, generally operating on an unconscious level, which develops and unfolds throughout a person's life.* It is based on decisions made early in childhood, reinforced by parents, justified by subsequent events and culminating in chosen alternatives which lead to an ultimate outcome.

A script's outcome may be constructive or destructive. Even a winner's script limits a person to a narrow path in life because it lessens autonomy and choice. The growing child makes basic script decisions from the messages he gets from the significant people around him. Some of these messages, verbal and nonverbal, are destructive and stem from unresolved problems in the parents. Some messages are misperceived because the child has not developed powers of judgment and discrimination.

Repetitive self-destructive patterns suggest tragic scripts and include such behaviors as suicide, alcoholism, violence, drug addiction, multiple marriages, crime, mental illness, obesity and recurrent physical illnesses (especially if they are preventable and treatable).

> A 25-year-old woman realized that she was following a tragic script by "eating myself to death." She weighed over 300 pounds and had recently had a severe coronary. Seeking love and affection, she became pregnant, which necessitated a therapeutic abortion for both physical and psychiatric reasons. She saw her slogan as "Underloved and Overfed."

In developing his script, the child absorbs many viewpoints relating to worth, lovableness, sex, work, responsibility, dependency, authority and countless other aspects of life. He makes basic decisions and acts accordingly as a winner or loser in life. Various life experiences, especially strokes and games, reinforce and further script decisions.

Negative script messages are called injunctions and originate in the Child ego state of the mother and father. They represent areas of unhappiness, confusion and conflict passed down from their own parents. The destructiveness of the script message depends on the time, intensity, duration, period of psychosocial development and possible neutralizing influences. Powerful injunctions which influence the child in a negative way include: Don't Be; Don't Feel; Don't Think; Don't Express What You Feel and Think; Don't Grow Up; Don't Be a Child; Don't Enjoy; Don't Succeed; Don't Be Who You Are; Don't Get Close; Don't Be Sane or Healthy.

These messages are especially harmful when given early, nonverbally and repeatedly to the little child. He may decide on a deep level such beliefs as "I will never trust"; I don't deserve to live"; I will never be able to take care of myself"; and "I am not safe when I show my feelings and thoughts."

Mothers and fathers also pass along messages from their Parent ego states called counterinjunctions because they often go against the negative messages (injunctions). They represent cultural ideas and conventional messages regarding success, manners, morals, work and the ways to please others. Counterinjunctions are generally verbally communicated and may represent whole family and cultural orientations. Examples are statements such as "Work hard"; "Keep trying"; "Be strong"; "Grow up, go to college, and get married"; and "Good, Better, Best. Never let it rest—'til the good is better and the better, best."

Effective parents give their children some direction from the Parent ego state to provide protection. They also communicate their permission and encouragement to the growing child in a loving way to: Be; Be You; Be a Child During Your Childhood; Grow Up When You Are Ready; Experience and Express Your Feelings; Develop and Share Your Thinking; Be Curious and Creative; Make It Your Own Way Because We Love You But Will Not Hold on to You When It's Time for You to Leave.

Figure 16-19 illustrates the script matrix.

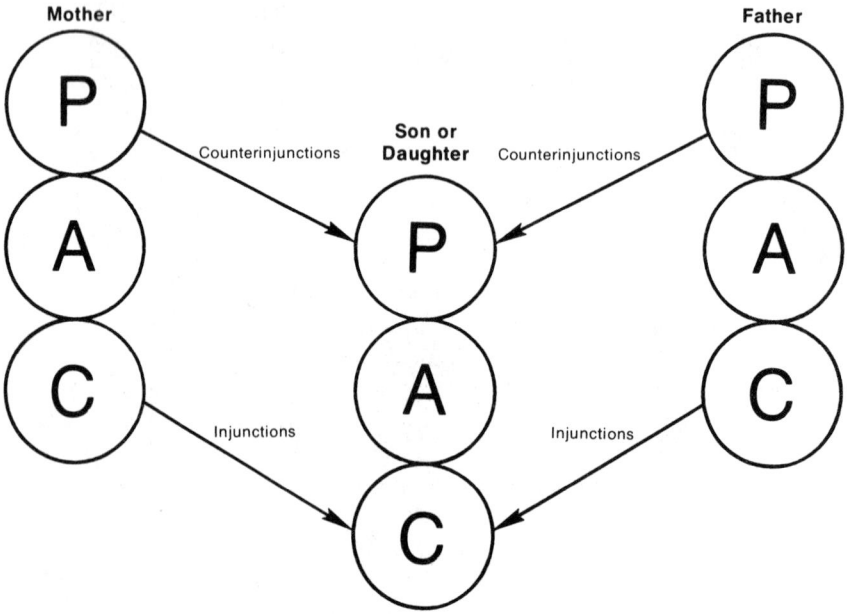

Figure 16-19. *Script Matrix*

In addition to the personal scripts which are developed by an individual in his family, there are broader cultural scripts. Specific messages, expectations and role behaviors exist for men and women in the American culture. Part of the effort of the Women's Liberation movement is to break through personal and cultural scripting to liberate all persons.

Women contribute to and perpetuate script behavior relating to the sexes. In a woman's workshop, this was illustrated by the following responses to the phrase, "Women are . . .": "weak, fragile, obedient, manipulative, illogical and polite. We women can be soft, nurturing, smart, but often suffer and come last." This group said that, "Men are . . .: important, thinkers, doers, logical, tough and the head of the family. They also need to be taken care of, need sex all the time, are unfaithful and never around when needed."

This group constructed their concept of the egograms of the typical American white woman and man as follows:

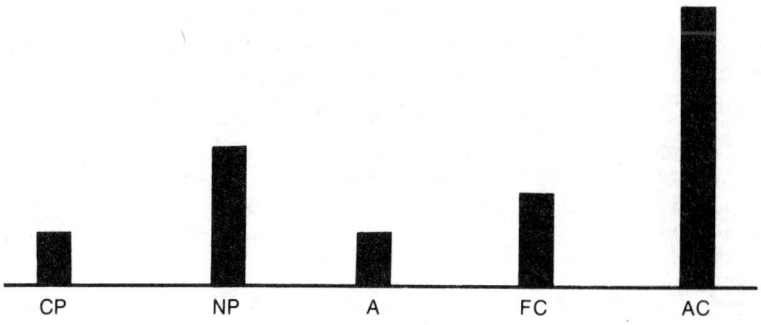

Woman

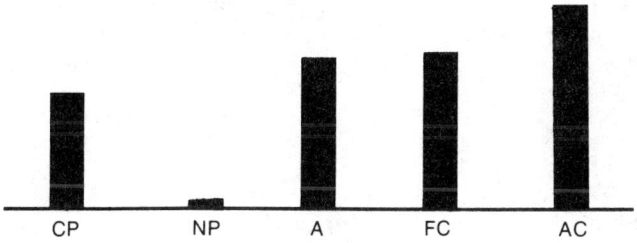

Man

Figure 16-20

Jerome and Terri White described the American cultural parenting of women and men and listed the differences in the messages they receive about how they "should" be and act as shown in Table 5.[14]

These script messages, passed along from generation to generation, have an impact on the personality development of individuals. This concept helps one understand the behavior and conflicts of the women and men who are nurses, doctors, other staff members, husbands, wives, sons, daughters and lovers.

Sex scripting is often part of banal scripts. A banal script is one that does not have a specific tragic or loser quality but is more of an everyday, humdrum existence with no clear beginning or ending. A person living out a banal script is described as a nonwinner with a stereotyped, rigid, boring life.

Colloquial names of banal scripts of men include: Big Daddy, Man in Front of the Woman, Playboy, Jock, Intellectual and Woman Hater. Common banal scripts of women include: Mother Hubbard (Woman Behind the Family), Plastic Woman, Woman Behind the Man, Creeping Beauty, Fat Woman, Guerrilla Witch, Tough Lady and Queen Bee. In addition to being the life stories of real people, banal, winner and tragic scripts are continually presented in books, movies, plays and television.

Table 5

Women	Men
Be passive	Work
Suffer	Take care of things
Be taken care of	Wear the pants in the family
Be emotional	Count as number one
Look good	Be waited on by women
Be a possession	Be a success
Nurture	Compete
Rescue	Look manly
Be a lady/wife/mother	Manipulate women
Don't feel sex	Sex is fun but dirty
Don't play	Be tough
Feel too much scared, sick, tired, sad	Be busy
Don't think	Collect things
Don't get needs met	Don't feel tender, sad, soft
Be busy	Fell angry, competitive, aggressive
Be seductive	Be sexual
Put everyone else first	Real men don't nurture

Application of the Concept of Scripts to Nursing Situations

Nurses usually are genuinely interested in the people who become their patients. They may come to know each other very well or may have only a fleeting glimpse of understanding. A nurse often wonders what happened to a person before, during and after an experience of illness. She questions how the parts of the human puzzle fit together and just what part she played in this patient's life.

A nurse may not be able to identify script behavior in patients who spend short periods of time in the hospital during acute illness. However, this experience may be a significant part of a person's life script. For instance, even the delivery of a healthy, wanted baby is full of possibilities related to the family balance. Marital conflict or compatability hinges on the scripts of the spouses and their ability to accommodate to each other.

The consequences of script behavior may bring a person to nursing services through physical illness, accidents, substance abuse, suicide attempts or emotional illness. Longer term patients, such as those seen in public health, rehabilitation, geriatric and psychiatric settings, often show script behavior which may complicate or facilitate recovery.

How a person faces death is related to his script. Some dying people are serene; others are enraged. Some people die before their seemingly allotted biological time ends; others linger on and on. In psychotherapy some questions help the patient to live his life more fully and to prepare for his death. Some examples are:

How do you expect to die? When? How old were you when you developed these ideas?

> What would be written on your tombstone if you died today? What would you like to be written? What do you imagine your family and friends would say at your funeral?
>
> What can we do to sustain you during your last days?
>
> What can you tell me about your life experiences? What do you want to leave behind?

Most people are very uncomfortable in considering their own mortality.

In addition to applying the concept of scripts to understanding patients better, the nurse applies it to herself. Hogie Wyckoff described a life script which she called NURSE.[15] It pertains to many women (and men) who were scripted into this helping profession. The following elaborates on the nurse script.

Life Course: The person living this script is a professional Rescuer who works in an institution that exploits her and pushes her beyond her limits. Her initial motivation comes from the desire to help others, but eventually caring becomes oppressive to her. She is taught to intuit the needs of others and then expects them to reciprocate. She is unable to ask directly for what she wants and needs and, therefore, usually does not get it.

Too much Rescuing leads to disappointment, anger and retaliation. She actively Persecutes or withdraws into a hurt, detached Victim position.

A person with a NURSE script plays "Ain't It Awful" about doctors, hospitals, patients and the nursing profession. She feels unable to take any effective action to better her condition through individual or collective action.

A tragic outcome for some people with a NURSE script is that they end up being patients themselves. This may be through neglect of physical health, injury on the job or the abuse of drugs or alcohol used to keep going.

Counterscript: Her initial enthusiasm wears thin as she encounters the realities of the everyday working world. She feels the drain of giving much and getting little back. She finds a nice man (who may be a poor medical or law student), marries and supports him. He eventually becomes self-supporting and leaves her.

Injunctions and Counterinjunctions: The person with a NURSE script is influenced by such injunctions and counterinjunctions as: don't express what you feel or think; don't be a child; don't enjoy; don't succeed; don't challenge men; don't take care of yourself; don't ask for what you want and need; don't make it; take care of others first; work hard; be independent; be strong; sacrifice.

Decision: When very young, she decided that the way to take care of herself was to take care of others. She is "good." She always considers the needs of others before her own; she is not "selfish."

Mythical Heroines: Her heroines are Clara (or Sue) Barton, Florence Nightingale, June Gale and Wonder Woman—long-suffering, courageous, unappreciated, effective but martyred women.

Somatic Aspects: The person with a NURSE script develops back injuries, varicose veins, bad feet, obesity, alcohol and drug abuse, emotional crack ups and dropping out of nursing because it is too exhausting and unrewarding.

Games: The NURSE plays the following games: Why Don't You?—Yes, But; Ain't It Awful; If It Weren't for You; Blemish; I'm Only Trying to Help.

Therapist's Role in the Script: He tells her to keep up the good work, cooperate with the doctors and take care of others. He may prescribe medication which are either "uppers" or "downers." And, under certain circumstances, he may tell her his troubles because she is so nurturing and a good listener.

Antithesis: To stop living a NURSE script and to start being a real, autonomous person who may also function as a nurse, the individual needs to reevaluate the current situation in light of past experiences and future expectations. She needs to identify her own needs and wants and find ways to have them met. She must get out of the Rescuing position to avoid the eventual switch to Victim or Persecutor.

To stop living a NURSE script, the nurse must take care of her own needs first. This will free her to be much more effective in her ongoing job. Later, she may mobilize her Parent and Adult ego states to join with other nurses to put down exploitation. She can work with other nurses, physicians and patients to identify mutual and separate needs and responsibilities.

As a professional woman the nurse is often capable and confident in taking care of others from either a Parent or Adult position. But this is often done at the expense of taking care of herself. She has difficulty taking care of her own Child ego state, which is evidenced by her lack of fun things to do, difficulty taking time off and reluctance to ask for and get nurturing strokes for herself.

A nurse may experience conflict between professional/work responsibilities and personal/home/family life. She may seriously wonder if being a professional nurse means that she must be single. Jean Elder pursued the idea that many women operate under the script injunction of "Don't be satisfied."[16] They are scripted to struggle with an "either/or" dilemma—either don't feel or don't think; either don't be close or don't make it; either don't be a child and have fun or don't grow up and figure things out.

This orientation leaves a woman in the dilemma of either getting married and having children or becoming a successful but lonely single professional. Some women attempt to resolve the conflict by vacillating between the two and continuing to feel unsatisfied, bored and tired. A positive resolution is for the woman to act on the reality that she can have both satisfying, close relationships with others and a meaningful, contributing professional life.

CONCLUSION

Transactional analysis provides a conceptual framework in which to understand human behavior and human communication. In any clinical situation, the nurse can apply her understanding of ego states, transactional analysis proper, strokes, time structure, basic life position and scripts. In applying this theory, she will be able to design and carry out more effective nursing interventions.

In specific settings, the nurse may participate in advanced education and training in the practice of transactional analysis in order to function as a primary therapist. Although she may not use TA as psychotherapy, she can use the concepts to provide better care for patients, families, coworkers and herself.

REFERENCES

1. Sanford, F. H.: The behavioral sciences and research in nursing. Nurs. Res. 6:56, October 1957.
2. Harris, T. A.: I'm OK—You're OK: A Practical Guide to Transactional Analysis. New York, Harper, 1967, pp. 4-11.
3. Ibid., p. 18.
4. Ibid., p. 20.
5. Dusay, J. M.: Egograms and the "constancy hypothesis." Trans. Analysis J. 2, 3:37, July 1972.
6. Harris, I'm OK—You're OK, pp. 95-96.
7. Spitz, R.: Hospitalization: genesis of psychiatric conditions in early childhood. Psychoanalytic Study of the Child. 1:53-54, 1945.
8. Steiner, C. M.: A fairytale. Trans. Analysis J. 9, 36:146, October 1970.
9. Berne, E.: Games People Play: The Psychology of Human Relations. New York, Grove Press, 1964, pp. 16-20.
10. Berne, E.: Transactional Analysis in Psychotherapy. New York, Grove Press, 1961, p. 98.
11. Berne, Games People Play, p. 48.
12. Ibid.
13. Karpman, S. B.: Fairytales and script drama analysis. Trans. Analysis J. 7, 26:39, April 1968.
14. White, J. D., and White, T.: A transactional analysis psychohistory: human personality as a resultant of family adapting and scripting and the ongoing influences of cultural scripting. Mimeo. Copyright 1974.
15. Wyckoff, H.: Sex role scripting in men and women and Banal scripts of women. *In* Steiner, C.: Scripts People Live. New York, Grove Press, 1974, pp. 165-222.
16. Elder, J.: Either/or. Trans. Analysis J. 7, 1:35, January 1977.

ADDITIONAL READINGS

Appell, L., et al.: Transactional analysis: improving the nurse/patient relationship. Pt. 2. J. Pract. Nurs. 25:18-19, August 1975.

Babcock, D. E.: Teaching caregivers to win. Trans. Analysis J. 5, 4:392-95, October 1975.

———: Transactional analysis. Am. J. Nurs. 76, 7:1152-55, July 1976.

Berne, E.: Principles of Group Treatment. New York, Oxford University Press, 1966.

———:Sex in Human Loving. New York, Simon and Schuster, 1970.

———:What Do You Say After You Say Hello? New York, Grove Press, 1972.

———:Beyond Games and Scripts. New York, Grove Press, 1976.

Dusay, J.: Egograms. New York, Harper, 1977.

Dzik, R. S.: Transactional analysis in crisis intervention. JOGN Nurs. 5, 1:31-36, June 1976.

Ellis, J.: TA Talk Terms and References Used in Transactional Analysis. Fort Smith, Ark., Child and Family Consultants, 1974.

———: TA Tally: A Quick Reference of Articles in the Transactional Analysis Bulletin and Journal 1962-74. Fort Smith, Ark., Child and Family Consultants, 1974.

George, J. and Gowell, E.: Transactional analysis in sensitivity groups for students of nursing. Nurs. Forum. 12, 1:82-95, 1973.

Goulding, R. and Goulding, M.: Injunctions, decisions, and redecisions. Trans. Analysis J. 6, 1:41-48, January 1976.

Gowell, E. C.: Transactional analysis strategies for dealing with pain. J. Psychiatr. Nurs. 12, 5:25-30, September/October 1974.

Hesterly, O., et al.: How to Use Transactional Analysis in the Public Schools. Little Rock, Ark., Hesterly, 1974.
Hover, D. E.: Mental health consultation with public health nurses, using transactional analysis as a tool. J. Psychiatr. Nurs. 14, 6:15-19, June 1976.
James, M. and Jongeward, D.: Born to Win. Reading, Mass., Addison-Wesley, 1971.
———: et al.: Techniques in Transactional Analysis. Reading, Mass., Addison-Wesley, 1977.
Jongeward, D. and Scott, D.: Women as Winners. Reading, Mass., Addison-Wesley, 1976.
Justice, R. and Justice, B.: Shifting symbiosis in abusive families. Trans. Analysis. J. 6, 4:28-36, January 1976.
Kambly, A.: The ABC's of PAC: An Introduction to Transactional Analysis. Ann Arbor, Mich., University Service Agency, 1971.
Kerr, C.: TA and sex-therapy for women; non-orgasmic scripts. Trans. Analysis J. 6, 4:28-36, January 1976.
Klingleil, G. A., et al.: Concepts of transactional analysis and anxiety with persons in crisis. J. Psychiatr. Nurs. 13, 6:5-10, November/December 1975.
Lee, I.: Are we rescuers . . . or victims? Nurs. 77, 7:94-6, October 1977.
Levin, P.: Becoming the Way We Are. Sacramento, Calif., Jalmar Press, 1974.
———: Sex roles: an added dimension to script theory. Trans. Analysis J. 7, 2:121-26, April 1977.
———, and Berne, E.: Games nurses play. Am. J. Nurs. 72:483-87, March 1972.
Peterson, G.: Feelings and sickness. Trans. Analysis J. 6, 1:73-77, January 1976.
Schiff, J. L., et al.: Cathexis Reader: Transactional Analysis Treatment of Psychosis. New York, Harper, 1975.
Smyth, L., Barter, M., Lopez, T., and Lotspeich, A.: Transactional analysis. Paper written for a course on theoretical Foundations of Nursing, Sacramento State University, Spring 1977.
Spence, M.: Group work with old people. Trans. Analysis J. 4, 2:35-37, April 1974.
Steiner, C.: Games Alcoholics Play: The Analysis of Life Scripts. New York, Grove Press, 1971.
———: Scripts People Live. New York, Grove Press, 1974.

ST. PETER'S HOSPITALS.
TEACHING DIVISION.
THE SHAFTESBURY HOSPITAL.
LONDON, W.C.2.